Primary Care in the UK

D0299457

Also by Stephen Peckham

Managing Public Involvement in Health Care Purchasing (with Carol Lupton and Pat Taylor)

A Public Health Model of Primary Care: From Rhetoric to Reality (with Pat Taylor and Pat Turton)

Also by Mark Exworthy

Professionals and the New Management in the Public Sector (edited with Susan Halford)

Primary Care in the UK

Policy, Organisation and Management

Stephen Peckham
and
Mark Exworthy

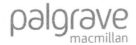

© Stephen Peckham and Mark Exworthy 2003
Foreword © Geoffrey Meads 2003

All rights reserved. No reproduction, copy or transmission of
this publication may be made without written permission.

No paragraph of this publication may be reproduced, copied or
transmitted save with written permission or in accordance with
the provisions of the Copyright, Designs and Patents Act 1988,
or under the terms of any licence permitting limited copying
issued by the Copyright Licensing Agency, 90 Tottenham Court
Road, London W1T 4LP.

Any person who does any unauthorised act in relation to this
publication may be liable to criminal prosecution and civil
claims for damages.

The authors have asserted their rights to be identified as
the authors of this work in accordance with the Copyright,
Designs and Patents Act 1988.

First published 2003 by
PALGRAVE MACMILLAN
Houndmills, Basingstoke, Hampshire RG21 6XS and
175 Fifth Avenue, New York, N.Y. 10010
Companies and representatives throughout the world

PALGRAVE MACMILLAN is the global academic imprint of the Palgrave
Macmillan division of St. Martin's Press, LLC and of Palgrave Macmillan Ltd.
Macmillan® is a registered trademark in the United States, United Kingdom
and other countries. Palgrave is a registered trademark in the European
Union and other countries.

ISBN 0–333–80068–0

This book is printed on paper suitable for recycling and
made from fully managed and sustained forest sources.

A catalogue record for this book is available
from the British Library.

10 9 8 7 6 5 4 3 2 1
12 11 10 09 08 07 06 05 04 03

Typeset by Aarontype Limted, Easton, Bristol, England
Printed and bound in Great Britain by
Creative Print & Design (Wales), Ebbw Vale

To Anna, James, Catherine and Nicholas
(SP)

To my parents
(ME)

Contents

List of Illustrations

Tables

Figures

Boxes

Foreword

Primary care has a particular political significance. At best its services represent an extension of the care we would hope for from our best friends or closest family relatives. Its relationships can be genuinely precious. In the United Kingdom there is an enormously rich and long legacy of popular television series, heroic novels, radio drama and, above all, local folklore and all give testimony to the value of these relationships. Governments which seek to change this cultural inheritance of primary care clearly do so at their peril.

Yet for a decade and a half this is exactly what UK governments – both Conservative and Labour – have sought to do. Not surprisingly, given the deeply personal value attributed to general medical practitioners in particular, they have not espoused policies that have directly targeted change in the relationship between the professional and the patient. Indeed the political claim is invariably that the reform agenda is designed only to strengthen and build on this relationship. Given the profound popular symbol of trust that general practice still constitutes, no other rhetoric would be acceptable. Which has left successive political administrations with only the indirect change agent mechanisms of organisation and management at their disposal. And historically, because of the strength of the individual professions in UK primary care where general practice has been the title of the building, service and the practitioners, it is the organisational and managerial capacity that has been its weakest feature.

How this shortfall has been addressed is the subject of this book. Given the scale of the changes involved and the political significance of the subject it is a text which is long overdue. The reasons for this delay are not hard to discern. The speed and scale of still continuing transformational change are daunting. There is still a dearth of relevant material for the serious student to draw upon. Systematic studies are scarce and anecdotal but non-generalisable stories plentiful. Above all, on the one hand there is the ever-growing local diversity of organisational and managerial models in the UK, while on the other central policy documents about primary care become every more standardised and eerily consistent in conformity with the modernising requirements of the 'New NHS'. It takes not a little intellectual courage to examine, from a contemporary academic perspective, the organisation and management of primary care today.

I suggest that we should therefore approach this book with a sense of gratitude and appreciation. At last there is an authentic book of reference, with breadth and depth, which describes and analyses the extraordinary years in which primary care in the UK has moved from an amateur small business outfit, in which even the mention of money was immoral, to a multibillion pound corporate enterprise crucially responsible for not just the complex formal and informal service infrastructures of communities, but also for the ways in which the strategic institutions of secondary care and strategic initiatives of public health are shaped at the level of the new devolved nation-states.

That this transformational change is incomplete is self-evidently true. Indeed the advent of yet another wave of new primary care organisations and primary managed care programmes in 2002 bear witness to what is a truly revolutionary process. The narrative will be out of date before the ink is dry. The numbers, especially given the notorious delays in central collations of family health services data returns, will never quite tally with the narrative. The general conclusion invariable differs from your local experience. The social scientists' resources are an anathema to those conditioned in the positivist scientific disciplines of medicine.

The criticisms, accordingly, are as easy to imagine as the credits for Mark Exworthy and Stephen Peckham. Neither they nor the readers should be in any way deterred. Today primary care in its organisation and management is politics. Ambivalent reactions are part of the territory. The authors have done us all a great service by taking on such a contentious political subject. Given its constantly changing character we can, with certainty, be sure there will be further editions. There will need to be, and we should look forward to them eagerly.

GEOFFREY MEADS
Visiting Professor
Centre for Primary Health Care Studies
University of Warwick, and Professor of Health Services Development
City University, London

Preface

Our interest in primary care comes from both our involvement in primary care research and the fact that policy interest in primary care has grown in tandem with our research careers. Primary care in the UK has evolved, and continues to evolve, as our research careers have developed and we feel that the need for careful description and insightful explanation is in many ways long overdue.

The origins of this book lie in a number of research collaborations in which we were involved whilst we were based at the Institute for Health Policy Studies (University of Southampton). Initially, we were supported by the Wessex Research Consortium (1991–95) which conducted various research projects related to primary care development on behalf of a number of Health Authorities in the Wessex Region. Although we have since moved on to different institutions, we have continued to be involved in research collaborations; our interest in and research on primary care have remained although they have taken different directions. Collectively, our research has covered a breadth of topics which has proved an excellent grounding for this book.

The topics which this book addresses draw on our personal interests and research and development work we have been involved in. Conducting research over these last few years has enabled us to witness an amazing set of developments across the UK, a period which has seen the primary care occupy a central position in the health policy arena and indeed the wider public policy sphere.

Though grounded in research and academic communities, we have engaged closely with clinicians, managers and policy-makers. Throughout, we have occupied a position on the boundary between research and policy, a position which aids the two-way transfer of information and ideas. This book embodies that; it seeks to offer students, researchers, practitioners and policy-makers insights from across the interface.

A major reason for writing this book was to provide a comprehensive text which addressed the key issues affecting primary care in the UK. Many health policy books provide excellent coverage of health policy generally or specific functions. Yet, it appeared to us that none took a specific focus on the nature and direction of primary care. In particular, there was a need to examine primary care using the frameworks and concepts of policy analysis. Given the importance of the subject across the NHS and other agencies, the relatively small literature in this field was significant.

The book provides a comprehensive assessment of the state of primary care in the UK in terms of policy, organisation and management. We have sought to balance depth and breadth of topics; inevitably there have been trade-offs between these – for example we do not cover community dentistry, pharmacy or ophthalmology nor do we provide in-depth analyses of community-based specialties such as mental health or learning disability services. We hope that it offers new perspectives to seasoned practitioners and an entrée into the field for students. For both, the book offers a collation of different literatures, research evidence and accounts of policy developments from a range of various sources.

To meet the changing needs and demands of students, researchers, practitioners and policy-makers is a tall order but we trust that this book is sufficient for these (and other) audiences. Our approach has been underpinned by an awareness that the rapidity of change in the policy environment means any book will soon be out-dated. The approach of drawing on a range of literatures and presenting frameworks is designed to offer an enduring method of understanding and explaining primary care in the UK.

In the course of our research and writing this book, we have become indebted to many colleagues and collaborators. We are grateful to our colleagues from the University of Southampton, University of the West of England, Oxford Brookes University, LSE and University College, London, and to those with whom we have collaborated.

In our various projects, we thank those who have given their time to be interviewed or consulted. We hope that this book goes some way to explaining why we sought their views.

We have tested out our initial ideas for sections of this book with a number of individuals including clinicians, managers, policy-makers and academics. Although the book is immeasurably better for their constructive comments, the final responsibility lies with us. Finally, the key to a good text is that is is well structured and readers can find what they are looking for. To this end, we would like to thank the reviewers for their useful comments, our editor, Keith Povey, and the indexer Michael Dickinson-Heary.

Stephen Peckham
Mark Exworthy

Abbreviations

ADSS	Association of Directors of Social Services
AHA	Area health authority
BMA	British Medical Association
CEO	Chief executive officer
CHC	Community Health Council
CHI	Commission for Health Improvement
CHS	Community health services
CM	Complementary medicine
CMO	Chief Medical Officer
COPC	Community oriented primary care
CPHVA	Community Practitioners and Health Visitors Association
CPPIH	Commission for Patient and Public Improvement in Health
DHA	District health authority
DHSS	Department of Health and Social Security
DMUs	Directly managed units
DN	District nurse
DH/DOH	Department of Health
FCE	Finished consultant episode
FHS	Family health services
FHSA	Family health services authority
FPC	Family practitioner committee
GDP	Gross Domestic Product
GMC	General medical council
GMS	General medical services
GP	General medical practitioner
GPFH	GP fundholder/fundholding
HA	Health authority
HAZ	Health Action Zone
HCHS	Hospital and community health services
HImP	Health improvement programme
HMOs	Health maintenance organisations
HV	Health visitor
LA	Local authority
LHG	Local health groups
LIFT	NHS Local Improvement Finance Trust
LIZ	London Initiative Zone
LSP	Local Strategic Partnership
MPC	Medical practices committee
NED	Non-executive director

NHI	National health insurance
NHS	National Health Service
NHSE	National Health Service Executive
NHSME	National Health Service Management Executive
NICE	National Institute for Clinical Excellence
NPCRDC	National Primary Care Research and Development Centre
NPM	New public management
NSF	National Service Framework
OAT	Out-of-area treatment
OHE	Office of Health Economics
PAL	Patient Advisory Services
PAM	Profession allied to medicine
PATCH	Planned Approach or Primary Action Towards Community Health
PCAP	Primary Care Act Pilots
PCG	Primary care group
PCO	Primary care organisation
PCT	Primary care trust
PHCT	Primary health care team
PI	Performance indicator
PMS	Personal medical services
PPP	Public–private partnerships
RCGP	Royal College of General Practitioners
RCN	Royal College of Nursing
R & D	Research and development
RHA	Regional Health Authority
SAFF	Service and Financial Frameworks
SNMAC	Standing Nursing, Midwifery Advisory Committee
SPCT	Scottish Primary Care Trust
SRB	Single Regeneration Budget
SSD	Social services department
StHA	Strategic Health Authority
TPP	Total purchasing pilot
UK	United Kingdom
UKCC	UK Central Committee for Nursing, Midwifery and Health Visiting
WHO	World Health Organisation

PART I

Primary Care:
A Policy Perspective

The first five chapters of this book focus on describing and defining the context and parameters of primary care from a policy perspective. We explore why primary care has become of such specific interest and develop a number of key themes in relation to why the interest in this area of health care has grown. We also set out key approaches to policy analysis used in this book and examine the nature, development and organisation of primary care in the UK.

CHAPTER 1

Primary Care in the UK: the Context

Introduction

Primary care now plays a central role in the UK National Health Service (NHS) and has become a major focus of health policy. The changes introduced by the Labour Government from 1997 have significantly shifted health care policy from an emphasis on secondary care to placing primary care at the centre of health care development, commissioning and public health. These changes to the health care system in the UK came at the end of a sustained period of health care reform in the 1990s, not only in the UK but also in many other developed countries. As we enter the twenty-first century, it is timely to review this policy movement towards primary care and to examine why the role of primary care in health care systems has become so important.

Specific policy interest in primary care in the UK has been slow to develop, but since the mid-1960s, it has become a central feature of governmental health and social care policy-making and action. At the same time there has been a re-evaluation of primary care in terms of its organisation and role. This book sets out to explore the reasons for such a re-evaluation and the shift towards primary care within the UK. It aims to provide a policy perspective upon primary care as a distinct element of the UK health care system. In taking this perspective, the book seeks not only to suggest answers as to why primary care has become so important but also to discuss how primary care developments engage with wider health policy issues such as management and organisation, interagency working, public health and public participation.

This chapter explores the first of these issues by discussing the reasons why primary care has become such an important focus of UK health policy generally and the NHS specifically. It starts by charting the growth of primary care services and then goes on to identify what has led to the growth in services. It ends by identifying a paradox in primary care between an increasing integration of primary care within the NHS and an increasing emphasis on diversity at a primary care level. Within UK health policy such a paradox is not new as there have always been tensions between government control at the centre to ensure universality and fairness and freedom at the locality to develop services according to local circumstances. While such tensions have remained, much else has been changing with many traditional structures being challenged creating shifts in power within the health care system.

In this book, we have been explicit in declaring the broad analysis of policies and activities that distinguish primary care from general practice or community health services (see, for example, Moon and North 2000; Ottewill and Wall 1990). However, in choosing a term such as primary care, we are also faced with its ambiguity and a need to define more precisely our field of interest. The focus of this book is, therefore, on both policy and practice and the interface between them. An explicit policy approach is adopted to illuminate changes in health care and to identify both the developing nature of primary care and the context within which this is taking place. The framework for such an approach is discussed more fully in Chapters 2 and 3. As indicated above, we start by examining why primary care has come to be seen as so important within the UK health care system.

The Growth of Primary Care in the UK

Central to the organisation of primary care services in the UK are general practice and community health services. Since the Second World War, there has been an enormous expansion of these services. From the 1960s there has been a steady increase in the workload and, consequently the numbers of staff. Today primary care is a major employer with, in England, Scotland and Wales, over 100 000 people now working in general practice with over 40 000 additional members of the primary health care team (PHCT) who also work in, or with, practices (see Tables 1.1, 1.2 and 1.3).

Despite the small increase in number of GPs, there has been a significant increase in the proportion of female GPs (from 27 per cent in 1991 to 36 per cent in 2001). This feminisation of general practice is reflected in the increasing proportion of female GP Registrars (who now constitute 46 per cent). Another

Table 1.1   General Practice Workforce

Description	2001	% change since 1991
GPs – number of practitioners	30 685	+1.0
Average list size	1841	−5.4
Practice Staff – number	104 300 (64 998 wte)	+35.1 (+33.4)
Practice Nurses	11 163	+27.2
Administrative and Clerical Staff	51 390	+35.1
Practice staff (wte) per Unrestricted Principals and Equivalents	2.3	+21.1

Source: DOH, 'Statistics for General Medical Practitioners in England, 1991–2001'. From DOH website, www.dohgov.uk/public/sb0203.htm accessed February 2002.

Table 1.2 Numbers of Primary Health Care Team Staff, England and Wales, 1996

	Job Title	WTE	Number
1	Practice Nurse	10 402	18 892
2*	Physiotherapist	90	350
3*	District Nurse	8 570	n/a
4*	Health Visitor	9 668	n/a
5*	Dietician	n/a	4 310
6*	Occupational Therapist	n/a	18 665
7*	Clinical Psychologist	n/a	2 500

Note: * Figures do not necessarily refer to posts just within the primary health care team.
Sources:
1, 2: Department of Health, *GMS Statistics for England and Wales 1996*. London: DoH.
3, 4: Dept of Health, *Health and Personal Social Services Statistics for England 1996.*. Figures are for England, 1994. London: DoH.
5, 6: Council for Professions Supplementary to Medicine. Figures are for UK, 1997. London: DoH.
7: Estimate based on membership figures of the British Psychological Society, 1997. London: DoH.

change has been the number of salaried GPs (137 in 2001), which is largely due to the introduction of Personal Medical Services (PMS).

The workload in general practice has also been increasing. In total, general practitioners in the United Kingdom carry out about 293 million consultations each year, an increase of almost 50 per cent since 1975 and 23 per cent since 1985 (Office of Health Economics 1997). Women tend to consult GPs more often than men. In 1995 there were almost 180 million consultations by women and almost 115 million by men (*ibid*.). Since 1975, the number of consultations per GP has risen by just over 14 per cent to 8896 consultations *pa* in 1995 (see Table 1.4). Seventy-eight per cent of people in England and Wales consulted their general practitioner at least once during the year 1991/92. This compares with 71 per cent of people who saw their doctor at least once in 1981/82. On average, each person saw a general practitioner five times during 1995 (See Table 1.5). Females are, however, more likely to consult than males (six and four respectively).

The evidence for a growth in the size and workload of primary care is therefore very compelling. However, why did this growth occur? Was it a planned development of primary care or did it simply grow by responding to circumstances such as increased health need? While neither of these scenarios provides a complete answer it is surely worth exploring the reasons for such growth. It has already been stated that there was little policy interest in primary care in the first 20–30 years of the NHS and thus we must look to other

Table 1.3 Practice Staff in England and Wales, 1992 and 1997, and Scotland 1998

Job Title	England & Wales 1992	England & Wales 1997	Scotland 1998[p]
	Whole time equivalent		
Fund Manager	–	1 677	–
Management & Admin	6 409	–	834[1]
Practice Manager	–	7 094	–
Secretarial & Clerical	13 300	–	3685[2]
Secretarial	–	6 157	–
Receptionist	20 717	–	–
Receptionist/Clerical	–	30 899	–
Computer Operator	1 195	2 287	190
Other Admin	–	3 396	–
Practice Nurse	9 450	10 724	968
Dispenser	1 065	1 213	26
Physiotherapist	77	94	–
Chiropodist	10	27	–
Interpreter/Link Worker	24	58	–
Counsellor	174	253	–
Comp. Therapist	–	10	–
Other Duties	661	710	801
Total Number of Staff	53 082	64 599	6504

Notes: [p] Figures for Scotland provisional as at 1 April 1998.

explanations for both the growth of primary care and the interest of national policy-makers.

Before exploring this wider context it is useful to examine why this growth in services occurred. A number of key factors can be seen to have contributed to this growth:

Table 1.4 Estimated Number of NHS Consultations per Unrestricted Principal, UK, 1995

	1975	1985	1990	1995	% change 1975–95
0–4	609	852	989	815	34
5–15	785	737	781	685	−13
16–44	2889	2903	3580	3010	4.1
45–64	1916	1891	2151	2008	4.8
65–74	907	833	891	934	2.9
over 75	674	813	879	871	29.2
All[1]	7780	8030	9269	8896	14.3

Note: Totals include consultation where age was not recorded.
Source: Office of Health Economics (1997, table 4.21).

- The increasing availability of medical cures and technology such as beta-blockers, anti-depressants, improved surgical techniques and a wider spectrum of antibiotics meeting rising demands but also generating demand;
- Rising need for community-based care to support people with long-term health problems;
- Increased access to health care in the post-war period following the introduction of the NHS and development of family practitioner services;

Table 1.5 Average Number of NHS GP Consultations per Person per Year, by Age, GB 1972–1995

All persons	1972*	1983	1991	1995
0–4	4	7	7	7
5–15**	2	3	3	3
16–44**	4	4	4	4
45–64	4	4	4	5
65–74	4	6	6	6
>74	7	7	6	7
Total (all ages)	4	4	5	5

Notes: * 1972 figures relate to England and Wales.
** These age-groups were 5–14 and 15–44 in 1972.
Source: OPCS, *Living in Britain: Results from the 1995 General Household Survey*, London: ONS, 1996, table 7.20, p. 112.

- Search for cost-containment strategies (especially outside primary care);
- Shifts in the location of care from the secondary to the primary care sector from both a cost-incentive perspective and because hospitals were becoming more specialised and technological with an emphasis on shorter patient stays (Taylor 1991).

These issues may also provide an explanation of why the government has been taking an increasing interest in primary care. However, an examination of policy suggests that the government's interest in primary care grew from the mid-1960s with the Family Doctor's Charter, the introduction of the general practitioner training schemes, from 1970, and then in the 1980s with *Agenda for Discussion Primary Health Care* (DHSS 1986a) and *Promoting Better Health* (DHSS 1987). Until the 1960s there was little attention paid to the structure and organisation of primary care services and it was relatively left to develop in its own way. While there were major exceptions with the changes to general practice initially arising from the Family Doctor's Charter and GP training and education (Moon and North 2000) and the incorporation of community health services into the NHS in 1974 (Ottewill and Wall 1990), much of the pattern of care remained the same. Policy thus remained largely static. The policy focus in this period was predominantly on the development, management and organisation of acute health care services (see for example Ham 1999; Klein 1995). This situation in the UK was reflected in many other developed countries such as in Europe, New Zealand and North America – for example, in the USA the numbers of registered family practitioners actually diminished. Yet, the 1990s demonstrated a marked change in the focus of health policy with an increasing interest in the structure of primary care, its role within the health care system and its contribution to improving population health. A critical feature of these reforms was the establishment of internal or planned markets in health care which has received wide debate. (Le Grand *et al.* 1998; Ranade 1998; Saltman and Von Otter 1992). The reforms of the early 1990s are widely seen as presenting a new paradigm in health policy (Saltman and Figueras 1997). In this book we will be exploring whether the changes to primary care also represent a new paradigm for primary care policy which begs a number of key questions:

- Why should this increased policy interest in primary care happen in the 1990s?
- Why has primary care often been promoted as a panacea to the ills of health care systems including secondary care?
- Why has there been a shift away from a medically dominated primary care service to an interdisciplinary and intersectoral one?
- Why has primary care become of such importance in both institutional and technical health care policies for tackling health problems?

It is these questions which this book seeks to answer. We focus on developments in the UK and yet the wider reform processes are under way in other countries. The UK thus provides a backdrop for such debates on primary care. In the remainder of this chapter we seek to understand why primary care has become such an important focus of health care policy both in the UK and in other countries. Importantly, the chapter will draw on a range of (academic) disciplines to explore primary care which thereby sets the context of future chapters. Later in the book we will draw together theory, policy and practice relating to key elements of primary care.

Why has Primary Care Become Such an Important Policy Focus?

The rising interest in primary care policy has been a widespread and international phenomenon. Its importance within international health policy was first highlighted by the World Health Organisation's declaration of Alma Ata in 1978 (WHO/UNICEF 1978). This was a response to the need to develop health care systems in non-developed countries which were relevant to health care issues, appropriate in terms of the use of technology and affordable (Macdonald 1992). Yet, in many developed countries, including the UK, the use of the term primary care was very limited. One indicator is in its use by policy analysts and writers. Using a combined search strategy of 'primary care' and 'primary health care' on MEDLINE and the Social Sciences Citation Index (SSCI) shows the increasing usage of the terms in the literature (see Table 1.6). Of particular interest is the increase in usage in the social sciences literature.

In the UK, primary care assumed greater prominence within the development of primary health care teams from the 1960s, but particularly in the 1970s and 1980s (Ottewill and Wall 1990; see Chapter 8). However, policy remained directed specifically at either general practice or community health services; it invariably failed to capture the entirety of primary care. This situation was mirrored in other developed countries such as the USA and Canada

Table 1.6 References to Primary Care or Primary Health Care in Databases

Year	Number of articles in Database	
	MEDLINE	*SSCI*
1971–1980	521	–
1981–1990	520	1365
1991–2000	1563	9095
2001–2002 (Apr)	1206	1468

where the main focus has been on family medicine. Yet, in the UK, the 1990s saw a spectacular rise in the use of the term primary care within health care policy. Where did this use of the term primary care come from? Why did it develop? What does primary care encompass? During the 1990s, governments of developed countries across the world discovered (and some rediscovered) primary care and took more interest in policy development and service provision. This interest has a specific manifestation in the policy and organisational changes in the UK (discussed further in Chapters 4 and 5). It was also evidenced elsewhere in the introduction of reforms in New Zealand (Malcolm and Powell 1996), the maturing of managed care approaches in the USA (Robinson and Steiner 1998) and stronger interest in Western Europe about the role of general practice and primary care organisations (Fry and Hodder 1994; Peckham 1999).

The reasons for the growth in interest in primary care and its policy dimensions are many and varied. A simple review of UK health policy demonstrates little interest in general practice and community health services. As Moon and North (2000: 13) argue:

> the current status that general practice enjoys as a speciality within medicine and the influence that GPs wield are in sharp contrast with its origins and much of its history, during which general practice was overshadowed by the more prestigious branches of medicine.

Traditionally, the sidelining of general practice and community health within UK policy is seen as a by-product of the establishment of the NHS in 1948. The settlement (between the government and the medical profession) ensured that governments would focus on the secondary and tertiary sectors and that GPs would be semi-detached from the NHS (Klein 1995). Two consequences of the establishment of the NHS were the independent practice status of general practice, outside the mainstream NHS administration, and the retention of community and public health services within local authorities (Ottewill and Wall 1990; Timmins 1995; Klein 1995). For the UK, this tended to push policy interest in these areas to the sidelines, though not ignored. There has been, for example, a continuing debate within the UK about the relationship between community health and hospital services (Ottewill and Wall 1990) and since the 1950s an interest in the development, quality and role of general practitioner services (Moon and North 2000) (see also Chapter 4). Klein (1995) has suggested that, in the last 20–30 years, health policy has been marked by an increasingly crowded policy arena with more stakeholders (e.g. managers and patient organisations). This 'congestion' applies as much to primary care as any other part of the health policy spectrum. He argues that this leads to a veto of change and a preponderence to the status quo. However, as Glendinning (1999) has noted, the interest of government in primary care services rapidly escalated from the mid-1980s. This interest has grown for a number of reasons, not least the coincidence of several trends including:

- broader changes in the delivery of health care services associated with the 'crisis in health care' and the 'crisis of the welfare state' (Ham 1992; Starfield 1998);
- an interest in the organisational relationship of general practice to the NHS as the key to managing activity (Starfield 1998);
- a desire to extend managerial control over primary care and, following the failure of earlier cost-control measures, to engage general practitioners in financial management (Glendinning 1999);
- the growth of the 'new public management' and consequent changes in approaches to the management and organisation of public services particular to curb expenditure, contain demands and increase efficiency and effectiveness;
- changes in patients' expectations about being treated more promptly and closer to home;
- a fragmenting medical profession with changing professional expectations – especially for GPs – towards more flexibility in their working arrangements and career choices;
- the rise of professionals as managers and a desire to control the gatekeepers to the NHS as general practice was seen as the last untouched bastion of clinical and medical autonomy;
- an increasing emphasis on localisation and community-based services.

While identified as separate contributors to policy and organisational changes there are clear interrelationships between these areas.

Key Themes in UK Primary Care Policy

We present a number of themes in order to map the primary care landscape in the UK. These themes provide an overarching perspective of societal, organisational and political forces which apply to the chapters which follow. They are:

- responses to the crisis in health;
- the role of general practice in the health care system;
- managerialism and financial control;
- changing patient expectations;
- changing professional expectations; and
- localisation and community.

Responses to the 'Crisis in Health'

In the 1970s there was an increasing recognition of a growing number of problems and issues facing health care systems in developed countries. While labelled as a 'crisis', this was not one incident but the coming together of a range of factors. Many of the features of the 'crisis in health' were visible in all industrialised countries and had their roots in concerns about the rapidly escalating costs of health care (Saltman and Von Otter 1992) and other factors (Ham 1992) including:

- Demographic changes – the UK has an ageing population while at the same time a reduction in the proportion of the population of working age, leading to an increasing demand for health care at a time when health systems will be limited in their ability to respond to this demand;
- Epidemiological transition comprising a move from infectious diseases to concern with chronic conditions;
- Concern with social factors – the biomedical or curative approach to health is being questioned with a search for a broader approach which takes into account social factors, recognises the harmful effects of the environment and shifts the emphasis to prevention of ill-health;
- Continuing concerns about inequalities of health and the recognition of their deep-seated nature;
- The ever-widening gap between demands made on health care services and the resources which the government is prepared to make available.

The response to the 'crisis' involved a recognition that changes in the epidemiology and demographics of disease required a different approach from one which focused on the delivery of acute care. Thus, in dealing with chronic illness and supporting older people, the role of general practice and community health services became more central. In the UK, the response was to place greater emphasis on the development of general practice and primary health care teams. This led to an increasing engagement of government and the NHS in developing the quality and role of primary care (DHSS 1986a; DHSS 1987; Ottewill and Wall 1990). There was also a retrenchment with an initial focus on high spending hospitals but a recognition that control also needed to be exercised over the gatekeepers to the NHS.

In the UK, general practitioners have traditionally adopted a 'managed care' approach being both first point of contact for health care for the majority of the population, providing immediate health care to individuals and families and making referrals to secondary care (Fry and Hodder 1994). As Starfield (1998) notes, the UK system of general practice is the most universal and comprehensive system in the world. For example, GPs have a critical role to play in dealing with long-term chronic illness. Similarly, the UK has one of the most comprehensively developed community health services which has increasingly become integrated with general practice. This integration interestingly combines both primary medical care and primary health care. Thus the need to address changes in disease management from mainly acute episodes to the management of chronic disease places a greater burden on primary care and perhaps led to the 'rediscovery' of the GP's role.

The Role of General Practice in the Health Care System

General practice has a long history within the UK health care system (discussed further in Chapter 4). GP medical practice has its roots in community-based medicine. However, developments in health care systems in most developed countries during the last century led to a decreasing emphasis on community medicine and an increasing emphasis on hospital-based medicine. In the UK, and to a certain extent in New Zealand, Canada and parts of northern Europe, the GP has traditionally played an integral role in the organisation of health care systems, notably as gatekeeper to secondary care. However, it was only in the UK that this was applied both universally and comprehensively across the whole population through the registering of patients (GP lists/rostas).

It was this pivotal role of the GP as manager of care and gatekeeper of the NHS which became more formally recognised in the 1980s and 1990s, particularly with the introduction of fundholding, and more recently primary care commissioning. The supposition was that primary care purchaser/providers will have more incentive to reduce referrals and secondary health care costs by managing patient care more effectively. It was also assumed that primary care can be developed to provide more cost-effective care than hospitals by improving local community-based services and introducing new home-based services. There is some evidence to support this but overall research suggests that cost saving through shifting services to primary care and developing primary care commissioning may not be realised (Gordon and Hadley 1996; Godber *et al.* 1997; Le Grand *et al.* 1998; Peckham 1999).

Of particular relevance here are the international comparisons of health care systems which have demonstrated that countries with stronger primary medical care systems with limited direct patient access to secondary care have lower overall health costs (Fry and Hodder 1994; Starfield 1998). Thus, in reviews of USA managed care systems commentators have questioned the appropriateness and transferability of the potential health improvements and cost savings as the UK, and other European countries, have more developed primary medical care services (Saltman 1997; Robinson and Steiner 1998). In the UK, the system, established in 1948 and providing universal free access to health care via GPs, has served well by providing large benefits for low costs. In addition, the management and payment arrangements for GPs (based on capitation payments for registered patients topped up through fees and allowances) have ensured that consultation rates remain low compared with countries such as the USA and Canada and have maintained lower overall health costs partly because of the limitation of access to specialists and sub specialists (Starfield 1998).

Managerialism and Financial Control

Within the history of the NHS, one recurrent theme has been the need to deal with an increasingly complex area of the public sector. Given the relative dominance of professions in policy-making, administrative or managerial policies were remarkably feeble for the first 30 or so years of the NHS. Real interest in the way the organisation of the NHS was managed became particularly relevant in the 1970s in response to a slowdown in the expansion of the public sector, the desire to control health care expenditure and the introduction of new approaches to public finance management. The focus of these attempts at managerial control focused on the hospital sector with cost centre budgeting, the Resource Management Initiative, the introduction of general management and the development of the NHS internal market (Klein, 1995). While these reforms impacted on community health services and on quality improvements in general practice, it was not until the further reforms of 1991 were introduced that GPs were to become more involved in resource management issues. The impact of such explicit managerial strategies has been questioned (Harrison *et al.* 1992) although they represent an additional component of primary care policy.

Central to such managerial strategies was the redefinition of primary care as purchaser and providers on the basis that, being closer to and more aware of patient needs, primary care practitioners (initially GPs) have more incentive to reduce referrals and secondary health care costs by managing patient care more effectively. It is also assumed that primary care can be developed to provide more cost-effective care than hospitals by improving local community-based services and introducing new home-based services. Perhaps, more importantly, the growing organisational interest in primary care has more to do with the pervading managerialist agenda across the NHS. The introduction of changes in the 1990s (especially the GP Contract, and the development of primary care organisations (PCOs)) has brought GPs and other practitioners within budgetary control measures for hospital and community health services (Moon and North 2000). With this has come an increasing emphasis on managerial accountability and performance management. The introduction of Primary Care Groups (PCGs) and Trusts (PCTs) in England and their counterparts in the other UK home nations (during the late 1990s) represents an extension of these developments on a comprehensive and universal scale (Glendinning 1999). The reforms of the early and late 1990s were both aimed at reducing variation in practice between areas, addressing the problem of fragmentation and finally bringing all GPs under the managerial ambit of the NHS (Moon and North 2000). These issues are discussed further in Chapters 6 and 8 where we explore the extent to which managerial approaches have been not only adopted to the control of primary care but also adopted by some primary care professionals.

Changing Patient Expectations

General practice has generally enjoyed a high degree of public confidence and support. The first patients' survey in 1998 found that of the 80 per cent of respondents who had seen their GP in the last year most had found services to be satisfactory and that GPs made the right treatment choices. Practice nurses enjoyed similar levels of satisfaction (DoH 1999a). Over the past few years, there has been no marked increase in GP consultations and no significant shift in services from secondary to primary care (Rogers *et al.* 1999). However, there have also been changes in the way people are using primary care services. One area that has seen a significant rise in demand is for out-of-hours services (Hallam and Craig 1994). There have also been rises in the number of consultations for specific population groups such as very young children, and for specific diseases (Rogers *et al.* 1999).

Among GPs there is a widely held perception of patients being more demanding but the evidence for this is somewhat mixed (Hayter *et al.* 1996; Rogers *et al.* 1999). That patients are making different demands on general practice is clear but the way general practice and other primary care services are providing services to patients is also changing. Referrals have risen over the past 30 or more years because of clinical and technological advances. There is more intensive community support, particularly in areas such as child health and cancer treatment and support. Patients are also being discharged earlier from hospital with intensive community nursing support. At the same time there have been wider changes for individuals in other service sectors where 'consumerist' patterns have been changing rapidly. This has consequent effects upon primary care as it forces a reassessment of service provision such as the organisation and delivery of out-of-hours services.

There has also been a wider questioning of the role and power of professionals with patients showing less deference and also a willingness to challenge their decisions (R. Smith 1998). Patients will no longer offer their (unquestioning) loyalty to primary care or its practitioners; exit and voice may become much more apparent (Hirschmann 1970. See Chapter 7 for a further discussion of Hirschmann). The growth of patient and user groups and the increasing access to information places patients in a different context than say 40 or 50 years ago (Lupton *et al.* 1998). Alongside these developments there has been a growing recognition that the role of the patient is changing from one which is a passive recipient to one as informed partner. This concept of partnership between practitioner and patient involves a whole-patient focus, a high degree of knowledge of the patient, caring and empathy, trust, appropriately adapted care, *patient participation and shared decision-making* (Leopold *et al.* 1996). The increased availability of information for patients coupled with higher expectations is perhaps one of the biggest changes in recent years but it is doubtful whether patients will use such information (Marshall *et al.* 2000). It is likely that this trend, encouraged by NHS policy, will continue but will also be supported by the growth of new technologies such as access to the Internet, video consoles in GP surgeries and a growth in consumer health information services, such as Help for Health (based in Winchester), and helplines such as NHS Direct. Patients in the surgery are more likely to be able to obtain relevant information before consulting their general practitioner (Hardey

1999). There is also growing evidence to demonstrate that patient involvement is likely to lead to an improved clinical outcome (Coulter 1997).

This 'partnership' contrasts with traditional views about the patient–doctor relationship which have been more focused on the patient presenting their illness to the professional doctor who diagnoses and validates the illness (D. Lupton 1994). This relationship can be seen as paternal in nature and also as one in which the patient is passive. Such changes provide enormous challenges for primary care practitioners and for GPs, in particular. However, the need to make such changes was widely acknowledged within policy documents in the late 1990s, such as *Patient Partnership* (DoH 1996c) and the White Papers *Primary Care: Delivering the Future* (DoH 1996a), *The New NHS: Modern, Dependable* (DoH 1997) and *The NHS Plan* (DoH 2000). Perhaps more importantly, such changes were seen as being necessary by the medical profession itself (Toop 1998; Gillam and Pencheon 1998) which was also undergoing rapid change.

Changing Professional Expectations

The second half of the twentieth century saw enormous changes in the practice of primary care. The training and education programmes available to primary care staff have grown enormously, often from a low level; for example, education and research programmes in general practice and specialist training courses for community nursing have developed rapidly since the 1960s (Boaden 1997). The professional development of existing staff and the challenges of 'new' professional groups have been catalysts for changing expectations. In addition, the organisational changes in the health service and general changes to working patterns in the NHS and the wider workforce have also contributed to this (Pringle 1998). The professional configuration of primary care has changed substantially in the last 20 years with a consequent impact upon ways of working between and within professions. Changes in professional boundaries, workload, accountability and location have resulted.

In terms of patient consultations, there has been a small increase and on average each general practitioner carried out 152 consultations per week in 1992/93. This had increased from 146.73 in 1989/90. The significant change has been in the mix of type of consultation, with telephone consultations becoming increasingly important, largely because of out-of-hours consultations by telephone.

As Table 1.7 shows, while the average number of consultations remained constant in the UK during the 1990s, the proportion of home visits decreased and telephone, surgery and clinic visits increased. GPs, supported by government policy in the mid-1990s, opted for more deputising services or co-operatives to handle out-of-hours services including opening clinics and surgeries and requesting patients to telephone in and/or visit surgeries rather than GPs visiting patients.

Table 1.7 Number of Patient Consultations per Week by Type, Great Britain, 1989/90 and 1992/93

Type of Activity	1989/90		1992/93	
	No.	*%*	*No.*	*%*
Surgery	117.87	80.33	107.50	70.70
Home visiting	22.30	15.20	19.20	12.60
Clinics	6.56	4.46	6.70	4.40
Telephone	N/A	N/A	18.70	12.30
Total	146.73	100	152.10	100

Source: Doctors and Dentists' Review Body. *General Medical Practitioners' Workload Survey 1992/93. Final Analysis* (London: DoH), Table D5.

For GPs it was this transition to the use of out-of-hours services which created a major transformation in working practice and was directly related to frustrations with running practices as 365-day, 24-hour services: 'the main reason it's done is because GPs are fed up with their on-call' (GP quoted in Rogers *et al.* 1999: 29).

From the mid-1950s the increasing professionalisation of general practice involved concerns about the quality of care and the development of services. This ultimately led to larger practice sizes and the development of practice teams (see Table 1.8). The trend to multi-partner practices has been consistent since the 1960s. Between 1991 and 1997 the fall in the number of single-handed practices (212) has almost been matched by the increase in the number of partnerships of seven or more GPs (187). Overall there are now nearly 140 fewer partnerships than in 1991 but also more GPs have meant lower average list sizes.

The development of larger practices as business units – especially through the extension into health care purchasing – rather than the more traditional practitioner partnerships has provided new organisational contexts for general practitioners, and later on, community nurses. GPs were no longer simply independent practitioners but members of practices with organisational and managerial responsibilities. This shift was stimulated by the introduction of the Allowance Schemes for practice staff, and later, the 1990 GP Contract and the developments in primary care commissioning in the 1990s. New horizons were opened up for GPs and managers in primary care creating new primary care entrepreneurs who were often the driving force behind organisational and policy developments in the 1990s (Glennerster *et al.* 1994; Meads 1996). The shift of GPs and, post-1998, primary care nurses into organisational management in primary care organisations represented a clear milestone in primary care developments and demonstrates the shift in professional expectations of

Table 1.8   Number of Partnerships by Partnership Size, England and Wales, 1991–1997

	Number of partnerships of													
	Single Handed		2		3		4		5		6		7/+		Total
Date	No	%	No	%	No	%	No	%	No	%	No	%	No	%	Partner-ships
1991	3059	32	1972	20	1602	17	1259	13	875	9	528	5	382	4	9677
1992	2993	31	1955	20	1569	16	1208	13	860	9	559	6	406	4	9646
1993	3017	31	1930	20	1558	16	1270	13	891	9	560	6	461	4	9687
1994	2954	31	1933	20	1494	15	1270	13	917	10	574	6	503	5	9645
1995	2924	30	1898	20	1441	15	1285	13	932	10	604	6	512	5	9596
1996	2863	30	1876	20	1423	15	1257	13	933	10	645	6	535	5	9531
1997	2847	30	1884	20	1377	14	1263	13	953	10	645	7	569	6	9538

Note: Percentages are rounded to 100.
Sources: DoH, *GMS Statistics for England and Wales, October 1991; 1992; 1993; 1994; 1995; 1996; 1997.* London: DoH.

many GPs away from a purely medical role. However, such trends have often been felt unevenly within the primary care professions; these developments did not affect everyone everywhere.

Medicine is often considered the archetypal profession in the sense that it has secured such a high degree of autonomy in its regulation, operation and evaluation. This autonomy is often called clinical freedom in health care settings (Harrison 1999). Professions have varying degree of 'success' in protecting their occupational group from the incursions or attentions of other professions or managers, a process known as social closure (Flynn 1999). The experience of general practice in securing autonomy is somewhat mixed. On the one hand, medicine has been the most effective profession at securing such closure and yet, as generalists working in primary care, GPs have perhaps been more susceptible to competing claims from nurses and therapy professions than other medical specialities (Exworthy *et al*. 2002a) (see Chapter 8). On the other hand, general practice has arguably secured autonomy by virtue of the semi-detached position that it negotiated for itself at the outset of the NHS. Policy shifts since then have, in the words of Klein's (1990) famous analogy, altered the position of the partners in the 'politics of the double bed.' The 'contract' between the government and the (general practice) profession – in which the former provides the resources and freedom for the latter to deliver an electorally popular welfare service – is thus in a constant process of being re-made.

A number of consequences flow from such autonomy of GPs and the relative lack of autonomy for other primary care professionals. First, they are in a superordinate position *vis-à-vis* clinical colleagues although they are, at the same time, *de facto* members of the primary care team. Second, operating as small businesses, GPs employ primary care staff including practice nurses, some paramedical staff, practice managers and receptionists. These two factors stress the relative power of GPs. Third, GPs have traditionally guarded the process and outcomes of performance assessments such as clinical audit. Usually, only fellow GPs have been allowed to assess the clinical performance of their colleagues. However, since practices 'compete' for patients, the assessment of work performance by fellow GPs or even the profession was cursory or non-existent. The managerialisation of general practice has begun to ensure that clinical performance is no longer the preserve of GPs alone, a move being hastened by the scandals concerning Drs Ledward, Neale, Shipman and those at the Bristol Royal Infirmary. Nurses' work has been assessed more closely than GPs. Fourth, the deference that patients and the public had towards doctors is declining. Aided by advances in information technology, their willingness to criticise GPs is making some GPs defensive in their attitudes and style of practice. These factors are combining to ensure that general practice is no longer an isolated and unfettered area of medicine and the NHS.

Localisation and Community

The final key area which has been closely associated with developments in primary care has been the issue of localisation. This is often seen as being hand in hand with decentralisation and has been identified as a key element in recent reforms in the UK (Hudson *et al.* 1999b; Hudson 1999b) and also in other countries such as Canada (Rachlis and Kushner 1994; Armstrong and Armstrong 1999) and New Zealand. General practice has always been a localised service with decision-making autonomy. Since the establishment of the NHS there has been a concerted policy to ensure a geographical spread of GPs across the country overseen by the Medical Practitioners Committee, who made allocation judgements based on equitable distribution, and thus avoiding major discrepancies in list size or distribution of GPs (Exworthy 1994a). This is in marked contrast to countries such as Canada and the USA (Fry and Hodder 1994).

The localised nature and universal geographical coverage has been one of the key strengths of UK general practice. There are two distinctive elements to this locality focus. The first is the decentralist nature of health care organisation (owing to professional autonomy and discretion), although this is occurring within a more centrally regulated framework (Mohan 1995, Powell 1998). In health care systems, general practice and the wider primary care service have been seen as being ideal structures within which to incorporate decentralised organisations. Further, in the UK and New Zealand, area-based approaches to health care have been developed from initial reforms promoting primary care-led purchasing (Peckham 1999). The second is the emphasis on links with local communities. There is a perception that as general practice is a local service it is closer to the community and, therefore, best placed to understand patients' and the community's needs (Myles *et al.* 1998). This approach appears also to have been adopted at a policy level, certainly by health authorities who canvassed the views of GPs as proxies for communities and by the government who are drawing GPs more and more into decision-making (Le Grand *et al.* 1998; Lupton *et al.* 1998). Above all, however, this view is often held by GPs themselves, despite contrary evidence of their abilities to represent the views of the communities within which they are located (Hudson *et al.* 1999b).

In the UK suggestions for the development of more area-based primary care were first developed before the Second World War with the idea of local health centres – building on the ideas of the Dawson Report discussed in Chapter 3. However, owing to the pressure applied by the medical profession at the creation of the NHS in 1948, the eventual model of 'primary care' developed at a local level was marked by independent general practitioners working with local authority community health staff. This tension remained, with community nursing being developed on a mainly area basis and GPs working to practice lists. The tension came to a head with the Cumberlege Report on community nursing in 1986 which recommended area-based nursing teams rather than practice-based ones (DoH 1986b). However, GPs mounted a sustained attack on these proposals and the government eventually backed practice-based teams (Ottewill and Wall 1990; Exworthy 1994a). However, localities remained an enduring approach to health care organisation and many Health Authorities developed such locality approaches, especially in the post-reform era of the internal market in 1991, and by the mid-1990s primary care purchasers were also exploring larger multi-practice groups covering geographical areas. With Total Purchasing, GP Commissioning Groups and finally universal primary care groups being implemented throughout the UK in the late 1990s the pendulum has swung decisively towards locality arrangements for the development of health care (Hudson *et al.* 1998). This is likely to continue with primary care trusts.

Research evidence has suggested, however, that the formation of the new PCOs throughout the UK had little to do with local community factors and owed more to GP relationships in fundholding, existing health authority boundaries in relation to PCGs (Hudson *et al.* 1999) and for PCTs the need to align organisations with local authority boundaries. In many ways, the new PCTs are akin to old health authorities in form and function. Moreover, as they grow in size, they are starting to search for locality focus. As Strategic Health Authorities begin in 2002, PCTs will be under greater pressure to manage both the efficiencies (generated by the economies of scale) and ensure a locality outlook.

Understanding Primary Care: Integration, Diversity and Changing Boundaries

The interaction between these multiple factors has cumulatively provided the impetus for policy interest in primary care. These factors highlight three crucial tensions in primary care: integration, diversity and changing boundaries illustrated in Figure 1.1. These recur throughout the book and we shall revisit them in the final chapter.

The key tensions demonstrate how changes in policy and organisation tend to work within this paradox. Policy has supported greater diversity and differentiation within primary care while at the same time pursuing a strategy of integration into the NHS. Likewise, diversity and integration have necessarily shifted the boundaries of primary care and its constituent professions, organisations and relationships. These themes are not necessarily mutually exclusive and, as will be discussed in later chapters, UK primary care policy has sought to reconcile these parallel policy tracks. They will probably continue to do so for the foreseeable future. These seismic shifts in primary care resonate with broader public and social policy changes in the UK. There are clear parallels in education and local government, for example (Powell, 2002).

Taken together, a number of these contextual changes relate to postmodernist analyses of welfare services (Loader and Burrows, 1994). In particular, integration, diversity and shifted boundaries are central to many debates about postmodernism (Giddens 2001; Petersen and Lupton, 1996; Pinch, 1997). The discussions in this chapter demonstrate that primary care (its policies, organisation, services and practitioners) has been responding to both internal and external context. Elements of the changes in primary care are associated with a postmodern analysis including: the fragmentation of services; the decentralisation of organisation; the blurring of traditional roles; and the blurring of responsibilities between stakeholders (including lay people). Primary care has always been difficult to organise along Fordist lines given autonomous professionals working with a range of social and medical problems. Yet, primary care (and especially general practice) has been noted for its professional hierarchy. In recent years, Fordist organisations (characterised by centralisation, standardised production and consumption) have been replaced by post-Fordist models of decentralised and dynamic forms. The effects of such changes elsewhere have shifted the (internal and external) boundaries of primary care as it becomes integrated into the mainstream NHS and as it both tackles and fosters diversity. Old traditional structures are being challenged and there have been shifts in the relationships between different practitioners in primary care, between other NHS and public services, changing relationships with patients and the public, and changing organisational structures.

Yet, these changes need to be set within the wider context of UK health policy which has emphasised integration through the use of techno-bureaucratic solutions, which are favoured by the Labour Government (Harrison 2001). This includes more central direction to the shape of health care services

Themes	Integration	Diversity	Changing boundaries
The wider model of primary care	More embedded in the NHS Role for nurses on PCO boards and executive committees	PCG/PCTs/LHGs/ SPCTs autonomy Different models of PCO – geographical, organisational and functional differences	Merger of boundaries between health and social care Public health role in PCOs
Managerialism	Stronger contractual relationship between primary care organisations and health authorities Stronger emphasis on regulation and performance management – role of NICE and CHI	Individual PCO freedom to decide resource allocation within PCO – i.e. Between practices	Clinicians' role in management Private sector involvement Managerial care in primary care
Changing patient expectations	National standards of care Equity	Meeting individual/ local community needs Local involvement/ responses	Patient as expert Overlap between 'informal' and 'formal' carer roles
Partnership	Health Improvement Plan as blueprint for service development and delivery Local Strategic Partnerships Integrated providers, Health Act partnerships – Care Trusts	Range and nature of partnerships will vary Historical legacy	Closer links with Local Authorities Organisational complexity increasing (primary–secondary care interface) Fluid organisational boundaries
Changing professions	Emphasis on clinical governance and reduction of variation in standards of practice constrained autonomy PMS changes e.g. salaried GPs, nurse led Incorporating professions	GPs retain independent contractor status – mixed independent and salaried status Contractual arrangements for nurses vary Roles and responsibilities between professions vary – Walk-in Centres	New professions and professional roles Skill mix and substitution/ delegation Private sector employment

Figure 1.1 The Policy Paradox: Incorporation and Differentiation in Primary Care

Themes	Integration	Diversity	Changing boundaries
Localisation and community	Population focus (not just registered patients) Increasing size of PCOs Looking upwards and outwards (to regulators and inspectors)	Focus on patients and practice list Practices encouraged to adopt neighbourhood approaches particularly for public health activity Developing local solutions – include actions by others (HAZ, SRB)	Stronger public health focus in PCOs Coterminosity in LHGs

Figure 1.1 (*continued*)

(through national (clinical and organisational) standards, regulation and increased performance management). Thus, tensions are introduced into the health care system which appears to demonstrate, on the one hand, a post-modern leaning towards diversity while, on the other hand, retaining a strong Fordist sense of structure and control over the apparatus and organisation of health care services.

Conclusion

This chapter has examined some of the reasons why primary care has become so central to health care policy in the UK, and also in many other countries. The enormous growth seen in UK primary care is a response both to changing circumstances and to policy initiatives. The dividing line between these is often very blurred. Undoubtedly primary care is more complex both in terms of activity and organisation than it was at the inception of the NHS in the late 1940s. However, it is also clear that the changes in primary care, which began as a quiet revolution, have rapidly built up a quickening pace of change. Primary care has attained central place in current policy and in organisational and managerial changes in the UK. This centrality can be not only seen as a response to changing external circumstances about how health care can be more efficient and effective, but also arises from changing patterns of professional working and patient demand.

At the turn of the twenty-first century, primary care is still in rapid transition in common with many other aspects of the NHS. The Labour Government, returned for a second term of office in 2001, is determined to push through its modernisation of the NHS. PCOs form the basis of organisational change across the UK. The precise form of these PCOs will vary between the devolved territories but it is likely to generate tensions between decentralisation and centralisation. Thus, primary care represents and is emblematic of many of the reform processes currently operating in the UK. Primary care is also a central component of that reform.

The book is divided into three main parts. This first part (Chapters 1–5) defines our approach to policy and primary care before presenting a descriptive account of the historical and present organisations of primary care. The second part (Chapters 6–11) deals with individual components of contemporary primary care in the UK. These components examine the activities and functions of particular aspects. The third part (Chapter 12) revisits our three themes (integration, diversity and changing boundaries) and provides the basis for a set of scenarios for primary care in the UK. These scenarios offer some potential directions in which primary care might travel.

CHAPTER 2

Policy Perspectives on Primary Care

This book adopts a viewpoint of primary care in the UK in which policy perspectives are central. Many other books explore the issues of primary care but not from a policy perspective; likewise, there are many health policy books but most do not focus on primary care. We hope to rectify this by providing an explicit link between policy and primary care. Though we draw on evidence from a wide range of sources, the thread which runs through each chapter is a focus on the structures and processes by which decisions about, for example, the allocation of resources within the NHS, the strategy for interagency collaboration and the direction of primary care organisations are made and applied. The consequences (intended or otherwise) of such decisions also fall within our remit.

This perspective seeks to describe, understand and explain how policy is formulated and implemented. In effect, this is the lens through which primary care is viewed. Others will take different perspectives depending on their ideological and disciplinary standpoints. This book is neither concerned with, for example, clinical service delivery nor specific managerial techniques, and similarly, it does not draw on one discipline such as sociology or economics.

This chapter explores the nature of policy and provides an introduction to our approach to policy analysis. It sets out a range of approaches and concepts which we use within the book in order to explore and assess primary care in the UK. Use is also made of policy models and concepts in relation to the specific themes which are explored in individual chapters. In short, this chapter provides the 'methodology' for the book.

Primary care provides both the object and process of policy in the UK; that is, primary care is seen as a focus of policy – the purpose and goal of policy – but also the mechanisms or means by which objectives are to be met. Moreover, primary care can be viewed as an area of health care, an activity undertaken by professionals and lay people, and a form of organisation to be structured and managed. Policy has been and is directed to all three of these. Whilst Hogwood and Gunn (1989) have argued that one of the main precepts of policy is that there is clarity in both definition and purpose, it is perhaps the imprecise nature of primary care that makes the policy approach adopted in this

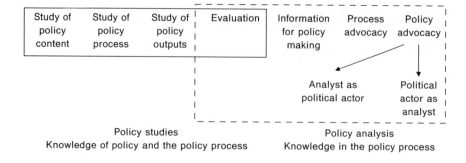

Figure 2.1   Studying Policy

book more meaningful. The study of policy encompasses a broad range of approaches which range from an analysis of policy content to advocating particular policies (see Figure 2.1).

The focus of this book is mainly concerned with the left side of this spectrum – the study of content primary care policy, policy processes and outputs. Our intention is to provide readers with knowledge of policy and the policy process as it pertains to primary care such that they can apply the models and frameworks to their own context and as new policies emerge. Inevitably, a book such as this is out of date as soon as it is published in terms of the specific governmental and organisational policies being pursued. However, the policy perspective offered here provides a means of understanding and explaining previous, current and future policy developments. By doing so, the book is intended for students, practitioners and policy-makers to enhance their 'knowledge in the policy process' – the right side of the spectrum. Hence, our research *of* policy can also provide research *for* policy.

The next section explores the nature of policy and discusses our approach to an analysis of primary care policy in the UK. We also discuss the management and organisation of primary care and further clarification is required as to why these elements are incorporated in our study.

Defining a Policy Perspective in Primary Care

Students of health and social policy in the UK could be excused for thinking that health policy is only about the NHS, albeit with some discussion of public health and social welfare before the NHS or in the context of Beveridge. Yet can this really be all there is to health policy? The NHS is clearly the main emphasis of health and social policy texts published in the UK and perhaps we should be forgiven for our attachment to such a cherished and undeniably important institution. It is also true that a discussion of primary care in the UK would necessarily focus on the NHS as this is how we would understand its development in the post-war period. However, our approach is one which is based within health policy rather than simply NHS policy.

Clearly both the terms *health* and *policy* require further definition. In examining the state of health policy in the UK what becomes immediately clear is the limited definition and focus of both these terms. Policies devoted to 'health' can be seen in a variety of ways including the delivery of health services, improvements to individuals' and populations' well-being, and as activities which affect the health of individuals and populations. It is thus more than just the study of the policies of the Department of Health or the organisations of the NHS. 'Health policy' is multi-faceted and yet it is often portrayed in simplistic terms. Hogwood and Gunn (1989: 13–19) reveal this complexity and present different ways of thinking about policy *per se*:

- policy as a label for a field of activity;
- policy as an expression of general purpose or desired state of affairs;
- policy as specific proposals;
- policy as decisions of government;
- policy as formal authorisation;
- policy as a programme;
- policy as output;
- policy as outcome;
- policy as a theory or model; and
- policy as process.

We will be drawing on most of these uses of policy in the following chapters. However, these merely describe uses of the word policy. Definitions of policy bring together a range of ideas that focus on the notion of policy as process and action but which also incorporate decisions and non-decisions. In this sense, policy can be both implicit and explicit. Policy also encompasses inaction in the sense that it is decided not to do something or even that issues are considered as either not a problem or not amenable to a policy intervention. For Walt:

> Health policy embraces courses of action that affect the set of institutions, organisations, services and funding arrangements of the health care system. It goes beyond health services, however, and includes actions or intended actions by public, private and voluntary organisations that have an impact on health. (1994: X4–5)

This inclusive approach suggests that health policy should be concerned with issues which affect people's health. To deal with this diversity and complexity, it is useful to draw on three dimensions of health policy, as defined by Walt (1994) (also see Ham (1992)):

- Content;
- Process; and
- Power.

We are concerned with all three of these elements within this book. Content is the object of health policy and health policy analysis. Content can be further subdivided into technical policies and institutional policies (Janovsky and Cassels, 1996). Current UK health policy is embracing such an approach with a growing interest in public health and the role of private and public agencies; note, for example, public health strategies (DoH 1999b) and National Service Frameworks such as for Mental Health or Older People (DoH 1999c; 2001a). Recent work on health inequalities and health impact assessment demonstrate this further. While such moves are welcome, this work still focuses very much on institutional arrangements rather than areas of health. In this book, our concern is with the area of health policy and as such we are as interested in the nature of the institutional arrangements of primary care (its organisation and management) as objects of policy. In this sense we can view primary care as both an 'end' of policy and a 'means' – traditionally the two concerns of public policy (Hill 1997; 1998). However, it is not sufficient simply to view primary care as an area of study for, as Walt, Janovsky, Ham and other health policy analysts have argued, we need to place more emphasis on process. As Wildavsky (1979) reminded us, 'policy is a process, as well as a product'. Policy is an activity, and as Walt's definition of health policy (above) demonstrates, this involves intentions and actions.

The policy process should not be viewed as straightforward for two reasons. First, the notion that policy process moves from intention (as manifest by strategy documents and proposals) to action (in the form of action plans or the activities of managers and practitioners) is inadequate and misleading. Second, the policy process is sometimes described as 'messy' denoting that it is not linear or rational. Moreover, it often has no definite start or end point – only a middle (John 2000). Most policies are formulated and implemented in pre-existing situations such that most decisions have already been made in previous time periods. Most funding decisions, for example, consider only marginal changes to funding levels rather than a fundamental reassessment of allocative principles. Hence, there is invariably little scope for major change. This incremental perspective was highlighted by Lindblom (1959) who argued that the policy process was often static and only punctuated by short periods of dynamism. He coined the term 'disjointed incrementalism' to describe such situations. Furthermore, the policy process is marked by (positive and negative) feedback loops, occurring as a result of often unintended outcomes; hence, the process rarely reaches completion.

The policy process concerns decision-making and evaluation of alternative options. Despite policy strategies and plans, much of the policy process takes place out of sight – it is not easily observed by the public or researchers. Whilst there are some notable empirical studies of the health policy process (e.g. Flynn *et al.* 1996; Griffiths and Hughes 2000), much analysis draws heavily on the use of concept, theories and models. This is the focus of the next section.

Dimensions of Policy in Primary Care

Given the volume of literature relating to the study and analysis of health policy, it is a fruitless task in this chapter to provide anything more than a thumbnail sketch of some of the key concepts. The purpose here is thus not to offer a comprehensive guide but rather to highlight a selection of theories and models which, we believe, are most applicable to the study and analysis of primary care in this book. More comprehensive guides can be found elsewhere. The following texts provide general interesting and analytical approaches to the topic: Ham and Hill (1993), John (2000), Rhodes (1997), and Hogwood and Gunn (1989). Others are more focused on health policy: Ham (1992), Green and Thorogood (1998), Klein (1995) and Baggott (1998).

We present three broad topics to explore a range of theories and models applicable to primary care: interest groups and stakeholders, central–local relations, and implementation within which there are a number of themes.

Interest Groups and Stakeholders

Pluralism

It is axiomatic that there are multiple interest groups in UK health care including the general public/taxpayers, patients, doctors, nurses, paramedical professions, managers, politicians and civil servants, to name but a few. Pluralism implies that these stakeholders can affect policy, as Ham and Hill (1993: 28) summarise:

> No group is without power to influence decision-making, and equally no group is dominant. Any group can ensure that its political preferences and wishes are adopted if it is sufficiently determined.

However, each group is not homogeneous but comprised of hierarchies and niches. In the policy process, these groups (and subgroups) have varying levels of influence. Hence, the inequality between and within groups enables some groups to use the policy process and its outcomes to enhance their position (John 2000). Moreover, the state is not a neutral arbiter in this process; it privileges particular groups and interests, either implicitly or explicitly. Pluralism generates a fragmented policy process and is thus associated with incrementalism and muddling through, as stakeholders exert their varying degrees of influence (Lindblom 1959). In cases where no single group is dominant, Lindblom (1965) argued that decision-makers co-ordinated their behaviour through adaptive adjustments, a process termed partisan mutual adjustment (Harrison *et al.* 1990).

Policy communities and networks

Building on the notion of pluralism, it is possible to argue that most policy processes do not take place in isolation but in groupings of differing interests. Certainly a key development over the past 20 years in the UK has been the development of a strong primary care policy community with new national representative organisations (e.g. NHS Confederation and NHS Alliance) joining traditional professional groups such as the RCGP, RCN, and CPHVA. These policy communities and interests (Hill 1998) denote the often close interactions between policy-makers and others, whether at national or local levels. It is thus important to identify, explain and understand the values, ideas and practices of such communities and networks. As a classic example, Heclo and Wildavsky (1974) in their study of the policy community examined the interactions between Treasury civil servants and their colleagues in other Whitehall departments.

Rhodes (1997), among many others, has identified the multiplicity of stakeholders within different policy sectors such as health, education or transport, involving public and private interests. 'Although decision-making bodies have some room for manoeuvre, they usually depend on each other, and thus form close dependent relationships within a policy sector' (John 2000: 83). Sabatier (1991), among others, has argued that policy formulation and implementation emerges from the formation and maintenance of coalitions of interests. Many communities and networks are marked by close, ongoing relations between stakeholders which can generate high levels of trust and dependence. It can also bring about detailed knowledge of other stakeholders. Hence, a degree of embeddedness can result. This may be manifest in, for example, GP patterns of referral to secondary or health authority commissioning decisions (Exworthy 1998a).

Networks illustrate how policy-making (particularly in health care) can often involve bottom-up processes. Close relations between network members can provide the basis for learning from each other, thereby anticipating or obviating government policy. Such policy learning and development is often more effective since it has been grounded in experience. Commissioning developments in the 1990s demonstrate such policy learning arising from experimentation with different models in the absence of, or before, formal government policy.

Two types of community or network have been distinguished: issue and policy networks. Issue networks are oriented around specific issues and, as a result, tend to comprise loose and open connections between a shifting group of actors. Policy networks tend to be marked by a stable and limited group of stakeholders who enjoy shared responsibility and high degree of integration. Unlike issue networks, most policy-making occurs in policy networks. However, networks are, by definition, not institutions (as organisations are) but affiliations of interests. This makes the definition and identification of networks problematic.

Structural interests in health care

Alford's (1975) theory was originally deployed to explain local reform processes in the city of New York in the 1970s. It has, however, also been extensively applied to the NHS (Ham 1992; Harrison *et al.* 1990; North and Peckham 2001). While problems have been identified in its application to the UK (North 1995), the theory is helpful in focusing attention on embedded structured interests underpinning political processes within the health services and in providing a lucid framework for analysis in later chapters of this book. It is worth, therefore, exploring the notion of structured interests a little further.

Alford identified three interest groups – the professional monopolisers, the corporate rationalisers and the community – reflecting dominant, challenging and repressed interests in health care respectively. These represent the key stakeholders, visible or otherwise, in health care politics. Compare these interests with those of, for example, Lindblom (1977) (namely, group representatives, policy-makers and citizens) or the 'iron triangle' comprising the US Congress, executive agencies and producer interests (see John 2000: 79). Dominant structural interests are those maintained by the existing structure of social, economic and political institutions. For Alford, professional monopolisers, exemplified by the medical profession, comprised the dominant structural interests. The power of the professional monopolisers was both reflected in and secured by the law and practices of both public and private institutions. Various interests were represented within the profession and would be affected differently by reforms, but the diverse types of medical practitioner shared a common interest in preserving professional autonomy. When that autonomy was threatened, the different subgroups of the profession were able to unite to mount a common defence. Alford argued that the political and cultural hegemony which medicine enjoyed was not a product of societal consensus but, rather medical power operated to legitimise the profession's position. (The notion of power is discussed in the next section.)

The challenging interests of corporate rationalisation were represented in such groups as hospital administrators and government health planners. Their objective was to extend control over the work of professional monopolisers and contain costs but, writing in 1975, Alford was not optimistic that reforms would challenge the latter's institutionalised control of the system. The third category – repressed structural interests – represented the medically indigent who could either not afford health care or were neglected by patterns of provision.

Their voices were not heard, because 'no social institution or political mechanisms ... ensure that these interests are served' (Alford 1975: 15), thereby
meaning that they had to muster enormous political and organisational energies
to overcome their disadvantaged position. Alford viewed no one group as being
isolated from the other two. Alliances could form where the possibility of mutual
benefit arose. In particular, the professional monopolisers and corporate rationalisers could develop mutually advantageous alliances to exclude community
interests. However, alliances did not guarantee power-sharing and could result
in the exploitation of the weaker partner such as in the colonisation of patients'
groups by doctors and other professionals (Wood 2000; Jones *et al.* 2002).

Primary care represents a particular challenge to Alford's analytical model as
there is less clarity in relation to the three interests he identifies. Recent developments in primary care policy and organisation only serve to make this situation
more complex (North and Peckham 2001). The integration of primary care into
the corporate structure of the NHS, increasing diversity of primary care actors
(to include social services, nurses and allied health professionals) and the fluidity
of boundaries both within health and between health and other agencies (such as
social services) clearly raises problems for a strict application of Alford's thesis.
However, it serves as an approach to analysing interest groups alongside broader
concepts of structure and agency that are important in understanding both the
content and process of primary care policy.

Power

To understand the content and process of primary care policy requires a focus
on the dynamics of power for, as Walt (1994) argues, health policy is about
power. A focus on power is concerned with how issues are raised in the policy world, who is involved in making decisions and those factors influencing
policy implementation. An analysis of power is necessary to understand, for
example, the continuing development and implementation of primary care
policy innovations over the last decade, including GP fundholding, 'a primary
care-led NHS', primary care groups and primary care trusts. The discussion
of power has been a notable omission in much recent policy analysis of primary care, an exception being Williams (2000). Although a shift in power was
often identified and associated with the quasi-market reforms of the 1990s, the
nature of power in primary care was rarely analysed. The *apparent* shift (in the
balance of power) from secondary care to primary care was not as straightforward as many presumed (Godber *et al.* 1997).

Much current health policy focuses on the overt exercise of power in terms of
decision-making at individual or organisational level. Power is often seen as the
(observable and measurable) ability to control resources or determine policy
decisions (Evans and Exworthy 1996). This Weberian notion of power (Clegg
1989) implies a zero-sum situation; one person or group can only increase their

power at the expense of another losing power. Nurses, for example, could *only* gain power at the expense of doctors.

Two further sets of theories can be identified which demonstrate power as a more complex and subtle concept (Evans and Exworthy, 1996). First, the structuralist approach views power as largely ideological with power being maintained through mechanisms of control which are contested by subordinate groups. Lukes' (1974) three-dimensional theory of power illustrates this. The first dimension concerns the explicit 'conflict over values or course of action' (Bacharach and Baratz 1970: 24). In the second dimension, power is exercised by limiting the scope of action to certain alternatives; here, non-decision-making takes place whereby issues and/or interests are excluded from the (policy) agenda and policy process (Harrison *et al.* 1992). The third dimension involves the shaping of perceptions, preferences and expectations by those 'in power' such that others may not be conscious of such an exercise of power. As Hunter (1994: 16) argues: 'The use of power in this sense can occur in the absence of actual, observable conflict'. Hence, non-decisions are difficult to observe as there is nothing to see. Structuralist approaches have also been employed in the political economy of health (Doyal 1979).

The second theory, the Foucauldian approach, views power as more diffuse, localised and invisible (Evans and Exworthy 1996). The approach sees power located in relationships between individuals or groups; hence, it is not held by a few 'powerful' people but is dispersed in the routines and practices to which we are all subjected. It is thus more fluid and dynamic. Foucault (1973) saw power as closely linked to knowledge. In medicine, for example, this knowledge enabled doctors to exercise power through scientific medicine.

Foucauldian analyses of power provide a useful way of thinking about the use and distribution of power within the policy process. However, as discussions in later chapters will demonstrate, the ability to use power is shaped by institutional forces and the ability to use power actively. Giddens (2001) has characterised this as the relationship between structure and agency. Agency relates to the individual (or possibly organisations or interests) whereas structure is the political, economic and societal context within which agency is exercised. Agency is not just about intentions but the capability to act; individuals must be able to perpetrate an event. The concept specifically relates to the power possessed by human agents and their ability to achieve certain effects. Structures are characterised by inertia to change and can be institutional structures such as organisations or professions, or prevailing interests, customs or ideology. Dietz and Burns (1992) have applied this framework to the policy process arguing that to be effective policy actions need to change material or cultural conditions, must be intentional, be sufficiently unconstrained and that the policy actor possesses the ability to observe the consequences of the action and be reflexive in evaluating actions. In other words, the exercise of power must be observable. To this end it is worth keeping Lukes' three views of power in mind when assessing the extent to which policy actors can influence the policy agenda.

Central–Local Relations

The size and complexity of health care systems and organisations necessarily generate tiers and levels. For the NHS, the tiers range from central government to individual agencies. The relations between these tiers – often termed central–local relations or inter-governmental relations – characterise the nature of the system itself. However, unlike other institutions, the NHS is marked by a high degree of political involvement and a highly professionalised workforce. Such features have shaped the creation and evolution of the NHS. Hence, this section is concerned with the ways in which the tiers of the NHS interrelate.

Frenk (1994) has described four levels of the policy process – the systemic, programmatic, organisational and instrumental:

1. The systemic level is that which shapes the health system overall: policy on the shape of the NHS or public health;
2. The programmatic level is concerned with deciding health priorities and resource allocation at the macro level, such as HA decisions on funding for children's services or mental health;
3. The organisational level is concerned with the way health services operate, such as the organisation and management of PCOs and their relations with other providers;
4. The instrumental level is where management policy is 'made' and relates much more to implementation of services.

(These levels are used to structure the discussion in Chapter 4). While there is some separation between these different levels of policy process, in reality aspects of each of these levels can be seen operating at both national and local spheres. More importantly, with political devolution in the UK, new governmental spheres have been introduced affecting the nature and location of policy-making. Certainly, decisions about the overall strategic direction of the NHS are taken at a national level but it is also true that organisational policy is made nationally. This reflects an apparent dichotomy. On the one hand, over the last decade, much of the development of primary care policy has been pioneered at a local level by practitioners and managers because central policy development has lagged behind local developments and because much central policy has only provided only a broad framework. On the other hand, governments have become more interventionist in terms of national standards, regulation and funding.

Central government policy-making has often sought to introduce a 'transmission belt' from the centre to the periphery, thereby providing a degree of command and control over the NHS. Such a strategy serves the political saliency of the NHS and aids cost containment. Indeed, the notion that a bedpan dropped on a hospital ward should reverberate around the corridors of Whitehall (articulated by Bevan at the outset of the NHS) still has some applicability. However, Mohan (1995) and Powell (1997) among others have questioned whether the transmission belt (translating central policy into local action) is, or ever was, effective. For example, the strength of central–local relations has served to create the notion of a *national* health service, whereas local decision-making makes uniformity unlikely. Claims of 'postcode rationing', for example, undermine the notion of uniform health service provision; instead they reflect the NHS's organisational decision-making structures.

The balance in central–local relations is not simply shaped by local decision-making structures such as health authorities. Many governments, especially in recent years, have sought to decentralise decision-making away from Whitehall and intermediate tiers. This decentralisation has been associated with the introduction of general management throughout the NHS (in the 1980s) and the creation of more discrete organisational units (such as NHS Trusts). Decentralisation has sometimes been taken further, devolving responsibility within organisations (Burns *et al.* 1994; Exworthy 1994a). In primary care, this has often been linked to improve health needs assessment, to respond to locality issues and to engage better with the public.

Decentralisation is often seen as a 'good thing', empowering local practitioners and reducing bureaucracy. Whilst these may be laudable aspects of decentralisation, the consequences should not be overlooked. For example, decentralisation can be seen as a strategy whereby blame for system failures is devolved whilst credit is centralised (Mohan 1995). Thus, discontent can be isolated and questions about the system itself become invalid. Moreover, the undercurrent of decentralisation necessarily involves centralisation. The principles upon which power is decentralised, resources are allocated and performance is assessed become crucial aspects of the decentralist approach.

These relations are further complicated by the nature of health care itself and its professionalised character. First, the indeterminacy of health and health care interventions necessitate a degree of discretion for clinicians. This uncertainty and the interpersonal nature of health care makes the management of clinicians problematic. Guidelines, regulation and other techniques have only partly challenged clinical freedom. Second, professionals' decisions relating to diagnosis, treatment and/or referral reflect the societal power conferred upon them. However, this complicates the central–local relations such that a great deal of latitude within the health care system resides at local levels, at the clinician–patient interface rather than formal *de jure* policies contained within strategy documents. Lipsky (1980) argued that practitioners – 'street-level bureaucrats' – enjoy discretion over resources. Thus their decisions effectively become the *de facto* policy of the organisation. For example, the official policy may be to reduce health care costs but unless practitioners adjust their decision-making, such a policy is likely to flounder.

> Users of services invariably experience government through [street-level bureaucrats], and their actions often are the policies provided by the government as a result of the substantial discretion allowed them in the execution of their work. (Harrison *et al.* 1992: 9)

This is the essence of professional autonomy, often called clinical freedom in the NHS. Such autonomy provides the basis for a certain amount of discretionary behaviour by clinicians. Harrison (1999) argues that clinical autonomy has 'figured fairly prominently' in government policy (51), an approach reinforced by the formal organisation of the NHS. In primary care, GPs were able to secure independent contractor status when the NHS was formed whereby they were largely free from external intervention. Harrison (1988) has also argued that the practice of (local) management has often colluded with (rather than challenged) medical autonomy.

Implementation

Conditions for effective implementation

A distinction between policy formulation and its implementation is often used in the policy literature and in policy documents. However, these distinction can be overstated, not least because of the effect of street-level bureaucrats who formulate *and* implement in their daily decisions. Among others, Hill (1997) has argued that policy formulation and implementation are so closely intertwined that they are often seen as indivisible. However, it is legitimate to ask: how can policy implementation be promoted? What factors accelerate or hinder implementation?

It should be becoming clear from earlier discussions that the existence of *de jure* policies stated in official documents, reports and plans does not necessarily mean that they will be implemented, as intended, when they reach the clinician–patient interface. As shown above, the discretion of street-level bureaucrats implies that a system's or an organisation's policy is effectively the decisions of its practitioners. Such discrepancies denote a wider concern with implementation more generally within the policy literature. This top-down approach to implementation has often been termed the implementation gap or implementation failure (Dunsire 1978; Pressman and Wildavsky 1973; Wolman 1981; Harrison *et al.* 1992). The gap or failure indicates the difference between intentions and actions. However, more recent research on implementation has criticised such top-down approaches because ideal implementation is rarely (if ever) achieved and objectives often change in mid-course (Rothstein 1998). These approaches often use a list of factors which apparently foster more effective implementation (Gunn 1978; Wolman 1981) (see Box 2.1).

Box 2.1   Gunn's 10 Preconditions for Perfect Implementation

1. External factors do not impose crippling constraints
2. Adequate time and resources are available
3. At all stages, the combination of resources required is available
4. Policy is based on a valid theory of cause and effect

> 5. There is a direct connection between cause and effect, with few (if any) intervening variables
> 6. Only one agency has responsibility for implementation
> 7. There is a shared agreement about the policy's objectives
> 8. The order of tasks to meet objectives is specified
> 9. Communication between stakeholders is perfect
> 10. Persons in authority can guarantee compliance of subordinates
>
> *Source*: Gunn (1978).

Clearly, in most cases, many of these preconditions cannot be assured with any degree of certainty. Nonetheless, drawing on the basis of Gunn's approach, it can be seen that implementation in a complex environment such as the NHS or specifically primary care can become highly problematic.

Implementation models

As a response to the limitations of these preconditions, a number of models have been developed which seek to provide a more analytical perspective than just the vertical dimension – from the government to an individual organisation, for example. Such an approach is more rounded, recognising the 'horizontal' or lateral partnerships that develop at central government or at the local level. Such a perspective has become increasingly important in recent years given the policy emphasis on joined-up government and interagency collaboration (Kavanagh and Richards 2001; Clarence and Painter 1998, see also Chapter 9).

Here we focus more closely on implementation models and in particular upon the notions that policy consists of a number of 'streams' which must be joined in order to facilitate implementation (Challis *et al.* 1988; Webb and Wistow 1986). Kingdon's model based on 'windows' (rather than streams) has also been used to examine how components of policy are applied (Kendall 2000; Kingdon 1995). Both the stream and window models have been used to describe and explain progress in social policy and other fields. Here we compare the policy streams models (Powell and Exworthy 2001) and the policy windows model (Exworthy *et al.* 2002a).

Policy may be seen in terms of three 'streams': policy, process and resource. The *policy stream* refers to the policy objectives which must be clear and agreed. The *process stream* refers to the means and mechanisms by which objectives will be realised; these must be effective and feasible. The *resource stream* refers to the finance, staffing and time which must be available to ensure the mechanisms are adequate. Failure to connect these streams may lead to conflict between stakeholders. The 'success' (or otherwise) of the policy may thus become disputed and may lead to claims that policies are simply rhetorical or symbolic (Edelman, 1971).

Though similar, Kingdon's model examines how issues get on to the policy agenda in the first place and how they become translated into policy (Kendall, 2000). The various streams must be connected before the 'policy window' opens. This model is useful in explaining how opportunities for policy formulation and implementation are created and destroyed. The *problem stream* comprises evidence of the nature of an issue which becomes defined as a problem amenable to policy interventions. This evidence might be crisis incidents, research results, patient feedback or performance indicators. The *policy stream* consists of proposals, strategies and initiatives to address the problem. These often pre-date the problem being recognised and circulate in a 'primeval soup' awaiting their identification. This requires a critical mass of stakeholders to appreciate the merits of the policy. The merits must include an accordance with (political or organisational) values, a technical feasibility and a recognition of future constraints. The *politics stream* comprises party politics, organisational power struggles and interest groups. These three streams may be connected by natural cycles (such as elections), crises or the actions of a policy entrepreneur, an individual or individuals who invest their reputation, status and time in joining the streams in order to open and keep open the policy window. Natural cycles, complacency or the entrepreneur's departure might force the window to close.

The diversity arising from policy implementation has been addressed by a number of policy models that consider the role of context. Here, context applies to the national or local conditions within which the policy is implemented. Such conditions might be social, economic, political or cultural. Pettigrew *et al.* (1992) argue that policy outcomes can be explained by the interaction between inner (local) and outer (national) context, policy content and policy process. The model advanced by Pawson and Tilley (1997) is perhaps more straightforward as it considers policy outcomes as the interaction between context and policy mechanisms. Their 'formula' has been widely adopted:

$$C \text{ (context)} + M \text{ (mechanisms)} = O \text{ (outcome)}$$

In these models, the impact of policy is not simply a reflection of the aims and objectives of policy; rather context has a significant bearing.

It is thus clear that policy formulation and implementation are not simply processes applied *to* primary care but emanate *within* primary care itself and hence it is important to consider organisation and management as part of the policy process as well as the policy content and context. Thus, practitioners and managers should not be viewed simply as passive recipients of policy formulated by central government. They can equally be seen as active participants in the ways in which policies become translated from intention to action.

Governance

The introduction of new public management (examined in Chapter 5), private sector involvement in public services, the emphasis on interagency collaboration and the emergence of more complex policy networks have complicated the policy process. These new processes of governing are termed 'governance' (Rhodes 1997). In recent years, this complexity has increased to the extent that Skelcher (2000) has coined the term 'congested state.' Similarly, Rhodes (1997) has described the differentiated polity in which multiple agencies are involved in policy formulation and implementation because of the 'functional and institutional specialisation and fragmentation of policies and politics' (7).

As Rhodes (1997) and John (2000) have argued, networks have made the policy process more problematic, largely because of the need for interaction and interdependence between network members. Such interaction is marked by unequal resources between stakeholders, notably between professional and lay members. Coalitions between groups are often required to effect change but the strength of such coalitions depends on network membership. Policy networks (such as the civil service) are more stable or entrenched than issue networks (which form around particular concerns). The ability to steer networks is invariably limited; the use of decentralised management and performance indicators (among other measures) has led to the claim that successive governments have sought 'more control over less' (Rhodes 1997: 16).

Emergent policy: a new paradigm?

Within the UK over the last 50 years, Harrison and Wood (1999) argue that there has been a distinct change in the way that policy is formulated and implemented. From the inception of the NHS to the 1970s, the dominant approach to policy development provided a detailed 'blueprint' based upon a clear notion of policy ends and means. This approach is manifest, for example, in the establishment of Royal Commissions or detailed planning bodies such as for the Hospital Plan (MoH 1962) and the 1974 reorganisation (DHSS 1971). By the 1980s, policy became much less detailed as implementation gaps and failures become ever more apparent. Harrison and Wood (1999) argue that, over the last ten years, policy formulation has provided a broad outline with scope for detail during the implementation phase. The policy guidance for GP fundholding schemes and PCGs illustrates this emergent approach. Rather than the blueprint, current policies tend to lack detail, allowing for local innovation. Local variations and diversity are a necessary consequence of this approach unless clear parameters (relating to overall objectives) are set by government.

There may be a number of reasons for this including: the effect of new governance across the public sector; increasing complexity of the organisation of health care; difficulties in ensuring policy compliance (due to multiple stakeholders); and the need to develop quick responses. These factors explain, for example, the 'becalming' of UK health policy during the operation of the internal market of the 1990s (Wainwright, 1998). However, one consequence of the emergent policy is that there is now a renewed emphasis on the interrelationships between policy formulation and implementation (Hill 1998; Exworthy *et al*. 2002a). This has particular relevance to the development of primary care policy. The extent to which the factors shaping UK primary care have been the result of predetermined policy changes or the result of (local) circumstance is not always clear.

The 'emergent policy' paradigm does not provide an overarching or wholly convincing thesis. It may be applicable under certain circumstances and/or at certain levels. For example, it could be argued that government policy is marked by both prescriptive *and* emergent features. For example, whilst 'beacon' and 'pilot' sites have been widely adopted (allowing for emergent policy), other areas are tightly controlled through performance management. The emergent policy paradigm can therefore be located within a strand of social policy which focuses on the convergent and divergent effects of particular policies. For example, under (political) devolution in the UK, a divergence between devolved territories might, at first, be anticipated but, as will be shown in Chapter 4, there are grounds for arguing that there may be a convergence over time. Previous policy provides a template which both constrains and liberates current policy options; policy thus emerges from a specific context (Immergut 1992; Tuohy 1999). The degree of latitude that an emergent policy offers is termed path dependency (Wilsford 1994).

Conclusion

Primary care can never demonstrate its complete uniqueness from broader health and social care (Gordon and Hadley 1996; Godber *et al*. 1997; Starfield 1998). This defining feature provides a distinct weakness in trying to analyse primary care policy as it would appear that primary care remains an elusive and malleable concept. Yet, for most practical purposes, primary care policy can be viewed as an explicit object of policy and by the actions of those involved in primary care. Primary care is thus both the object and subject of policy, or alternatively it is the means and ends of policy. It should thus not be surprising that, from a policy perspective, there are multiple dimensions to its analysis. Some of these have been examined in this chapter, including the role of stakeholders, inter-governmental relations and implementation. From these flow the organising themes of the book: integration, diversity and changing boundaries. These will recur throughout the book and will be revisited in the final chapter. The themes encapsulate the opportunities, dilemmas and apparent contradictions of UK primary care.

The aim of this chapter has been to provide frameworks for the remaining chapters. Discussion in this chapter has shown that there are different ways of viewing and interpreting primary care policy. We have drawn on the models and concepts which will inform our analysis in subsequent chapters and especially those which focus on specific dimensions of primary care in action (Chapters 5–11). Our review of policy has necessarily been selective and there are other frameworks upon which other analysts and practitioners may draw. The value in our approach, however, is to provide a way of understanding and explaining not just past or current policy but also future policy.

CHAPTER 3

Primary Care: Definitions and Applications in UK Policy

Introduction

This chapter explores the different definitions that have been applied to primary care across a range of literatures and how the term has been used in practice within the UK and also within policy. The discussion will draw on UK and international literature, identifies different models of primary care and is set within the wider debate about the medical and social models of health. While the debate between the medical and social model of health is not new, it is important that the problems of definition and the tension between the two models, in current context, are understood as they have significant implications for the definition of primary care as well as the policy, organisation and management of primary care in the UK.

However, as suggested in Chapter 1 a major problem in analysing primary care is the lack of clear definitions and the interchangeability of terms used to describe primary care, including: primary medical care; primary health care; community medicine; family medicine; and general practice. Often policy described as primary care is actually about general or family practice. Even in texts it is not always clear as, for example, in Starfield's (1998) book on primary care, which is predominantly focused on primary *medical* care although placing this within a wider population health perspective to explore the contribution of primary medical care to health. Notwithstanding these problems, the discussion of definitions does have value as it clarifies and frames discussion about primary care. Therefore, in this chapter we introduce a definitional framework identifying key differences between individualistic and collaborative primary care and between reactive and proactive approaches to care (Peckham *et al.* 1996; Taylor *et al.* 1998). This framework is then applied to the UK situation and how developments in policy have defined primary care.

It is also important to identify the nature of UK primary care policy. As discussed in the previous chapter there is a range of different ways of thinking about policy. In particular we may view policy as both *means* and *ends*. This is an important distinction and in analysing primary care policy in the UK it is clear that primary care has been both the means of change within the UK health system and also as an policy end itself. At the same time the nature of primary care has itself changed, to some extent reflecting the shift from primary medical to primary health care. Such changes have led, on the one hand, to a diversification of what constitutes primary care with a blurring of organisational and professional boundaries and, on the other, greater integration of primary care within the NHS. Again these thematic changes result from policy makers interest in primary care as a means of change within the NHS and as an end itself in the type of primary care service being developed. These changes and themes are explored in more detail in the following chapters but it is useful to reflect on how these have emerged within UK policy development. Thus UK policy presents a paradox as to the role and nature of primary care, but which may also explain the current pre-eminent status of primary care within the policy arena.

Primary Care: the Term

Before exploring why the role of primary care has become so important in developed countries we first need to examine the term itself and to define our use of it. In policy, primary care is the term generally used in the UK – although its exact meaning is often very unclear or at best is used to describe what is often only a specific part of primary care services. In examining the growing use of the term, Summerton (1999) has described Primary Care as a portmanteau concept 'a favourite of politicians and [it] can be viewed variously as a set of activities, a process, a level of care or even a strategy for organizing the health care system as a whole' (604). The first major use of the term was in the Dawson Report of 1920 which defined three levels of health service: primary health centres, secondary health centres and teaching hospitals (see Chapter 4).

This definition or separation of levels provided the basis of both the functional sectoring of health care systems (primary, secondary and tertiary) and the geographical pattern with community, district and regional levels. These concepts have significantly influenced the pattern of health care systems in many countries (Starfield 1998). This basic sectoring of health also helps us to visualise people's contact with health care services and to explore the relationship between the various levels or sectors. However, in order to complete this visualisation it is also important to include self-care – those episodes of ill-health which are dealt with by the person who is ill or by their family or immediate community without recourse to a health specialist (although it may involve purchasing propriety drugs or other treatment for self-administration). This relationship can be pictured as a triangle, as shown in Figure 3.1.

The breadth of the triangle represents the episodes of ill-health and we can immediately see that most episodes of ill-health are catered for within the self-care section of the triangle. The next section is primary care which deals with the second largest section of the triangle. As you move towards the point passing through secondary care and then to tertiary care the number of episodes of ill-health dealt with in each portion decreases. Within the NHS,

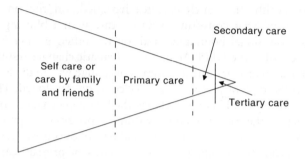

Figure 3.1   Levels of Health Care

some 90 per cent of contacts are in primary care with 10 per cent in secondary and tertiary care. This clearly demonstrates the tapering effect of passing through the levels of a health care system, with tertiary care provided to only a minority of patients while primary care deals with most episodes of ill-health that come into contact with a health care system. This is, of course, only a general model but adequately portrays the situation in most industrialised countries. However, in some countries this is not true, a point we will return to later in this chapter and also in Chapter 12. Thus, the triangle can also represent flows of patients from self-care to primary care, from primary to secondary and secondary to tertiary care. At each boundary a number of decisions are made which vary according to individual circumstances but also relate to the organisation, structure and nature of the health care system. For example, in the UK there are significant barriers of entry into secondary care based on the universality of general practice and the referral system. This contrasts with countries in Europe such as France and Germany, and also the USA where there is more direct access from self-care to secondary care.

Within the UK context it also worth identifying one other feature of the structure as portrayed by the triangle. If you were to place another triangle representing cost over Figure 3.1 it would be a direct mirror of it with the point (showing least cost) overlapping the self-care section and the broadest band (showing the most cost) overlapping secondary and tertiary care which are the most expensive parts of the health care system in the UK, although dealing with the fewest episodes of care (see Figure 3.2) (Kennedy 1999; also Chapter 5).

While this visualisation is useful it does little to help us define primary care as it does not allocate functions to each sector, nor does it describe the relationship between sectors. While recognising that there appears to be a positioning of primary care between self-care and other sectors of health care systems it tells us little about the way patients might utilise primary care or what the role of this sector is within the overall system. Thus we need to explore the term in other ways starting with an examination of terms.

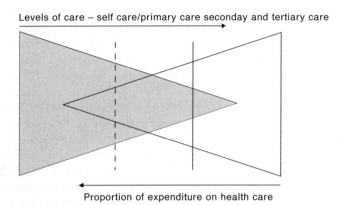

Figure 3.2 Relationship of Health Care Expenditure to Levels of Care

As well as primary care, two other terms are used – often interchangeably; these are Primary *Medical* Care and Primary *Health* Care. Primary Medical Care generally refers to general practice or family medicine – that is, primary care delivered by general medical practitioners. In this sense it is very specific in its use. Conversely, Primary Health Care is a much broader concept 'a reorientation of all health services towards the health needs of communities, both local and national' (Macdonald 1992:14). Like Primary Medical Care, Primary Health Care has a specific use (see Macdonald 1992; Duggan 1995). Other commentators and policy-makers have often used the terms interchangeably (see Gordon and Hadley 1996) to describe developments. More recently the term 'primary managed care' has become increasingly used in relation to the experience of USA health maintenance organisations and GP commissioning in the UK (Robinson and Steiner 1998). In the UK, primary care also comprises community health services including community nursing, professions allied to medicine, community paediatrics, adolescent psychiatric services, etc. Like Starfield (1998), we have opted to use the term 'primary care' to describe our field of study – i.e. inclusive of primary medical care, primary health care, general practice, etc. However, unlike Starfield, we wish to explore the relationships between primary medical care and primary health care. This distinction will become clearer as the book proceeds and is an issue returned to in the last chapter.

From a UK perspective, it is perhaps most appropriate that the term 'primary care' is used as this is most commonly referred to in UK policy documents. For example, in the mid-1990s the development of a primary care-led NHS was predominantly policy about the organisation and development of general practice and GP commissioning (NHS Executive 1994; NHS Executive 1996; DoH 1996a; DoH 1996b). In the UK, the dominant use of the term 'primary care' has, however, tended to obscure the fact that government policy has been mostly concerned with general medical practice. This confusion has often been transferred to discussions of primary care which are predominantly about general practice (see for example Boaden 1997; Rogers *et al.* 1999). This could, therefore, be more properly defined as primary medical care. This focus on general practice or family medicine within primary care policy is reflected in other countries such as Canada and the USA. In a recent article, Iliffe (2001) has characterised primary care as the industrialisation of family medicine. Yet, as discussed in this and later chapters in this book, the experience of primary care in these and many other developed countries has been much broader than medical services. In the UK, for example, there is a long and rich history of community nursing and community medicine (Ottewill and Wall 1990).

The term 'primary care' continues to be used within government policy, yet its conceptual coverage has undergone significant changes. The other main use of the term has been a negative one used to define NHS services which are not secondary care, that is primary care equals all that is not hospital care. These changes are explored more fully in later chapters but the key issue here is that the term 'primary care' is no longer so closely associated with general practice – a key change perhaps delineated by the shift from GP commissioning or fundholding (post-1991) to Primary Care Groups, Local Health Groups and Scottish Primary Care Trusts in 1998. New forms of primary care organisation are developing not only in the UK but also in other countries which serves to change our understanding of the term itself. Yet, the meaning of primary care may differ from country to country even though there are similarities and similar constituent elements. For example, primary care in the USA includes specialists such as internists and obstetricians, in Canada there is greater fragmentation of medical practitioner and nursing services, and in New Zealand there are attempts to fuse traditional primary/secondary care boundaries, though more recent reforms have focused on changes to the primary care sector (Devlin *et al.* 2001). What many of these developments share is the blurring of traditional professional and organisational boundaries – predominantly between doctors and nurses and different health and social care organisations.

For policy analysts, such as ourselves, the lack of clarity over the term 'primary care' presents an interesting question that we hope to answer within the following chapters. It is malleable according to the needs of different stakeholders an important facet of policy analysis. Our use of the term 'primary care' is, therefore, a way of setting an area of study that seeks to analyse specific policy issues relating to the development of policy without immediately attaching ourselves to the specific meanings associated with primary medical or primary health care. Finally, we have limited our focus to the discussion of primary care in the UK – with international comparisons restricted to other major developed countries. The purpose of comparison is primarily to contextualise our discussion and, therefore, comparisons with similarly developed health care systems are most suited to our purpose.

Defining Primary Care

Definitions of primary care come in all shapes and sizes perhaps appropriately if it is a portmanteau concept (Summerton 1999). However, this is not useful if our purpose is to study primary care policy and organisation. Starfield (1998: 8–9) defines primary care as:

> that level of a health service system that provides entry into the system for all new needs and problems, provides person-focused (not disease-orientated) care over time, provides for all but very uncommon or unusual conditions, and co-ordinates or integrates care provided elsewhere or by others.

This is a functional definition which seeks to identify the uniqueness of primary care by characterising a specific set of functions by which we can recognise it. However, there are other ways of conceptualising primary care including as a set of activities, as a level of care, as a strategy for organising health care and as a philosophy underpinning health care and health (Vuori 1985; Macdonald 1992). The concept of levels has been discussed above but it is worth briefly exploring these other conceptualisations. Primary care can be seen as a set of activities but it is difficult to see how many activities in primary care are different from those in other sectors of care or unique to primary care (Starfield 1998) – the exceptions may be the gatekeeper role in the UK and the fact that primary care practitioners deal with undifferentiated need (care is person-centred). This is particularly true as the organisation of care is changing very rapidly (Godber *et al.* 1997). The last two conceptualisations are interrelated and need to be explored more fully within the UK context.

In the UK there is a clear concept of levels of care which place general practitioners specifically, supported by other primary care workers at the heart of primary care. UK general practice has been described as:

> the single port of entry into the NHS, with the exception of A&E and special clinics ... 24 hour availability [for] first contact care, co-ordination and manipulation of local medical and social services ... gate keeping and protection of hospitals ... [and] long term and continuing generalist personal and family care. (Fry 1993: 3–4)

This concept of levels is also accepted in UK health policy where the NHSE has defined primary care as 'first contact, continuous, comprehensive, co-ordinated care provided to individuals and populations undifferentiated by age, gender, disease or organ system' (NHS Executive 1997: 8). With moves towards a primary care-led NHS (NHS Executive 1994), it would also suggest that primary care is seen as a strategy for organising health care and as a philosophy underpinning health care and health. However, it is clear that during the 1990s in the UK there was a definite tension between the development of a general practice or primary medical care service and the desire to broaden the context of primary care to embrace primary health care. We shall return to the definitional problems and the underpinning philosophies of these two approaches later in this chapter and in later chapters in the book. However, in order to do this we need first to explore more fully a UK definition of primary care.

Primary Care in the UK

There is no agreement in the UK as to what constitutes primary care (Gordon and Plampling 1996; Meads 1996). Over the years government documents have identified the primary health care team, but this also has varying definitions depending on who is included (Pratt 1995; RCGP 1996). In policy discussions the focus of primary care has, as suggested above, been seen as the general practitioner and the immediate primary care team in the surgery (NHS Executive 1994), but this view has been contested by many commentators (Thomas 1995; Gordon and Hadley 1996) and, with developments in primary care post-1991, challenged by the very nature of primary care in the UK (see Chapter 7).

In the mid-1990s in the midst of this changing context in the UK, Gordon and Hadley (1996) outlined some key characteristics of primary care which included:

- general practice which is offered by a generalist medical practitioner, involves teamwork, is first contact care, accessible, comprehensive, co-ordinated with a responsibility for its population and is activated by patient choice;
- community health services which support general practice, provide community specialists, support people with continuing illness and disability, work with people discharged from hospital, provide services for well people, provide choice for those without a GP and provide economies of scale;
- changing definitional boundaries between general practice and community health services (RCGP 1996) owing to new organisational structures which were developing through GP commissioning/fundholding and locality developments (Meads 1996).

Their work pre-dated further developments in the organisation and structure of primary care which had its roots in developments during the 1980s. These addressed issues relating to quality and health promotion in general practice (DHSS 1986a; DHSS 1987), changes to the GP contract in 1990 and the developments in the 1990s which grew from fundholding, its derivatives (e.g. multi-funds) and alternatives (GP and locality commissioning) (Meads 1996). Perhaps the key turning-point was the development of the concept of a primary care-led NHS (NHS Executive 1994) which placed primary care at the centre of developments in commissioning in the NHS. This development is discussed in more detail in Chapter 6. Of interest here is the conceptualisation of primary care which remained very specifically focused on general practice as purchasing organisations but which recognised the need to address organisational issues through the development of Total Purchasing, which moved more towards a geographical or population focus away from the traditional individual patient focus of general practice. More importantly, the 1990s saw the gradual integration of primary care into the NHS with increased financial and performance management while at the same time allowing for the development of a diverse range of organisational models.

Policy development in relation to primary care was intense in the mid-1990s with general political support for a primary care-led NHS, although with distinct political differences between the Labour and Conservative parties over the shape of the NHS in relation to the internal market. The broad agreement about primary care was important given the proposals outlined in the White Papers published in 1996 (see Chapter 4). Within these documents there was a clear vision regarding primary care which underpinned both political parties' views about the role of primary care in the NHS and how it would be encouraged to develop in the future. UK policy at this time was promoting primary care as the vehicle for delivering major change within the UK health system by incorporating primary care more within the NHS and within the resource management aspects of health care provision. At the same time the government had a vision of a more developed and expanded primary care system designed to better meet the health care needs of local populations. This marked a distinct change with previous primary care policy (e.g. DHSS 1986a; 1987) which focused more on developing the role of primary care in response to concerns about the quality of care and the range of care provided. It was the introduction of fundholding and the linking of general practice to resource control and greater involvement in health care system management – which marked the distinctive change towards primary care as a means towards health care system reform.

Choice and Opportunity: Primary Care: The Future (DoH 1996b) explicitly acknowledged the central role of GPs but extended this to dentists, pharmacists and optometrists and which recognised the implications for nurses, health visitors, midwives, therapists and managers. Throughout the White Paper, reference is made to the professionals and managers working in primary care. However, the first full definition of primary care came within the subsequent *Primary Care: Delivering the Future* (DoH 1996a):

> Primary care depends on the contribution of a wide range of professionals working together to meets the needs of all patients living in the community. At its heart is the family doctor and the general practice team of nurses, managers and, increasingly, other professionals. They need to work closely with community nurses, midwives and therapists to offer comprehensive and appropriate support to their patients. But primary care does not stop here – pharmacists, dentists and optometrists on the high street provide essential services as do social workers and housing officers from local authorities. (para 1.8)

The White Paper further set out the principles of good primary care (see Box 3.1) which to some extent laid a blueprint and developmental agenda that is still being addressed today. The White Paper established the basis for the Primary Care Act of 1997 (see Chapter 4) and while the predominant focus was on changes to general practice there were distinct sections on developing partnerships between general practice, the wider group of health care professionals working in the community and other organisations such as social services. There was also an emphasis on developing multi-practice primary care organisations, working with local communities and exploring new

---

Box 3.1 Principles of Good Primary Care

Quality
> Professionals should be knowledgeable about the conditions that present in primary care and skilled in their treatment and in contributing to their prevention
> Professionals should be knowledgeable about the people to whom they are offering services
> Services should be co-ordinated with professionals aware of each others' contributions (including inter-professional working) and no service gaps
> Premises and facilities should be of good standard and fit for their purposes, and equipment should be up to date, well maintained and safe to use

Fairness
> Services should not vary widely in range or quality in different parts of the country
> Primary care should receive an appropriate share of overall NHS resources

Accessibility
> Services should be reasonably accessible when clinically needed
> Necessary services should be accessible to people regardless of age, sex, ethnicity, disability or health status

Responsiveness
> Services should reflect the needs and preferences of the individuals using them
> Services should reflect the health demographic and social needs of the area they serve

Efficiency
> Primary care services should be based on evidence or clinical effectiveness
> Primary care resources should be used efficiently

---

models of practice. This White Paper set a number of themes which have remained consistent in government policy. These include the integration of a range of primary and community-based services into a more diverse framework for the organisation of primary care. At the same time policy focuses on developing partnerships between agencies, professionals and patients and carers challenging traditional role and organisational boundaries.

Cross-party agreement meant that many of the proposals continued to be developed by the Labour Government after 1997 laying the foundations for changes which occurred in the late 1990s and early the twenty-first century. Perhaps key to these changes was a broadening perspective of primary care which drew very much on the chief tenets of community care which placed the home or where people live at the centre of a model of care with the role of health care services being to help to maintain people in their own home – a model of care, epitomised in proposals for Care Trusts and integrated services outlined in *The NHS Plan* (DoH 2000). This focuses on the extended role of primary care services and suggests that there needs to be a greater co-ordination of services. It also brings out the tension between primary medical care and a broader model of primary care espoused in *Delivering the Future* (DoH 1996a). This tension remains at the heart of debates about continued developments in primary care.

In keeping with a long tradition in policy the Labour Government has also shied away from providing a definition of primary care. Current policy builds on the developments in the 1990s but sees primary care organisations very much at the heart of the NHS as the main focus for delivering or commissioning an extended range of care to its local community and also being responsible for improving public health. Here we see primary care policy promoting both *means* and *ends* arguments for the development of primary care. The structural reorganisation of the NHS in the twenty-first century involves the expansion of primary care organisations and services and the placing of increasing control over resource use in the hands of the new primary care organisations. While there are variations between England, Northern Ireland, Scotland and Wales on the extent of this dual focus, increasing the scope of primary care has become a central feature of policy development. Ironically such developments make a definition of primary care even more difficult to pin down – something we shall return to in Chapter 12.

It is the dual focus of primary care as both *means* and *ends* which underpinned *Shifting the Balance* (DoH 2001b). This document set the organisational blueprint for the NHS into the twenty-first century with the abolition of health authorities and regions in England, and the establishment of 28 Strategic Health Authorities overseeing PCTs. From 1997, the Labour Government sought to expand the nature and coverage of primary care, trying to shift from primary medical care to a broader model which integrates public health and social care. The organisational vehicle for these changes has been PCOs. These include PCGs and PCTs in England, PCTs in Scotland and Local Health Groups (LHGs) in Wales. Following the initial development of PCOs, public health and NHS policy has gradually defined a central role for primary care which, on the face of it, looks more like primary health care based on partnership and collaboration between agencies and with a public health focus (DoH 1999b; DoH 2000; DoH 2001b; Scottish Office 1998; National Assembly for Wales 2001). In addition, in the drive to improve access to health care, new developments such as Walk-In Centres and NHS Direct have been developed which add additional layers to our conception of primary care. Thus we are seeing the development of a more diverse range of primary care models in the UK. These developments are explored more in later chapters. However it is perhaps useful to explore the broader conceptual debates relating to primary medical care and primary health care and the way these relate to both the focus of a new system of health care and public health, and an attempt to improve people's health.

From Primary Medical Care to Primary Health Care

Macdonald (1992) has argued that the view of primary care in the UK is based on a biomedical model of health care – individual pathology and individual interventions – thus the emphasis is on the role of the doctor and the treatment of illness. He sought to develop a broad definition of Primary Health Care based on the Alma Ata declaration (WHO/UNICEF 1978) which expands the biomedical model, within a framework which embraces issues of access, equity, prevention and participation. He advocated moving to the macroscopic view which reflects the need to address structural causes of ill-health and thus use primary health care as both a strategy and philosophy to underpin health policy and action. He identified the main focus of primary care as microscopic with an emphasis on individual health treatments, seen in the following Royal College of General Practitioners definition of general practice:

> personal, primary and continuing medical care to individuals and families ... ([the doctor] will intervene educationally, preventively and therapeutically to promote his patient's health. (RCGP 1972)

Most commentators have applied the RCGP criteria of primary care specifically to services provided by the NHS. However, aspects of these criteria can apply to other approaches to health. In particular, many community projects display key characteristics of primary care including being accessible, continuing relationships, health promotion, support, rehabilitation, teamwork and choice. Community health projects cover a range of health-related issues and, organisationally, can be located in local authorities, within the community and voluntary sector and occasionally be found within the NHS (Kenner 1986). Likewise social workers and other social care professionals provide elements of these services which have a direct impact on people's health. Yet traditionally in the UK the activities of non-health professionals have been excluded from primary care and, as argued above, the focus has, up until recently, been on general practice and the general practitioner.

That this should continue to be so is perhaps surprising given the seemingly wide endorsement of the WHO definition of Primary Health Care. The World Health Organisation has also focused attention on participation by including it within its definition of primary health care.

Primary health care is essential health care based on practical, scientifically sound and socially acceptable methods and technology made universally accessible to individuals and families in the community through their full participation (WHO/UNICEF 1978).

Such a view suggests that people have the right and the duty to participate in the planning and delivery of their own health care. More recently this has been reinterpreted defining three sets of activity (WHO 1991):

1. a contribution by people to their own health and health care;
2. the development of organisational structures that are needed for participation to be effective;
3. empowerment of patients and their organisations and advocates, so that their voice is heard not assumed.

This more recent definition articulates both the individual and collective senses of participation and the range of activity within health care that people should be involved in. The WHO definition asserts that people have the right and the duty to participate in the identification, planning and delivery of their own health care. The recognition of the importance of participation represents the first key aspect of primary health care. In addition, as Meleis has argued, there is an implicit acceptance of the principle of equity between health workers, lay people and administrators; and the consideration of health within the larger context of the socio-economic and political structures (Meleis 1992).

This identifies two further aspects of primary health care:

- the notion of equity;
- the need for collaboration (to engage the broader context).

Macdonald (1992) and Tarimo and Creese (1988) identify these three dimensions (Equity, Participation and Collaboration) as the basic pillars of primary health care and point out that the international debate on primary health care has for two decades engaged with the challenges emerging from these principles. It is possible, therefore, to see a span of primary health care from the reactive medical practitioner or GP, through health service-based teamwork, to collaborative and participative primary health care. The key dimensions are participation and whether services are reactive or proactive as demonstrated in Figure 3.3.

The application of this wider approach to primary health care has been debated, to varying degrees, in this country (Macdonald 1992; Pratt 1995;

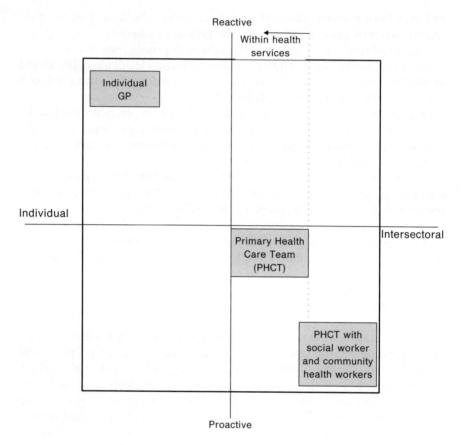

Figure 3.3   A Framework for Primary Care

Thomas 1995) but the concepts have not had any formal adoption. There are also many practical examples of primary health care which have moved beyond the reactive medical practice and which strive towards the WHO model, such as the West End Health Centre in Newcastle, as well as those that sought different approaches to primary health care – particularly in the 1990s – such as the Lyme Regis Community Care Unit (Robinson 1996), the Castlefields Practice in Runcorn (Colin-Thome 1996) and the Marylebone Centre in London (Pietroni 1996). More recently these principles have underpinned the development of Healthy Living Centres and Health Parks which form part of the government's strategy to develop a broader model of primary care within the UK. They also underpin community-based approaches to primary care advocated by the 'Peckham Health Centre' and Arts in Primary Care movements.

Alma Ata had a *radical* edge, notably in its explicit acknowledgement of the social, economic and political underpinning of health and ill-health. Moreover, documents which followed on the international scene drew on its perspectives, notably the Ottawa Charter on Health Promotion of 1986 to which Britain also subscribes (WHO 1986). But conceptually, Alma Ata's endorsement of the expression, *primary health care,* went further than the notion of *promoting* health in that it obliges policy-makers to hold together the preventive and treatment aspects of health care in one system. In the UK, since the system has not involved itself in this movement and had continued to separate these two wings of health care in practice, primary health care continued to mean primary *medical* care for many people, including policy-makers.

If the notions of participation, equity and intersectoral collaboration have been mentioned at all in the British context, they have generally relegated to the area of Health Promotion and in this way general practice avoids some of the conceptual challenges of Alma Ata mentioned above, namely the challenge of combining in one system the preventive and promotive aspects of health care systems with the treatment/curative aspects. The other challenge which is sidelined in this way is that of involving people in genuine decision-making concerning provision (see Chapter 9). This has allowed primary medical care to continue very much as before in isolation from these challenges presented by the 'pillars' of primary health care and the exciting initiatives which they foster. The challenges posed by Alma Ata to our ways of thinking and doing health care were, until recently, considered, if at all, as valid only in the Third World (Macdonald 1992).

Recent changes to the organisation and structure of primary care in the UK challenge this separation and organisational changes in the UK have brought the debate about the nature of primary care into sharp focus from both a policy perspective as well as in practice. This debate will be addressed in forthcoming chapters. It is possible, however, that the UK may have something to learn from the international debate about primary health care which will help inform UK developments.

The international debate on the three pillars of primary health care, participation, equity and the need to work with other sectors is therefore much more advanced. Involving people in decision-making of a significant kind (as opposed to asking them what colour they would like the reception room to be painted in), systematically finding out their needs and opinions and building on these, is a much more frequently debated dimension of health services in other countries than in the UK.

The international literature on participation in all kinds of service provision, including health care, reveals sophisticated analyses of the meaning of participation which have highlighted the danger of *tokenistic* and even *manipulative* forms of involving people in which the power in the relationship remains firmly in the hands of the professional (Arnstein 1969) and people are not genuinely involved (see discussion below and in Chapter 9). The notion of power is central in this international debate, with the United Nations Research Institute for Social Development reminding us as far back as the early 1980s that 'Participation is about power' (UNRISD 1979). The seminal work in the late

1970s and early 1980s of Cohen and Uphoff's team from Cornell University
had a focus on rural development. Nevertheless, their analysis applies to any
pursuit of participation. They offer a simple taxonomy based on the *kind* of
participation involved: in *implementation and in benefits* (relatively easy for
professionals to engage with and not particularly significant in terms of impact)
and in *decision-making and evaluation* (rather rare and more difficult for
professionals but representing the only genuine form of people's involvement)
(Cohen and Uphoff 1977; 1980). Power is also an issue within primary care
between professions and this issue is explored in Chapter 8.

More specifically in the realm of health care, the international discussion on
participation has deepened the challenge to health care workers:

> The training of health personnel to be promoters of CIH (Community Involvement
> in Health) requires a change in the medical paradigm. A health paradigm, such as is
> called for by CIH would involve a therapeutic relationship between health personnel
> and individuals or community groups in which there was a genuine effort to give
> power to the clients. (WHO 1991: 24)

In documents such as this it is acknowledged that people's participation in any
meaningful form of participation is difficult for health workers in general and
almost inevitably runs into problems arising from both the attitudes of these
workers and the structures of health care systems. In the UK there has been a
growing emphasis on participation since the early 1990s which has been
structured largely around health authorities, health care commissioning and
hospital service provision (Lupton *et al.* 1998). There is also a distinct tension
between involvement in services and involvement in public health. The
structures and processes being pursued in policy relate primarily to the
involvement in services but have been extended to cover primary care services
more fully (see Chapter 11).

Likewise, the notion of *equity* is now firmly on the agenda of health care
policy in many countries, partly as a result of the insistence of Alma Ata that it is
an essential dimension of primary health care and health care reform generally
(Saltman 1997). The international debate has sharpened since 1978 and it is
now common to find health policy documents acknowledging the need for the
entire health care system, including primary care, both to acknowledge disadvantage in society and its impact on health and to address that disadvantage
in order to attempt to restore this balance. In the UK the renewed emphasis on
inequalities in health (DoH 1998a; 1999b), the publication of the Acheson
Report (Acheson 1998) and the central place given to Primary Care Trusts
(in England) to tackle such inequalities (DoH 2001b) demonstrate the changing agenda in this area (see Chapter 11).

Linked to this we have the remaining 'pillar' of primary health care as
identified by Alma Ata: intersectoral working; this tends to be more commonly
addressed by those health care systems engaging with the broader definition
of primary care. Once the socio-economic underpinning of good health and

disease are acknowledged, the need to work with other sectors such as housing, social services and education becomes inescapable. When these dimensions of primary health care are ignored, there can be unfortunate consequences. Again in the UK this aspect is central to many of the developments within primary care, being a key principle which has developed considerably since the White Papers of 1996 to be enshrined institutionally within primary care organisations, as will be discussed in later chapters.

Primary care, therefore, can be defined in both narrow and broad terms. In attempting to analyse the concept it is useful to utilise a framework which recognises the broad range of primary care activity, one which incorporates both primary medical care and primary health care. This reflects the need to move away from a simple debate that places the medical model of health care against the social model which is perhaps unhelpful in furthering our understanding of policy, organisation and management.

However, at this point it is perhaps useful to characterise primary medical care and primary health care within the two models of health care – the medical and the social (Table 3.1).

The medical model of primary care is one characterised by a narrow focus on the individual, is provider-driven and emphasises clinical excellence. In contrast

Table 3.1 Primary Care Comparing the Medical and Social Models of Health

Social model	Medical model
Intersectoral: involving issues beyond the traditional boundaries of health such as housing, social services, education, leisure, community services	Intrasectoral: concerned mainly with traditional health (i.e. medical) boundaries: working together in a patient-centred team
The focus is on the wider community: addresses population health	The focus is on the individual or personal health within the context of their family/community
Represents *both* an individual and collective empowerment	It involves individual empowerment regarding making meaningful choices which positively affect one's own health
Needs and services are determined by the wider community including what is culturally and socially accessible and affordable	Needs and services determined by health providers
Concerned with essential care: the services the community cannot do without	Concerned with services within the medical context and focused on clinical excellence
Participation is based on a community development approach	Participation is more provider-driven

Source: Adapted from Calgary Regional Health Authority (1996).

the social model very much embraces the principles of primary health care identified above. The tensions between these models of health care resonate throughout this book and create a tension in the development of primary care practice and organisation in the UK (and other countries). However, it would be wrong to characterise primary care in such a bipolar way. It is not a case of either primary medical care or primary health care but rather how primary care can be developed to incorporate high-quality medical care within a primary health care model (Starfield 1998; Taylor et al. 1998). To this end it is more useful to view primary care across two continuum:

1. reactive – proactive;
2. individual – multi-professional and sectoral.

Using such a framework it is possible to map primary care as shown in Figure 3.3.

Such a transformation is central to attempts to develop primary care and thus many policy changes and local developments reflect such a change – with an increasing emphasis on public health and developing community services across agency and professional boundaries. In this sense primary care is very much the *end* of policy. However, it is also clear that such developments are also based on primary care as the *means* of policy to achieve other health policy goals. These include more patient-focused care, more community-based care, better resource management, improved public health and increased access to care. These issues are explored in more detail in later chapters.

Conclusion

Thus the focus of debate about the definition of primary care has been on its activity and the extent to which this is unique. However, as many studies have shown (Gordon and Hadley 1996; Godber et al. 1997; Starfield 1998), primary care cannot ever demonstrate its complete uniqueness from this activity alone. This provides a distinct weakness in trying to analyse primary care policy as it would appear that primary care remains an elusive portmanteau concept. Yet, we can observe primary care policy in real life through the use of primary care as an explicit object of policy and by the actions of those involved in primary care.

The aim of this and the preceding chapter have been to provide frameworks for the remaining chapters. The aim of discussing a definition of primary care is to explore its various facets not only as an object of policy but also as an area of policy concern. The discussion in this chapter shows, however, that there are different ways of viewing and interpreting primary care and primary care policy. We draw on the models and concepts put forward in this chapter to structure our discussion in the following chapters. We start, in Chapters 4 and 5 by examining the nature of primary care in the UK followed by an examination of primary care policy as a field of activity which defines an expression of general purpose as well as a set of specific proposals (Chapters 6 and 7). However, we move beyond this to explore a wider framework and policy implications which draw on discussions of power (Chapters 8 and 10) and debates about the very nature of primary care (Chapters 8, 9 and 11). It is true that our review of policy is selective and there are other frameworks upon which analysts and practitioners may draw. Indeed, other frameworks are offered in later chapters where we feel they have relevance.

As we shall explore in the following chapters of this book, it may be difficult to apply a clear definition of primary care as its boundaries are in flux and its nature is becoming more diverse but it is observable. There is no doubt that primary care is an important area of health care and one which has received, in recent years, a high degree of policy attention. To this end primary care is both an end and a means to providing high-quality health care and health services in the UK, although it is likely that primary care will remain defined by its activity and organisation. There may also be some value in keeping primary care definitions (and, therefore, primary care policy) vague and ambiguous as it allows government and others to shape the existing structure and systems. However, if these definitions or notions of primary care become too vague and ambiguous it will challenge the very notion of a separate primary care sector. In some areas this is already happening and thus one scenario is that the integration of primary care and blurring of health care sector boundaries will be the disappearance of a distinctive primary care sector – an issue we return to in Chapter 12.

CHAPTER 4

The Development of Primary Care Policy in the UK

This chapter outlines the historical development of primary care policy during the twentieth century. Primary care policy (as we know it now) did not exist in any recognisable form at the start of the twentieth century and so these last 100 years have seen the emergence of primary care policy as a distinct activity as well as the organisational and managerial infrastructure to support it in terms of professional groups and administrative agencies. The value of an historical perspective is especially relevant in appraising the current configuration of primary care. As Klein (1995) argues, many of the themes in the NHS, and primary care is no exception, are like an opera: the scenes and characters change but the story and the melodies remain remarkably consistent. There is, therefore, much to learn in analysing the development of primary care policy, organisation and management. The chapter provides a chronological overview of the main events and incidents. It considers a number of phases which characterise primary care up to the current arrangements (post-1997). Understanding this trajectory is key to explaining its current state across the dimensions explored in this book: integration, diversity and boundaries. This will therefore provide the context in which the current organisation of primary care is considered in Chapter 5.

A Chronology of Primary Care

To aid understanding and for ease of presentation, the chronology is divided into seven sections. These phases represent periods which were marked by particular features of policy development and/or broader societal change. Emphasis is given to most recent phases since these have had most direct and recent impact on the state of primary care. The chronology focuses obviously on primary care policy but takes a wider perspective in order to place these policy developments in the wider context of developments in the health care system. The key dates of this chronology are summarised in Boxes 4.1 to 4.7 at the end of the chapter.

Phase One: The National Health Insurance Act 1911

The nineteenth century and early twentieth century saw enormous developments in the fields of medical science and health care which shaped the growth of medical and nursing professions. There was no formal (*de jure*) policy towards what now might be considered as primary care. It is beyond the scope of this book to review these developments in their entirety (readers are directed to Abel-Smith (1964) for a more detailed discussion). However, it is worth highlighting a number of specific developments in this period which culminated in the 1911 National Health Insurance Act. These developments relate mainly to emergence of specific professions and the state of health and health care.

In the early nineteenth century the nascent medical profession was characterised by physicians, surgeons and apothecaries (Honigsbaum 1979: 2; Sibbald 2000: 15–16). Apothecaries were to form the bulk of general practitioners, the majority of their income being derived from drugs, and only after 1829 were they allowed to charge patients for giving advice. Although the 1858 Medical Act gave recognition to all doctors' qualifications, former divisions remained and were formalised by the 1911 legislation. The distinction between medical specialists and medical generalists was established at this time. Sibbald (2000) argues that medical specialisations were difficult to maintain outside urban centres and as such, 'practitioners [were] forced to practise generally' (15).

Friendly societies had been formed by workers in the nineteenth century to provide basic medical care by GPs, known as 'club' doctors. The societies grew steadily in the nineteenth century such that they covered one third of the adult working population (Honigsbaum 1979: 13). Club doctors needed the societies (despite some of their 'despotic practices') whilst they built up a list of private patients.

Parallel developments in nursing also occurred during the nineteenth century, although grounded in different circumstances. In response to social conditions in Liverpool in the 1850s, the philanthropist, William Rathbone, established a home nursing service which was to be based upon the districts (parishes) of the city for organisational purposes; hence 'district' nursing. (By 1868, district nursing had been established in London.) These developments roughly coincided with the Liverpool Sanitary Act 1846 which promoted preventive medicine. Similar developments in Manchester and Salford helped establish 'health visiting' in the 1850s. Though initially focused on providing information, these organisations employed women to visit homes and teach mothers how to look after their children. By 1905, health visiting had been established in 50 areas and by 1918 there were 3000 health visitors (Ottewill and Wall 1990: 32/33). Between the 1880s and 1910s many infant welfare centres were created in order to provide child health surveillance. One impact was a fall in the number of deaths from pregnancy from 5.49 per 1000 live births (1891–95) to 3.66 by 1918 (*ibid.*: 37). Similarly, the infant mortality rate in 1899 was 163 per 1000 live births (Honigsbaum 1979: 23).

In the first years of the twentieth century these (professional) developments and the continued (poor) state of the population's health prompted some to call for state intervention in health care. Webb, for example, in a report to the

Royal Commission on the Poor Law in 1908, called for a 'public medical service' or 'state medical service' (Timmins 1995: 108). Moreover, club doctors' dissatisfaction with the friendly societies reached a point where these doctors welcomed Lloyd George's Bill which introduced the National Health Insurance. State intervention in health care was thus accepted; capitation fees were increased in what was called '9 pence for 4 pence' because employers and the state contributed 5 pence to the 4 pence from the insured person. This enabled the NHI to extend to more people, about 15 million. Moreover, GPs could decide whether they would work for the NHI; hence they could decide to join the 'panel' of doctors administered by Insurance Committees (Honigsbaum 1979: 9). The 1911 Act enabled a relatively large proportion of the (male) population (though it was not comprehensive coverage) to gain access to free GP treatment under the panel system. The insurance enabling GP treatment was only available to manual workers and not their families. However, this system reinforced divisions within the medical profession:

> The general practitioner, operating usually on the small shopkeeper principle of running his own practice single-handed and relying on the income from capitation fees of his insured patients, was isolated from the mainstream of medicine'. (Klein 1989: 3).

The Act established a system which was not wholly run by the state (although it had been constructed by it) but neither was it a system of private practice (Honigsbaum 1979; Klein 1995). Though GPs' income came from insurance contributions, they retained freedom within the scope of Act. By 1920, three-quarters of GPs were on the 'panel' (Honigsbaum 1979: 111–12). Hospital treatment was not included within the NHI.

Phase Two: The Inter-war Period

The inter-war period was one of consolidation for the embryonic health service and of growth for what became primary care. It was also the time when policy towards primary care became more systematised. Four features of this period were noteworthy in this period: the creation of the Ministry of Health, the Dawson Report, the Local Government Act and the early but diverse calls for a national health service (including the 1926 Royal Commission).

The Ministry of Health was created in 1919. Although Honigsbaum (1979) identified some calls for a ministry in the nineteenth century, he argues that doctors were less than enthusiastic and were only interested when their economic position could be strengthened. Opinion shifted when doctors saw that the greater bureaucracy of the 1911 NHI Act did not limit their freedom. Moreover, the need for greater state involvement was heightened by the state of the population's health: 'for every 9 soldiers killed in the trenches [in the early years of the First World War], 12 babies died at home' (Honigsbaum 1979: 23). Also, the quantity and quality of medical care varied enormously (Ottewill and Wall 1990: 59). The creation of the Ministry was difficult because of the many agencies that were involved in health and welfare financing and provision, and the three sectors under which doctors practised (Poor Law, municipal and panel). The Ministry took on the responsibilities which had formerly been the remit of the Local Government Board and the powers of the Insurance Committees (formed under the 1911 NHI Act).

The Dawson Report was commissioned by the Medical Consultative Committee and concerned the future organisation of medical practice. The committee only produced an interim report in 1920 but it had a major impact on health care organisation, especially primary care, in the 1920s and thereafter. Doctors were concerned about the possible introduction of a salaried service after the Ministry was created but the Dawson Report allayed their fears, not by excluding the 'salary option' but by proposing an 'inter-locking network of health centres, starting with a form of first aid treatment at or near the patient's home' (Honigsbaum 1979: 67), a hierarchy of institutions would culminate in teaching hospitals (Klein 1989: 4). The Report defined a health centre as 'an institution wherein are brought together various medical services, preventive and curative so as to form one organisation' (quoted in Ottewill and Wall 1990: 57).

The Report's recommendations prompted no action (*ibid.*: 58) but, as Pater (1981) argues, 'they provided the outline of a national health service' (7). In terms of primary care, the Report suggested that domiciliary services for a district should be based on a 'Primary Health Centre', staffed by GPs in 'con-junction with an efficient nursing service and with the aid of visiting consul-tants and specialists' (Ottewill and Wall 1990: 57). One of the earliest primary health centres opened in Peckham (south London) in 1926.

The 1929 Local Government Act was another reform which addressed the complexity of health care provision. The Act transferred the health care functions (e.g. vaccinations) of the Poor Law authorities to county and county borough councils. It also unified preventive and curative medicine under the post of Medical Officer for Health. Other legislative and governmental changes reinforced the move towards a more unified health care system. For example, the 1902 Midwives Act allowed midwives' certification such that the term 'midwife' was reserved for those who had been trained. The 1936 Midwives Act developed their position by securing an adequate salaried midwifery service across the country. Previously, midwives had been self-employed or employed by voluntary organisations (Ottewill and Wall 1990: 34–5; 49). Similarly, health visiting became professionally established when its training was officially promulgated by health and education ministries in 1919; by 1930 only qualified health visitors could be appointed by local authorities.

During the inter-war period, various calls were made for a reorganisation of the health care system. For example, the Royal Commission on National Health Insurance in 1926 concluded that the ultimate solution will lie, we think, in the direction of divorcing the medical service entirely from the insurance system, and recognising it along with all other public health activities to be supported from general public funds. (quoted in Klein 1989: 5; also Timmins 1995: 108)

Also, the British Medical Association published proposals in 1930 for 'general medical service for the nation'. Revised in 1938, the plans included a comprehensive general medical service open to all (Ottewill and Wall 1990: 59). Klein (1989: 5) interprets the consensus which emerged around these calls for a national service as arising from the muddle of inter-war health care. The outcome of this confusion was either an extension of the NHI scheme or a public health model (akin to local authority provision developed in the nineteenth century).

These calls were not heeded by government until the late 1930s and early 1940s; the acceptance of them heralds the third phase of primary care policy, organisation and management.

Phase Three: The Genesis of the NHS (1940s)

A consensus had, Klein (1995) argues, developed from the various calls for a national health service in the 1930s but this consensus was 'marred' by doctors' fears of state control. It was not until the late 1930s and early 1940s that the government responded and its decision was forced largely by the Second World War. Ottewill and Wall (1990) sees two main responses from the government to the consensus and wartime situation: the Emergency Medical Service and the Beveridge Report. These and other developments culminated in the 1944 White Paper and subsequent legislation.

The Emergency Medical Service was established in order to co-ordinate municipal and voluntary services during wartime. Military personnel and civilians could use the service but it was oriented around the hospital (Honigsbaum 1979: 173). Although this highlighted inequalities in health care across the country (Ottewill and Wall 1990), it also proved that a national health service *could* be run (Timmins 1995). GPs' input into hospital care was largely ignored by the ministry. The clinical side of general practice was largely undisturbed by the war; the range of treatments was low and the quality of care poor, especially care administered under the panel system (Honigsbaum 1979: 173).

Among various other plans and proposals, two in particular cemented the move towards a national service: the plans by McNalty and the BMA. McNalty, the Chief Medical Officer, proposed, in 1939, that hospitals should be run as a national health service. The Emergency Medical Service was, in effect, the precursor to such a scheme (Timmins 1995: 109). Contextual factors supported this plan; voluntary hospitals were running into financial difficulty (which was significant because they were run mainly by GPs) and doctors were favouring national (cf. local) organisation. McNalty's plan, which Timmins argues was 'the one Bevan eventually adopted, was radical in that the state would become involved not simply as a supervisory body but also as an executive one'.

The BMA's Medical Planning Commission was created in 1940 to determine the nature of the health service after the war. It produced its recommendations seven months before the Beveridge Report, in 1942. Consultants, it argued, should be salaried whereas GPs should receive a mixture of basic salary, capitation fees and fee-for-service payments (Timmins 1995: 110). The scheme proposed was to cover the whole population but still to be insurance-based. The report was accepted by the BMA but the Beveridge Report overtook them. The 1942 Beveridge Report made recommendations about the social security system, to be supported by a national health service. As expectations rose, the government accepted Beveridge's proposals.

The White Paper *A National Health Service* (February 1944) was transformed into the 1946 National Health Services Bill. The White Paper advocated a service which was comprehensive and free. It proposed that GPs should be employed by a Central Medical Board which would control their geographical distribution. GPs would be encouraged to work collectively in local authority health centres. The White Paper enabled GPs to retain their private practice but offered no clear form of payment (other than 'the hint of salaries' (*ibid*. 1995: 112)). This and other proposals were attacked by the BMA, fearing further state interventions. The White Paper did not give doctors a role in any local administration (Honigsbaum 1979: 212).

Ottewill and Wall (1990) claim that the White Paper served to continue the debate about a national service since consultation followed for a year. This, according to Klein, helped GPs secure their right of veto, thereby maintaining the status quo. The 1946 Bill was marked by one key change from the 1944 White Paper. The Bill was extended to include voluntary and municipal hospitals, taking them out of local government responsibility. The new authorities, created to administer the national health service (i.e. regional boards and hospital management committees), were to have 'expert' members, not representatives; this meant doctors but not other health workers. Bevan's dismissive argument was that 'if the nurses were to be consulted, why not also the hospital domestic?' (quoted in Klein 1989: 21–2). The continuation of the Insurance Committees, renamed Executive Councils, would provide the organisation to which GPs would be contracted but were the 'part of the health service least amenable to planning initiatives' (Webster 1998: 127). This mollified their concerns of being either a local authority employee or subject to central control but also ensured the lack of a unified system (Honigsbaum 1979: 213). Some of the other GP-oriented proposals were changed during consultation: health centres would be experimental and GPs would be paid capitation fees, not salaries (Klein 1995; Timmins 1995). These debates were indicative of the way in which the medical profession was able to lever changes to the proposals but also the extent to which the profession was riven with differences between specialists and GPs (Webster 1991).

The outcome was the creation of the NHS on 5 July 1948, with a structure of regional hospital boards, hospital management committees and boards of governors to run hospitals, and Executive Councils to administer GP contracts. Local authorities still retained a role in the provision of community health services such as the school medical service, some home nursing, some health centres and ante/postnatal care (Ottewill and Wall 1990: 61; Timmins, 1995: 107). According to Ham (1985: 17), this tripartite structure was a 'representation of what was possible rather than what might have been desirable'.

Phase Four: The NHS in its Infancy (1948–mid 1960s)

The early years of the NHS were characterised by relative stability, as its foundations were allowed to consolidate, but also by effect of the 'separation of the [medical] profession' (Honigsbaum 1979: 299). A degree of political satisfaction at what had been achieved was evident. However, health was a low-ranking Ministry, not commanding a Cabinet seat for most of the period between 1951 and 1968, which may help to explain the regular arrival of ministers – six between 1951 and 1960 (Timmins 1995: 203).

Administratively, there was a great deal of work concerning the means (cf. ends) of the NHS; for example, in 1948–9, in terms of determining 'the fees to be paid to general practitioners for immunisations and vaccinations, the layout of the Health Service prescription book . . . [and] mileage allowances for rural practitioners' (Klein 1989: 43–4). In the hospital sector, new organisations needed to be created: 14 Regional Hospital Boards, 26 Boards of Governors for teaching hospitals, and 380 hospital management committees. Moreover, the ways of working needed a cultural change. Civil servants and administrators had to work alongside the individualistic (medical) professions in new capacities. As the Ministry was unable to direct the work of everything in the NHS, the sense of scale, as well as the impact of clinical freedom afforded professionals at the periphery, took time to be realised. In short, Klein (1989: 44) saw the 1950s as a period of 'maintenance rather than innovation' in the NHS (see also Lewis 1999).

For the profession, the separation between hospital doctors and GPs became entrenched during the early years of the NHS. Honigsbaum (1979: 301–3) places the responsibility for this situation upon the policy-makers who, in 1948, missed the opportunity to unite the two sides of the profession, and on the hospital doctors, who were trying to build up their service in quantity and quality.

A number of policy developments are worth highlighting here. First, costs of the NHS were rising faster than expected and charges were introduced for prescriptions and (further) dental charges. The Guillebaud Committee (1956) moderated concerns about the growing expenditure of the NHS. This leads into the second development – pay. Although the outgoing Labour Government in 1951 accepted a claim from the BMA for GPs' back pay amounting to 10 per cent of NHS spending (Timmins 1995: 205), the issue resurfaced by the late 1950s. The Royal Commission on Doctors' and Dentists' Remuneration (1960) examined the level of pay and the way in which it should be reviewed. They found that, between 1950 and 1959, average incomes had risen by 20 per cent but GPs' income had fallen by 20 per cent. (The same percentage fall applied to NHS administrators: Klein, 1989: 55). GP pay was determined by the 'pool system'. A set amount of money was allocated from which all GP payments were to be made. Once the overall size of the pool had been set, the Ministry was able to concede how the money was spent. The Commission recommended pay awards and a regular review. Pay was set to rumble on as an issue into the 1960s. In 1963, the BMA annual meeting called for pay increases for GPs in order to reduce the GP–consultant pay differential. Klein (1989: 87) argues that GPs' resentment at their being the profession's poor relation had 'broken into the open' over the pay issue.

Three other policy initiatives affected primary care. First, in 1952, the Central Health Services Council reported on obstacles to co-operation between hospitals, local authorities and family practitioner services. It identified cross-agency membership of committees, the exchange of papers between agencies and informal co-operation between agency officers as ways of fostering co-operation. It also recommended the creation of local joint health consultative committees (Ottewill and Wall 1990: 97). Secondly, the 1958 Local Government Act provided opportunities for local authorities to delegate the health care functions of their county councils to district councils, in order to ensure decisions were being taken as close as possible to patients. Thirdly, the concept of the primary care team was beginning to emerge as GPs began to be attracted by interdisciplinary working. This move was encouraged by the Gillie Committee in 1963. The wider team, it foresaw, would need larger premises than the traditional surgeries (Ottewill and Wall 1990: 127).

Phase Five: Growing Pains in Primary Care (1965–1979)

In this fifth phase, the NHS had become established as a national institution (Klein 1989: 62) but was beginning to experience dilemmas in its policy, organisation and management. The embryonic primary care was no exception to these dilemmas, symbolised by four issues.

The first issue concerned the 1974 reorganisation which had a major impact on the way in which community health services were organised. The 1960s had begun to generate a dissatisfaction with the tripartite era (founded in 1948), with 'the inefficiencies and jealousies' it created (Timmins 1995: 294). The Minister of Health (Kenneth Robinson) announced an administrative review in 1967, the outcome of which was the 1968 Green Paper. It proposed a single authority in each area (totalling 40–50) to combine the functions of Executive Councils, regional hospital boards, boards of governors and hospital management committees. (The Porritt Report in 1962 had recommended a similar structure.) The possible integration with local government structures was not resolved. A second Green Paper followed in 1970 (under the Minister, Richard Crossman) which resolved that the NHS should not be administered by local government but by 80–90 Area Health Authorities. General practice would remain separate, its finances coming directly from central government. By 1972, the White Paper had accepted most ideas from the 'second' Green Paper including the Family Practitioner Committee concept and an 'elaborate professional and advisory machinery' (Timmins 1995: 294). According to Webster (1998: 127) the change to FPCs made little difference to ECs' role.

The 1974 reorganisation, implemented by the incoming Labour Government, ushered in the 'unified structure'. Though Enoch Powell called it the final nationalisation of the health service (Ottewill and Wall 1990: 200/113), others saw it as the moment at which the ideology of (managerial) efficiency became predominant within the NHS (Klein 1989; Timmins 1995). However, the unification was a misnomer as it applied only to hospital and community health services. GP services remained separate. Unification was promoted as the reorganisation involved the transfer of community health services from local authority to (area) health authority control. This included many community nursing services. It was also in the early 1970s that social services departments were created. Professional rivalries surfaced between different services and between the then LAs' medical officers of health and social workers; relations between generic social workers (advocated by the Seebohm Report in 1968) and GPs were strained, according to Timmins (293). Moreover, organisational problems arose as hospital and community health services became enmeshed in consensus management. Despite problems, the reorganisation fostered better health service planning.

Associated with this period of reorganisation was a subtle change in terminology and commensurate impact upon policy. Webster (1998: 127) argues that, prior to 1970, little emphasis had been placed upon either the 'idea' or the 'term' primary care. However, after this, some changes were evident. For example, 'general medical practice' was increasingly seen as a medical speciality. For example, founded in 1952, the College of GPs was awarded the Royal Charter in 1967 (Pereira Gray 1992). Over time, primary care came to mean more than GP services.

Second, to understand the issue of GP pay, which resurfaced in the 1960s, it is vital to understand the context. General practice was considered as the poor relation in medicine and the NHS. As Timmins (1995) neatly argues, 'by the 1960s, new drugs, new technology and new techniques were making the hospital king' (218), implying that GPs were those who had, in Lord Moran's terms (quoted in Timmins 1995: 218), 'fallen off the career ladder'. The consequences were that GPs felt underpaid and undervalued, and many had begun to leave general practice.

The spark which ignited GPs' anger was the low pay-raise recommended by the pay review body in 1965. Resignations from the NHS were threatened and alternative representative groups were forming, reflecting the increasing divergence of views within general practice itself. (This has echoes of the May 2001 vote in which 86 per cent of voting GPs said they would resign if contract negotiations were not satisfactory.) One such – the Medical Practitioners' Union – formulated the 'Family Doctors Charter'. The BMA published the *Charter for the Family Doctor Service* in 1965. These, with some revision, were adopted in 1966 (Klein 1989: 87). The result was the introduction of the basic practice allowance (a form of salary) and the removal of the pool system of pay. Other measures included loans to encourage GPs into group practice premises, the attachment of nurses (and other local authority staff), postgraduate education and incentives to practise in 'under-doctored' areas (Timmins 1995: 223). The new GP contract also resulted in a 33 per cent pay-rise! As well as helping change the status of general practice, the 1965 crisis was significant because the new contract tied GPs more closely than ever before into the NHS; GPs became more financially dependent on the NHS as a result of the cost–rent scheme and other reimbursements.

The third issue arose from the first; the development of, and incentives for, practice premises enabled primary care to become more firmly established within the NHS. The development of health centres was rapid (Klein 1989: 88). In 1966, there were 240 GPs practising in health centres; by 1973, the figure had risen to 2500. This represented a rise from 1.5 per cent of GPs to 12 per cent in just seven years (Ottewill and Wall 1990: 127). The enabling factor had been the new GP contract in 1965 but, as the Harvard-Davies subcommittee on group practices (in 1971) recognised, the popularity of health centres reflected patient preferences and the need to accommodate the ever-expanding primary health care team (*ibid.*: 127). The appeal of health centres continued into the 1970s as, for example, the House of Commons' Expenditure Committee 'called for more health centres to be built on the grounds that they were far more suitable base for the development of primary health care teams than the traditional type of surgery' (*ibid.*: 285). However, the 1979 Royal Commission on the NHS argued that health centres were not always popular with GPs or their patients but recognised that they could be advantageous in deprived inner-city areas. A (Conservative) government circular in 1980 marked another change in policy towards primary care premises. The impact of the policy had been to increase the number of publicly owned premises. In prompting local reviews of this policy, the circular shifted the emphasis towards GP-owned premises. Ottewill and Wall (1990: 286) saw this as the 'privatisation of health centres'.

Fourthly, inter-professional working and co-operation among community health services staff were being fostered through specific initiatives. For example, the 1969 Maton Report on the management structure in local authority nursing services recommended that local authorities should appoint a chief nursing officer to co-ordinate health visiting, home nursing and domiciliary midwives (Ottewill and Wall 1990: 82). With support from government, most HAs followed this recommendation. Increased opportunity for collaboration would, it was hoped, improve service co-ordination and delivery. Whilst health centres might have facilitated such collaboration, the 1974 reforms scuppered local authority involvement.

Phase Six: 'Safe in Our Hands'? (1979–1990/1)

Given the volume of evidence (often from politicians' memoirs) and the rapidity of policy change in this sixth phase, the evidence presented here is divided into the general context of the period and the specific policy initiatives related to primary care.

i. Context

Published shortly after the election of the Conservative Government in 1979, the Royal Commission on the NHS marked a new era. It was commissioned by the previous Labour Government at a time when, as Klein (1995) vividly describes it, the demolition squads appeared to be moving into the monument of the NHS (104). The consensus which had formed the NHS was breaking down and conflict was spreading. The Commission favoured the existing system of health care funding (i.e. general taxation) but recommended that Area Health Authorities should be abolished, that chief executives should be appointed and that FPCs should be abolished (their functions being taken over by health authorities) (Klein 1989: 133; Timmins 1995: 385). Their foresight was fulfilled within five years for the first two but it took some seventeen years before the last was implemented.

The Conservative's public policy was one which sought to enhance the role of managerialism and managers at the expense of traditional interests (see Chapter 5). This generated hostility and conflict mostly from the medical profession. The stakeholders became greater in number and the debate was conducted at a greater volume. Thus, Klein (1995) suggests that 'the protagonists ... of the 1970s were beginning to lose their grip by the mid 1980s' (203). Specific developments such as the 1982 pay dispute weakened the power of vested interests and enabled the government to introduce controversial measures such as compulsory competitive tendering in hospital cleaning, catering and laundry.

One of the first Green Papers published by the Conservatives was called *Patients First* in December 1979. Criticising the rational planning of the 1970s, it proposed that the 90 AHAs be replaced by 192 District HAs. FPCs would remain and cover more than one DHA, a move which Ottewill and Wall (1990) and Klein (1995) considered contrary to integration within the NHS (see Table 4.1). Although FPCs became separate employing authorities, the

Table 4.1   Relationships Between DHAs and FPCs, 1982–85

No. of DHAs per FPC	Total no. of FPC areas	Total no. of DHAs (col. 1 × 2)
1	40	40
2	20	40
3	17	51
4	7	28
5	4	20
6	1	6
7	1	7
Total	90	192

Source: Ottewill and Wall (1990: 247).

decision marked an 'admission of defeat' that tackling general practice would generate conflict (Klein 1989: 138). 'Patients First' was the forerunner of the 1982 reorganisation. The introduction of DHAs illustrated the emphasis on localism – the notion underpinning decentralisation that services should be the responsibility of those delivering them.

A report commissioned by the London Health Planning Consortium (Acheson 1981) reviewed the state of primary care in inner London. It found that general practice (with many elderly, single-handed GPs working in inadequate premises) was poorly developed and primary care teams were poorly developed as a result; a high turnover of staff was often due to their high workload; and lower spending on community health services compared to other areas (see Ottewill and Wall 1990; Moon and North 2000; Chapter 7).

The 1983 election enabled the government to pursue its managerial agenda more forcefully. Budget cuts and efficiencies were sought from across the public sector including the NHS. These measures included further rounds of contracting-out and cost-improvement programmes. This was the context which prevailed when Roy Griffiths, a director of the Sainsbury supermarket chain, was commissioned in 1983 to report on NHS manpower, subsequently expanded to cover NHS management. The methods of the review illustrated the change which the government had wrought; professions and other interests were excluded. A small team of private sector managers collected no evidence and made their conclusions in a 24-page report (Wistow and Harrison 1998). They recommended that managers replaced administrators and that consensus management must be replaced with executive decision-making. The government's implementation of the report in 1985 marked the third major reorganisation in a decade (Timmins 1995: 410). (See Chapter 5.)

ii. Primary care policy initiatives

The 1980s witnessed a shift in health policy which increasingly placed attention on primary care. This shift had its origins in two aspects of the public policy. First, many of the managerial initiatives of the 1980s had only a peripheral impact on primary care. Compulsory competitive tendering, general management and other supply-side schemes were often directed towards hospitals. Where it did impact on primary care it was largely related to FPC activities, not the practitioners themselves. Secondly, GPs are the 'gatekeepers' to secondary services; they commit resources through their decisions to treat or refer. For the Conservative Government, the primary care sector, and especially GPs, represented 'an open-ended public expenditure commitment' (Klein 1989: 223).

However, the notion of tackling the financial costs of primary care in the 1980s was, according to Klein (1995), affected by previous governments' attempts: 'the financial costs of avoiding a confrontation with the medical profession over general practice might outweigh any political benefits' (223). Such confrontation was, however, considered politically feasible in community health services. As managerialism was thought to be the solvent for other problems, this strategy was pursued in primary care with attention initially turning to prescribing and organisational reform.

Prescribing accounted for almost half of the primary care budget and costs were rising at 5 per cent per annum in the 1980s. The government challenged the 'limited list' of drugs. In 1984, the initiative was launched to save £100 million but, indicative of the government's approach, no prior warning was given to the BMA; the Minister (Kenneth Clarke) would only discuss its implementation (Timmins 1995: 412). Some hospitals had already established their own limited list and some GPs wanted to confine the excess profits of pharmaceutical companies. 'The result, for all the GPs' fury, was a divided profession' (*ibid.*: 413). The limited list was introduced in April 1985. By doing so, it illustrated the power of the government to challenge clinical autonomy, *without* the consent of the medical profession.

The second tranche of the primary care policy at this time was organisational reform focusing on improving 'responsiveness' to patients. A report from the House of Commons' Social Services Committee on primary health care and the 1986 Green Paper on primary care focused policy attention on primary care. The Green Paper argued that primary care services had never been properly reviewed; it sought to 'make services more responsive, to raise standards of care, to promote health and prevent illness, to give patients widest possible choice, to improve value for money, to enable clearer priorities for FPS in relation to the rest of the health service' (Ottewill and Wall 1990: 416). The proposals were not 'desperately radical' (Timmins 1995: 415). They included a shift in GP income towards capitation fees, fees for immunisations, and an easier system for patients to change GPs. Timmins (1995) considered the whole raft of proposals as 'explosive' in the political context as they tried to generate competition between GPs (p. 415).

The Green Paper only addressed family practitioner services; the Cumberlege Report, launched on the same day that the Green Paper was published, considered community nursing. The Cumberlege Report (DHSS 1986b) proposed a structure for community nursing (mainly health visitors and district nurses) which was based on neighbourhoods between 10 000 and 25 000 population and headed by a single neighbourhood nurse manager. Though seen as a document which was supposed to bolster the status of the community nursing profession (Allsop 1986; Lewis 1999), it distinguished between core and peripheral community nurses (thereby undermining the unifying objective). It also generated opposition among GPs who saw neighbourhoods as duplicating their practice lists system and undermining their primary health care team. As such, some saw it as a controversial document. Some health authorities implemented their own neighbourhood nursing structure (Exworthy, 1994a) but the government only asked them to review the way in which community nurses were managed.

The Green Paper (to become the 1987 White Paper) asserted the government's policy of developing the primary health care team but it lacked coherence. Klein (1995) argues that there was a tension in the 1987 White Paper between managerial and the competitive strategies because it strengthened the role of the FPC and so ran counter to GPs' independent contractor status.

Working for patients

The momentum behind the primary care Green Paper 'evaporated' (Timmins 1995: 416) but many of the themes in the 1987 White Paper were later taken up in another White Paper in 1989: *Working for Patients* (DoH, 1989a). Under this 1987 primary care White Paper, free eye-tests and dental check-ups would be abolished to save £170 million. New GP contracts were also proposed. These planned savings were indicative of the state of NHS funding resulting in ward closures, cancelled treatments and a nurses' strike. The presidents of the three Royal Colleges petitioned the government for more money. The outcome of these events was a statement from the Minister (John Moore) that no review of the NHS was planned but that additional resources would be forthcoming from private sector collaborations (Timmins 1995: 458).

Famously, it was the Prime Minister who announced (on BBC's *Panorama*) a review of the NHS only six days after Moore's statement denying a review. It surprised everyone. The review began with hardly any parameters. However, it was significant that what had been precipitated by a funding crisis culminated in an organisational review (Klein 1989: 238). Funding was one issue which *Working for Patients*, published in January 1989, did not address. It was a 'reaffirmation' of the contract established at the inception of the NHS in 1948 (Klein, 1995) but it sought to extend managerialism and challenge institutional and professional boundaries. Though only an outline document (Timmins 1995: 465), the *Working for Patients* proposals included:

- an internal market through the separation of purchasers and providers;
- general practice fundholding;
- self-governing trusts status for providers;
- medical audit; and
- capital charging.

The concept of the purchaser–provider split (originally advanced by Enthoven 1985) applied most easily to hospitals and community units. The Minister (Clarke) feared that managers would be the only group of purchasers. Clinicians and especially gatekeeping GPs might remain untouched. However, clinicians lacked the financial skills, acumen and motivation to act as purchasers. Clarke solved the conundrum; whilst 'on holiday on a headland near Pontevedra in Galicia I came up with GP fundholders' (quoted in Timmins 1995: 464). Not only did GP fundholding incorporate GPs into the new structure but it also introduced a degree of competition among purchasers as health authorities also had a purchaser role. Fundholders would hold a budget for their patients to cover a limited range of treatments (initially, approximately 20 per cent of all treatments) under a certain cost threshold. GPs could choose whichever provider *they* thought best met the needs of the patients. Savings could be reinvested in the practice (although GPs' ownership of their practices raised concerns of probity). Emergencies were excluded from the fundholding scheme.

Concerns were expressed about the differential treatment that fundholding patients could receive, raising fears of 'two-tierism'. GPs' budgets were funded on historical patterns and were generally considered to be greater per patient than non-fundholders. Hence GPFHs, who were often the better organised practices previously, could secure treatments from providers once the health authorities' budgets had been exhausted, most evident towards the end of the financial year. Some feared that fundholding created incentives for 'cream-skimming' – the exclusion of high-cost patients from GP lists. No conclusive evidence was found for this (Lewis, 1999). (See Chapter 7.)

On 1 April 1991, 306 fundholding practices (involving 1700 GPs) were created (Timmins 1995: 471).

The publication of *Working for Patients* marked a watershed in primary care policy. Arguably, for the first time GPs were being brought centrally within the structure of the NHS. Though some practices were being offered new 'freedoms', GPs collectively were being increasingly subject to managerialism (Causer and Exworthy 1999). Hence, GPs and primary care were no longer an 'autonomous enclave' (Klein 1989: 223). The balance of power was also shifting towards (and within) primary care, away from hospitals (Exworthy *et al.* 1996). Through the internal market, GPs now had a new relationship with consultants (Lewis 1999); the latter now had to be responsive to the former. It reverted to the pre-1948 system whereby consultants in voluntary hospitals depended on GPs for referrals. Post-1948, GPs were dependent upon salaried consultants (Timmins 1995: 369). Although the intra-professional balance was shifting, the government was pursuing a 'divide-and-rule' policy in the medical profession. No longer was it granted special negotiating privileges; managerial considerations were given primacy. Though S. Harrison (1988) claims that managers were becoming agents of the centre, the government was transforming professionals (especially GPs) *into* managers (Causer and Exworthy 1999).

GP contract 1990

During this period, the GP contract had remained unresolved but it became inextricably linked with the proposed changes. The outcome of BMA–government negotiations over the new contract was rejected in a vote at a special GP conference. For Timmins (1995), this was significant: 'for the first time in the history of the NHS, the troops had proved more militant than the BMA's leaders' (468). Yet, the style of Kenneth Clarke was defiant: 'I do wish the more suspicious of our GPs would stop feeling nervously for their wallets every time I mention the word reform' (quoted in Timmins 1995: 467). It is not surprising that the government implemented the new contract anyway.

Traditionally, the GP contract has required GPs to 'provide a range of relatively unspecified general medical services for their registered patients and sets out the terms and conditions under which GPs will be reimbursed for providing those services' (Glendinning 1999: 117). It thus symbolised the state–profession concordat (as applied to GPs) established back in 1948; the 'politics of the double bed' (Klein 1989b). The contract was an inflexible and rudimentary device in achieving change in primary care but it mediated the interests of the profession and the state.

The 1990 GP contract marked a change in emphasis. It specified terms and conditions in greater detail and was much more managerial in nature. For example, it specified minimum standards and introduced payments based upon provision. For the most part, these were individualistic measures rather than a concerted attempt to re-focus general practice on the wider needs of the population.

Phase Seven: Primary Care at the Centre of Health Policy? (1990/1–1997)

The period from April 1991 onwards (when most of the 1990 NHS and Community Care Act was implemented) is the most significant period in primary care policy in the UK. By being at the forefront of policy, primary care symbolised the magnitude of the reforms being implemented. However, a policy transition was clearly evident between April 1991 and May 1997 (when a Labour Government was elected). The evolution of policy over this time represents a maturation of primary care to the point at which many of the

Labour reforms (described in the next chapter) were often 'natural' extensions to what had been implemented in the early and mid-1990s when the Conservatives held office.

GP fundholding, locality commissioning and TPP

The period 1991–1994 was marked by the creation and development of the internal market. GP fundholding, one of the central planks in the internal market, was extended each year. Additionally, more services fell within the remit of GP fundholding and significantly, in 1993, community nursing and other community health services were added to the scheme. (For a detailed review of the GP fundholding scheme, see Glennerster *et al.* (1994) and Chapter 7.)

However, as GP fundholding grew so did the criticism. Anecdotal and research evidence emerged of its impact; criticism centred on 'two-tierism' or, more precisely, inequalities in access. Though often expressed in terms of waiting times for elective surgery, the inequality was exemplified by the leverage that fundholders were able to exert over hospital and community health services. For example, consultant outreach services (Roland and Shapiro 1998) and other practice-based services (such as physiotherapy) were established in many fundholding practices. Whilst this was clearly of benefit to fundholders' patients, it was often done so at the disadvantage of the non-fundholders' patients.

Despite a plurality of purchasing models which developed in the early-mid 1990s (Mays and Dixon, 1996), the government pursued the concept of fundholding in the belief that its benefits were potentially available to all practices. The basic fundholding model was extended to create community, standard and total purchasing fundholders. Total Purchasing Pilots (TPPs) were announced in 1994 (NHSE 1994) and implemented in 1996. Arising out of existing fundholding schemes, the 53 TPP sites were given almost the entire HCHS budget for the patients. Whilst some made progress in further shaping hospital and community health services, many of the changes affected the delivery of primary care services (see Chapter 7 for a discussion of TPPs). However, the impending general election in 1997 becalmed the debate (Wainwright, 1998) and prevented the use of TPP experience more widely. TPPs were the high watermark of the fundholding initiative (Mays *et al.* 2001b).

Many of the initiatives were outward focused, rather than intent on reconfiguring primary care itself. For example, it could be argued that fundholding was a way of gaining greater leverage over secondary care (hospital) consultants. Fundholding and locality commissioning had left much of primary care untouched; reform was being conducted *by* primary care but not *for* primary care. This situation was addressed through a series of initiatives which shifted the emphasis of primary care policy.

Other primary care policy developments in the mid-1990s

The experience of the fundholding initiative(s) and the realisation that primary care could provide the basis for realising wider health policy objectives precipitated a reassessment of policy. The limitations of primary care (as then constituted) were becoming increasingly evident. For example, the 1990 GP contract had limited the integration of general practices into a network of primary and community health services, designed to meet the needs of the local population (Glendinning 1999: 122). Yet, there was a reluctance to amend further the GP contract, as it symbolised GPs' independent contractor status (Lewis, 1997). The result of this reassessment was a series of policy developments between 1994 and 1997:

Developing NHS Purchasing and GP Fundholding: Towards a Primary Care-led NHS (1994) (NHS Executive, 1994);
Health Authorities Act (1995);
Primary Care: The Future (1996) (NHS Executive, 1996)
Primary Care: Choice and Opportunity (1996) (DoH 1996b);
Primary Care: Delivering the Future (1996) (DoH 1996a); and
NHS (Primary Care) Act (1997).

Together, they represent the most concerted programme of policy reform directed specifically at primary care. Whilst primary care had been the focus of policy attention previously (such as in 1991), this was often in order to achieve other objectives (such as the creation of the internal market). The 1994–7 programme was to be much more far-reaching within primary care than hitherto.

a. Primary care-led NHS The NHS Executive 'letter' (EL(94)79) and accompanying booklet (published in October 1994) provided the philosophy underlying the initiatives which followed. It contained major proposals involving a:

- major expansion of options for GP fundholding ...;
- a continuing and important role for DHAs and FHSAs and for new health authorities which ... will replace them; and
- a stronger partnership between health authorities and all GPs (fundholders and non-fundholders). (EL(94)79)

The policy proposed three types of fundholding:

1. Community fundholding:

    - practices with more than 3000 patients
    - including: 'staff, drugs, diagnostic tests and most of the community health services in the standard scheme (excluding mental illness and learning disability services). It will exclude all acute hospital treatments (including outpatient attendances).' (EL(94)79)

2. Standard fundholding:

- practices with more than 5000 patients (previously 7000);
- 'an expanded and more coherent version of the existing scheme'. To include 'specialist nursing services and virtually all elective surgery and outpatients.' (EL(94)79)

3. Total purchasing:

- 'where GPs in a locality purchase all hospital and community health services.' (EL(94)79).

At the time, 4 projects were underway and a further 25 were planned.

The role of the HA in this modified system would involve strategy, monitoring and support. Though continuing to play a 'major role as direct purchasers', HAs would have the purchasing role derogated to GPs. Hence, these 'new' functions were part of the decentralisation drive. Moreover, the policy formally recognised the diversity of general practice and potential for different organisational solutions, an approach which was developed more fully later in the decade.

b. Health Authorities Act   Though focused on HAs, rather than primary care *per se*, the Act enabled the merger of FHSAs with DHAs to create (unified) HAs. Though some saw the merger as a 'takeover' of the FHSA, the result was agencies which, for the first time, placed the responsibility for primary care and HCHS under one organisation. Both also shared accountability to the regional health authorities. It is debatable, however, whether the merger resulted in a fundamental realignment of policy and management towards primary care since the new HAs were still grappling with the wider organisational changes wrought by the internal market.

c. Primary Care: The Future   This policy document, published in June 1996, presented the findings of a 'listening exercise which ... involved professionals, patients and others in a discussion about the future of primary care' (foreword). Covering general practice, pharmaceutical services, optometry services, nursing and therapy services, it identified five 'principles of good primary care' and for each, further principles were listed.

1. Quality

- 'professionals should be knowledgeable about the conditions that present in primary care and skilled in their treatment';
- 'professionals should be knowledgeable to whom they are offering services';
- services should be coordinated with professionals aware of each others' contributions ... and no service gaps'.

2. Fairness

- 'services should not vary widely in range or quality in different parts of the country';
- 'primary care should receive an appropriate share of overall NHS resources'.

3. Accessibility

- 'services should be reasonably accessible when clinically needed';
- 'necessary services should be accessible to people regardless of age, sex, ethnicity or health status'.

4. Responsiveness

- 'services should reflect the needs and preferences of the individual using them';
- 'services should reflect the demographic and social needs of the area they serve'.

5. Efficiency

- 'primary care services should be based on scientific evidence';
- 'primary care resources should be used efficiently.' (4)

Emerging from these principles was an agenda with seven 'themes': resources, partnerships in care, developing professional knowledge, patient and carer information and involvement, securing the workforce and premises, better organisation and local flexibility (49).

d. Choice and opportunity Arising from *Primary Care: The Future* (NHSE 1996) (and its equivalents in Scotland and Wales), the White Paper *Primary Care: Choice and Opportunity* (DoH October 1996b) proposed greater flexibility in 'meeting local needs', of using 'skills to the full' and creating 'employment opportunities' (1). This document proposed a series of pilots, mainly focused on new contractual arrangements.

> Ideas for alternative forms of contracting for general medical or dental service should be formulated locally and could come initially from, for example, GPs, dentists, NHS trusts, health authorities or health boards. (15)

In terms of general practice, the contractual options included:

- 'a salaried option for GPs, either within partnerships or with other bodies such as NHS trusts ...;
- practice based contracts ...;
- a single budget for general medical services, other hospital and community health services, and prescribing with the practice responsible for purchasing or providing services within it.' (5)

e. Primary Care: Delivering the Future   This White Paper (December, DoH 1996a) proposed 'a series of practical proposals for action to complement the opportunities presented by the legislation' (1). The many proposals presented in this document included:

- 'new employment and contract options in the NHS (Primary Care) Bill' (15);
- 'extension of the existing nurse prescribing pilot scheme' (15);
- 'NHS Pension Scheme open to practice staff . . .' (48);
- 'new cost rent schedules . . .' (48); and
- 'GP locality pilots.' (55)

These policy statements (c, d and e, above) were astute assessments of the advantages that primary care had already brought and the limitations which it posed on its own future development. Central among these was diversity (and inequality). On the one hand, general practice, as a key component of primary care, was characterised by its 'innovation and diversity' (*Primary Care: The Future* (NHSE 1996) Chapter 3) but, on the other, this exacerbated inequalities in the quantity and quality of care provided.

f. NHS (Primary Care) Act   The Act was given assent just before the May 1997 election and so represents the final stage in this review of primary care policy. However, it was a landmark in terms of the flexibilities which it facilitated though enabling the employment of salaried GPs and through the merger of GMS and HCHS budgets. Glendinning (1999) describes the Act as a 'watershed' as 'it offers a new organizational and financial framework' (125). The flexibilities were pursued through three types of pilot project:

1. salaried options: GPs would be employed by the HA under a separate contract;
2. PMS: contracts would be created between practices and the HA so as to improve the personal medical services within the cash-limited GMS budget;
3. 'PMS+': contracts would extend the 'PMS' pilots to cover personal medical services *and* a range of other services under a combined GMS/HCHS budget.

Each of the 94 projects took a specific focus in terms of the client group and/or geographical area they served. The nature of the projects meant that some served groups or were in areas which have been poorly served by primary care in the past, such as homeless people and inner cities. It should be noted, however, that the projects were voluntary and provision had been made to allow the participants to revert to their former organisational and financial arrangements should they so wish. (For a fuller description and discussion, see Walsh *et al.* 1999, 2001.)

Conclusions

This précis of primary care policy, organisation and management in the twentieth century has inevitably been partial. The 'history' described here has been one which has focused on the *de jure* policies and yet there are many *de facto* histories of primary care from the perspectives of practitioners, patients and policy-makers. No doubt, a different picture would emerge if these histories were presented. (See, for example, Widgery 1991 for a 'grass-roots' perspective of primary care or Pereira Gray 1992 from the general practice profession's perspective).

In short, the twentieth century saw the emergence of primary care as a specific area of health care, albeit dominated mainly by general practice. However, this process was accompanied by a formalised separation of the generalist model of primary care from the specialist approach of secondary care services. This separation was evident for the first third of the century and was formalised by the creation of GPs as independent contractors within the NHS. Yet, GPs' gatekeeping role was considered vital to the functioning of the NHS. In many ways, other primary care professions (especially community nursing) experienced a similar separation from the rest of the health care system by virtue of their distinctive professional developments in local authorities. The integration of GPs and community nursing became most apparent with the effective development of primary care teams from the 1960s onwards.

Although many saw the managerialism of the 1980s and the internal market in the 1990s as inimical to primary care teamwork, these two developments were arguably instrumental in placing primary care at the centre of health policy and in a pivotal role in the organisation and management of health care. It is no surprise therefore that the 1990s witnessed the most concerted attempt to shape primary care through policy reform, in part because of the pressures and needs elsewhere in the NHS.

As mentioned earlier, Klein (1995) uses the metaphor of recurring operatic melodies to signify the persistence of issues within health care politics. Most issues and themes have arisen in each of the phases described here and yet there has been a significant and often not so subtle change, especially over the last decade. Policy developments have intensified and expanded each of the three main themes of this book, namely integration, diversity and changing boundaries. In summary, these have specific manifestations which are explored in subsequent chapters. Policy has become less deferential to the professions. For much of the century, the government was wary about upsetting the professions (primarily medicine) given their status within society and the power which they wielded. However, with the rise of managerialism, policies have shaped the organisation and management of primary care in fundamental ways. This is resulting in a broader and more inclusive definition of primary care, a greater managerial role in what had been a professional enclave, and a more central role in meeting NHS objectives. Aided by an increasingly inquisitive and sceptical public, primary care has thus moved from the margins to the mainstream of health policy in the UK.

This chapter takes the evolution of primary care up to the May 1997 general election in the UK. Since the June 2001 general election provided the Labour Government with a second term of office, it is appropriate to consider the period since May 1997 as the current phase of policy evolution. Hence, the next chapter examines this phase and incorporates developments up to April 2002.

Box 4.1   Phase One: Chronology

1829	Apothecaries able to charge for medical advice.
1850	Rathbone establishes home nursing service in Liverpool
1858	Medical Act (establishing the medical register)
1862	Manchester and Salford Reform Association establish 'health visiting'
Mid-19th century	Rapid growth of the hospital, promoting the distinction between specialists and generalists (Honigsbaum 1979)
1891–95	5.49 deaths from pregnancy and childbearing per 1000 live births; by 1918, this had fallen to 3.66. (Ottewill and Wall 1990)
1899	Infant mortality rate was 163 per 1000 live births (Honigsbaum 1979)
1902	Midwives Act provides for certification of midwives
1911	Formation of panel system under the National Health Insurance Act

---

Box 4.2   Phase Two: Chronology

1919	Creation of Ministry of Health
1920	Dawson Report (proposing health centres)
1920	Three-quarters of GPs were on 'panel' system (Honigsbaum 1979)
1926	Peckham health centre opened
1930	BMA calls for a 'general medical service for the nation'
1936	Midwives Act secured national salaried midwifery service

---

Box 4.3   Phase Three: Chronology

1939	McNalty's proposal for a national health service
1940s	GPs' opposition to Bevan's plan for salaried service (Glendinning 1999)
1940	BMA's Medical Planning Commission created
1940	Emergency Medical Service created
1944	Beveridge Report published
1944	White Paper *A National Health Service* published
1948	NHS established
1948	Executive Councils formed

Box 4.4   Phase Four: Chronology

1952   Central Health Services Council reports on health and social service collaboration
1952   3/4 GPs worked single/dual-handed practices (Glendinning 1999)
1956   Guillebaud Committee report
1958   Local Government Act
1960   Royal Commission on Doctors' and Dentists' Remuneration
1963   BMA meeting calls for GP pay increase to reduce GP-consultant pay differentials
1963   Gillie Committee report encourages primary care team

Box 4.5   Phase Five: Chronology

1965   BMA's Family Doctor Charter
1966   New GP Contract
1966   240 GPs (1.5 per cent of GPs) work in health centres; in 1973, this had risen to 2400 (12 per cent)
1967   College of GPs receives its Royal Charter
1967   Minister announces review of the NHS; leading to Green Papers in 1968 and 1970 and a White Paper in 1972
1968   Seebohm Report proposes generic social workers
1960s/70s   Rapid development of health centres (Webster 1998)
1970+   Emergence of the term 'primary care (Webster 1998)
1974   Family Practitioner Committees formed
1974   NHS reorganisation
1978   WHO Alma Ata Declaration

Box 4.6   Phase Six: Chronology

1979   Royal Commission on the NHS
1979   Green Paper 'Patients' First'
1981   Harding Report (on primary health care team)
1981   Acheson Report (state of primary health care in inner London)
1982   NHS reorganisation
1983   Griffiths Report: NHS Management Inquiry
1985   General managers introduced into hospitals and community health services
1986   Cumberlege Report on neighbourhood nursing
1987   *Promoting Better Health* (DHSS 1987)
1989   White Paper *Working for Patients* (DoH 1989a)
1990   New GP Contract
1990   FPC transformed into Family Health Service Authorities
1990   NHS and Community Care Act

Box 4.7   Phase Seven: Chronology

1991   Introduction of GP fundholding and internal market
1993   Extension of GPFH to include commissioning community nursing
       (and other) services
1994   Less than 1/4 GPs worked single/dual handed practices (Glendin-
       ning 1993)
1994   EL(94)79: *Primary Care-led NHS*
1995   Introduction of Total Purchasing and other models of fundholding
1996   HA Act: FHSAs merged with DHAs to form health authorities
1996   Green/White Papers (*Primary Care: The Future* (NHSE 1996),
       Choice and Opportunity (DoH 1996b), and *Primary Care: Delivering
       the Future* (DoH 1996a))
1997   NHS (Primary Care) Bill
1997   '*The New NHS*' (DoH 1997)White Paper (and parallel White Papers
       in Scotland, Secretary of State for Scotland (1997) Wales, Secretary
       of State for Wales (1998) and NI, Secretary of State for Northern
       Ireland (1998)

CHAPTER 5

The Organisation of Primary Care in the UK

As the preceding chapters have shown, primary care in the UK is a complex policy sector that defies simple definitions. Its evolution is symbolic of the wider changes in health policy and society itself. Following on from where Chapter 4 finished, this chapter describes and analyses the current organisation of primary care in the UK. Attention is focused on the changes introduced by the Labour Government since 1997/98; these include the changes affecting primary care and those associated with political devolution.

The structure adopted for this chapter is Frenk's (1994) policy levels: the systemic, programmatic, organisational and instrumental. Frenk's approach is valuable here because it helps understanding of the interests operating at each level and the interactions between levels (say, between government and practitioners, or the professions and NHS Trusts). Though this section recognises the definitional debates presented in Chapter 3, it focuses on particular aspects that are considered crucial to explaining current primary care policy reform.

Systemic Level

The systemic level is comprised of the institutional arrangements for the regulation, financing and delivery of primary care. Hence, this level involves those decision-making structures and process that shape the overall health system; for example, decisions which determine the shape of the NHS or public health (Chapter 2). This section of the chapter also examines territorial differences within the UK in the light of political devolution.

National Differences within the UK

The UK is often seen as a paradox of four nations within one country (Exworthy 2001). Despite being a unitary state, public policy varies between England, Scotland, Wales and Northern Ireland. Though this variation is evidenced in many areas of public life and public policy, primary care is also subject to such diversity. The dual reforms in the NHS and in the devolution to

Table 5.1   Labour's Reform of the NHS by the Four Nations of the UK

Nation	Status	Title	Publication date	Cm
England	White Paper	*The New NHS*	Dec. 1997	3807
Scotland	White Paper	*Designed to Care*	Dec. 1997	3811
Wales	White Paper	*Putting Patients First*	Jan. 1998	3841
N. Ireland	Consultation	*Fit for the Future*	April 1998	n/a

Source: Exworthy (2001).

Scotland, Wales and Northern Ireland might lead to further variation between the four nations.

Following the 1997 election, the Labour Government placed emphasis on, *inter alia*, devolution of political responsibility to the UK's constituent nations through both devolution and modernising the NHS by abolishing the internal market. Although the new government stressed the need to return to a 'one-nation NHS', the proposals for devolution and the NHS indicated that the question of 'which nation?' was unanswered (Exworthy 2001; Boyne and Powell 2001). For example, Dixon and Mays (1997), writing soon after the election, argued that 'the notion of a one nation NHS emphasised so heavily by this government' (1640) was undermined by the capacity for national difference enshrined in the reforms. The principles were to be applied across the UK but 'significant differences' were expected in each nation (Wright 1998: 5).

Four policy documents were published in a five-month period which incorporated Labour's approach to the NHS (see Table 5.1).

Explanations for the impact of devolution on primary care are examined in Box 5.1. The specific policy reforms as they apply to each nation are presented later in this chapter.

Health and Health Care in the UK

Variations and inequalities are evident in health status and health care at a variety of geographical levels from the individual household to the nations and regions within the UK (Benzeval *et al.* 1995; Acheson 1998; Graham 2000).

In terms of health status, Table 5.2 shows that the variation is marked in, for example, perinatal mortality but not so much in infant mortality rates. The pattern of limiting long-standing illness does not match precisely with the pattern of infant/perinatal mortality.

It should be noted that the population of England (47.556 million in 1995) is significantly larger than Scotland (5.099 million), Wales (2.888 million) and Northern Ireland (1.578 million). Indeed, seven of the eight English regions

Box 5.1   Explaining Territorial Variations in UK Primary Care Policy

Administrative devolution has been a feature of UK health policy but, since 1997, political devolution has given greater freedom to devolved territories – Scotland, Wales and Northern Ireland. Though devolved experience is limited, it is possible to discern some possible directions by drawing on policy models and frameworks. Three are summarised here.

Purpose of policy: The means and ends of policy are often distinguished (Exworthy and Powell 2000). Those determining the ends of policy are often separated organisationally and geographically from those charged with the means of such policy. Central–local relations (or inter-governmental relations) exemplify the tension between policy ends and policy means. Thus, whilst primary care documents may look different in each country of the UK, differences may not be borne out in practice (Hunter and Wistow 1987). Policy variations between the four nations are tolerated if they relate to the means (Kellas 1975).

Policy types: Rose (1982) identified three types of policy applicable in devolved systems. Uniform policies apply equally across the UK and include foreign and defence policy. Concurrent policies have the same content in each nation but are administered by different agencies; they include health and education policies. Exceptional policies aim to meet specific needs of an area. Farrell and Law (1998) state that language policies in Wales are classed as 'exceptional'.

In terms of the NHS, concurrent policies (e.g. the abolition of GP fundholding) may have an exceptional impact. For example, the Scottish LHCCs 'hold budgets' and the three Island Health Boards retain a unitary structure. Also, the fundholding initiative has been retained in Northern Ireland.

Action space: This concept denotes the scope of independent action in each nation in different sectors. Economic policy exemplifies limited action space as each nation cannot pursue different economic policies. Health policy may be considered as an area of greater action space as some national variations are permissible. Action space is similar to the notion of high and low politics (Bulpitt 1983). Economic policy illustrates high politics in relating to the needs of the 'core' areas, spatially (Westminster) and sectorally (the economy), unlike health policy which is classed as 'low politics'. Primary care's action space is being renegotiated following devolution; policies are more closely scrutinised by Scottish Parliament/Welsh or NI Assemblies (and ministers). Representatives in devolved bodies may seek a clear separation from England/Westminster, using primary care as a vehicle. Primary care may shift to become 'high politics'. The final configuration of primary care policy will, however, reflect the 'disjointed incrementalism' in the territorial policy networks (Wainwright 1998).

Table 5.2   National Health Differences in the UK

1995/96	England	Scotland	Wales	N. Ireland
Infant mortality rate	6.1	6.1	6.1	7.1
Perinatal mortality rate	8.8	9.6	7.8	10.4
Limiting long-standing illness (% population)	19	20	22	19

Source: Office for National Statistics (1997).

Table. 5.3   National Health Service Differences in the UK

	England	Scotland	Wales	N. Ireland
GP consultations (% within last 14 days)	15	17	17	16
Average list size (no. of patients)	1887	1506	1730	1731
GP fundholding coverage (% population)	40	33	39	n/a

Source: ONS (1997).

have a larger population than the other three nations (CMA Medical Data 1996); only the Trent Region is smaller than Scotland.

In terms of health care, England has the largest average list size (Table 5.3) but this is not necessarily an indication of a healthier population, although the proportion of the population visiting the GP in the previous fortnight is the lowest of the four nations. It is difficult to interpret the connections between need, supply and demand, and between health status and health care (Rogers *et al.* 1999). Intervening variables might include the organisation of health care services in each nation, the influence of interest groups (such as the medical profession), social attitudes towards health and wider determinants of health.

Ministerial Responsibility and the Department of Health

Territorial responsibility for health and health care rests with the same ministerial departments. However, until recently, it is fair to say that these departments were primarily concerned with health services issues rather than health (such as health improvement) *per se*. This has changed somewhat in the 1990s with the publication of strategies for health improvement (DoH 1999b).

The Department of Health (DoH) is the responsibility of the Secretary of State for Health and is effectively the health department for England. However, it also takes responsibility for UK-wide issues and for international health policy issues (such as liaison with the European Union) (Hunter 1998).

Prior to political devolution, in each of the other three nations, responsibility for health and health care rested with the Secretary of State for each territory. Junior ministers usually took responsibility for particular aspects such as the minister for health and social services in Northern Ireland. Each health department had a structure of civil servants and professional advisers. The case of the safety of beef in 1999 highlighted the impact of differing structures; in this case, it was the discrepancy between different sources of medical advice. The English Chief Medical Officer believed that the beef was not safe whereas his counterparts in Scotland and Wales took contrary views. In future, such policy differences may become even more apparent as the respective administrations took responsibility for health (Calman and Smith 2001).

At the sub-national level, the relative populations shape policy-making processes and structures. For example, the size of England necessitates a regional structure. However, these Regions, as offices of the NHS Executive since 1996, did not have much leeway in independent policy formulation. Scotland, Wales and Northern Ireland have no comparable regional structure.

The funding of the Scottish Office was clarified in the 1970s by the Barnett formula and other formulae have since been implemented for Wales and Northern Ireland. Each of the territorial Offices gains from these; in 1995–6, Scotland was allocated 25 per cent more, Wales 18 per cent more and Northern Ireland 5 per cent more than England (Dixon *et al.* 1999).

Health and health care issues are given ministerial responsibility through the Department of Health (DoH). The Secretary of State, who has a seat on the Cabinet, is the head of the DoH. The DoH level is primarily concerned with:

- broad goals of health policy;
- negotiations with the Treasury for the share of government expenditure that will be devoted to health (mainly through the NHS);
- allocation of the overall NHS budget to various sectors;
- liaison with other government departments; and
- negotiations with the professions regarding policy proposals.

Several ministers of health report to the Secretary of State. The ministers have responsibility for various sectors such as public health or mental health. Although their remit varies from time to time according to the demands and needs of DoH and the government, primary care falls under the remit of a minister of health. Within the last 10 years or so, primary care has had several ministers which make continuity in and responsibility for primary care problematic. This is a wider issue of regular ministerial change associated with departmentalism (Kavanagh and Richards 2001).

The NHS Executive (NHSE) (formerly Management Executive, NHSME) was created to act as the executive agency which would implement the health policies formulated by the DoH. As an agency operating at arm's-length from ministers, it was supposed to be semi-autonomous. However, given the political saliency of the NHS, the NHSE and the DoH have become closely intertwined, blurring the division between formulation (strategy) and implementation (operation) (Klein and Day 1997; Osbourne and Gaebler 1992). Even the NHSE's headquarters location in Leeds was supposed to signify its (organisational) distance from the DoH in London.

The NHSE was headed by a Chief Executive and was divided into various directorates. The NHSE was responsible for the implementation of primary care policy, for example, in issuing guidance to PCGs. In 1996, the Regional Health Authorities (RHAs), which were semi-autonomous intermediary agencies, were incorporated within the remit of the NHSE and their names changed to Regional Offices (of the NHSE). Though the change involved RHA staff being transferred from the NHS to the civil service, it also signalled a more significant shift in terms of centralisation. Regional Offices were no longer semi-autonomous but became 'agents of the centre' in terms of disseminating guidance and directives from the centre (NHSE/DoH) and monitoring the performance of NHS agencies within the Region (on behalf of the centre).

In 2001, the document *Shifting the Balance of Power: Securing Delivery* (DoH 2001b) proposed that the 'Department of Health will change the way it relates to the NHS ... The Department of Health Regional Offices will be abolished and four new Regional Directors of Health and Social Care will oversee the development of the NHS' (DoH 2001b). Effectively this has entailed the amalgamation of the NHSE Chief Executive and Permanent Secretary (currently, as of 2002, Nigel Crisp). These structural changes 'will be complete by April 2003' (DoH, 2001b: 7) although many of the changes will be introduced in April 2002 (DoH, 2002a). (*Shifting the Balance of Power* has precipitated other changes elsewhere in the NHS; see below).

Resource Allocation and Expenditure Patterns within the UK

General Medical Services are generally provided by independent contractors. GPs are funded by a system of fees and allowances whereas dental and ophthalmic practitioners are funded by a 'fee-for-service' system. Pharmaceutical services are provided by pharmacists who are also independent contractors. Drugs are supplied under the NHS when prescribed by a GP and, as exemptions account for about 80 per cent of the prescriptions, drugs amount to about 10 per cent of NHS expenditure (Kennedy 1999: 144).

Publicly funded health expenditure is divided into two main areas: hospital and community health services (HCHS), and family health services (FHS). In 1993/94, HCHS expenditure accounted for 74.3 per cent of the total, with 22 per cent spent on non-cash limited FHS (Kennedy 1999: 144). The remainder was spent on DoH administration and central services (Robinson *et al.* 1994). Whilst acute services accounted for the largest single category in HCHS expenditure (45 per cent), FHS expenditure was dominated by spending on pharmaceuticals (51 per cent). Kennedy (1999: 144) estimates that, using a broad definition to include general practice and community health services, primary care accounts for 33 per cent of total FHS expenditure.

Table 5.4   FHS expenditure

	% of FHS expenditure, 1992/3
Pharmaceuticals	51
GMS	27
Dental	20
Ophthalmic	3

Source: Department of Health (1994).

In 1997/98, the costs of GMS in the UK was £3.36 billion (RCGP 1999a). This is a fourfold increase since 1949 even allowing for inflation. In 1996, GMS accounted for 8.9 per cent (in 1996) (*ibid.*). GMS is divided into:

- personal medical services (PMS) (payments to GPs);
- practice premises (rents and rates);
- fees and allowances;
- staff salaries and superannuation; and
- other expenses.

Only about 10 per cent of GMS budget was amenable to local flexibility because of national agreements. The schedule of payments for GPs is listed in the *Red Book*. Each GP is allowed to claim a basic practice allowance – a form of salary – which amounts to £8688 (full rate, for 1200 patients or more). However, over half of the payments to GPs are related on a per capita basis to their list sizes. (All payments are based on April 2001 figures; *Medeconomics*, 'Your pay', May 2001, 22(5), p. 69). Other 'items of service fees' are listed in the *Red Book*.

GPs' income has also been based upon bonus or target payments for the achievement of specified levels of childhood immunisations and cervical cytology which can account for 7 per cent of GP income (Kennedy 1999: 145). Other GP payments include direct reimbursements of expenses, whilst other expenses are met by GPs from their gross fees and allowances. Thus, an individual GP's income is not a straightforward matter based on such fees and allowances. GPs' gross income based on GMS was £107,300 (unrestricted principal) but the average intended income in 2001 was £56,510 (*Medeconomics*, 'Your Pay', May 2001, 22(5), p. 69).

Financing Health Care

In 1997, the UK spent 6.7 per cent of its gross domestic product (GDP) on health care. The NHS dominates health care expenditure in the UK; in 1997, it accounted for 85 per cent of total health care expenditure in the UK (EOHCS 1999: 49). The vast majority (about 94 per cent) of NHS expenditure is financed through taxation and national insurance contributions. The rest comes mainly from user charges (such as for prescriptions or dental care) (Robinson *et al.* 1994). The UK system of financing health care based on general taxation has the following advantages

- Funding health care is related to ability pay (and not to individual risk status as in private health care);
- Tax-based funding of health care is relatively cheap to administer;
- The growth in overall health care spending is easier to control than in private health care systems.

However, there are some disadvantages:

- Government control over health care spending has tended to result in lower levels of spending than other countries;
- As the NHS is (mostly) 'free at the point of delivery', it encourages patients to make more use of the service than they are willing to fund as taxpayers or voters (Buchanan 1965; Robinson *et al.* 1994);
- It is unclear how much of general taxation is spent on health care. Such 'ear-marking' or hypothecation has been advocated by some to ensure a transparency in government decisions. So far, the 'NHS ear-mark' has not been introduced.

These factors were recognised by the Wanless Report (2002) which was commissioned by the Chancellor of the Exchequer. Confirming the conclusions of his 2001 interim report, Wanless argues that:

> There is no alternative financing method to that currently in place in the UK which would deliver a given level and quality of health care either at a lower cost to the economy or in a more equitable way. (2002: 97)

Medical Practices Committee (MPC)

A systemic level mechanism which sought greater equity across the country was the MPC (in England and Wales) and its derivatives (in Scotland and Northern Ireland). Since April 2002 it is no longer in operation but there is a value in examining its methods and purposes. The MPC was established in legislation in 1948 as a way of ensuring a more even distribution of general medical prac-titioners in England and Wales. (Scotland and NI have comparable structures). However, it also had the effect of ensuring that the medical profession (here, GPs) has restricted the supply of GPs (Moran and Wood 1993: 135). The control of the distribution of GP workforce has led to accusations of 'unlawful restrictive practice' (Parson 1989) but these were probably unsustainable since the provisions of the Restrictive Trade Practices Act 1976 'simply do not apply to anti-competitive agreements affecting the way many health professionals provide services' (Miller 1992: 471).

Despite the many changes in primary care policy, the MPC had, until recently, changed relatively little (Moran and Wood, 1993); it still met monthly and considered applications by GPs to practise in particular areas (Exworthy 1994b). The MPC's powers were mainly negative, in the sense that they were only able to restrict applications on the basis of GP-population ratios (related to average list sizes) in certain areas. They had no other specific powers to influence the geographical distribution of GPs in relation to need or even the staffing patterns of other primary care professionals. The MPC determined each application on the basis of four categories (see Table 5.5).

It is difficult to attribute falling list sizes solely to the MPC but, in 1974, almost 50 per cent of GPs in England and Wales practised in open or designated areas. By 1980, this figure had fallen to one third and there were no areas classified as designated since 1986.

This categorisation is based on assumptions relating to the relationship between patient need and the workload of GPs. Both are notoriously difficult to determine (Stevens and Gabbay 1991; Jarman 1983). There have been adjustments in the average list sizes determining the MPC categories which reflect the general reductions in list sizes (by 10 per cent for unrestricted principals in the UK between 1985 and 1997 [RCGP 1998]). These changes in inter-professional working and deprivation or rural area payments have begun to affect the MPC's activities.

There have been some criticisms that the MPC has been inflexible to the changing needs of primary care and the general practice profession (Butler 1973; Exworthy 1994b). Though its legislative framework limited the scope

Table 5.5 MPC Classification

MPC area	Average list size	Definition	Applications to practise	% of all MPC areas (7/99)*
Designated	over 2500	Much less than adequately doctored	Encouraged	0
Open	2101–2500	Adequately doctored	Normally approved	2.7
Intermediate	1701–2100	Adequately doctored	Depend on local circumstances	46.9
Restricted	under 1700	More than adequately doctored	Normally rejected	43.1

Note: * Figures as of December 1993.
Source: MPC Annual Report, 1998/99.

for innovation, the MPC did respond to initiatives in London in the 1990s by suspending the normal classification in the 12 London FHSAs (hence the LIZ and London controlled areas). (In 1993, 106 or 7.3 per cent of MPC areas were under the jurisdiction of the London Initiative Zone or were 'London-controlled').

FHSAs were advised to devise 'local plans' (recognising demand and supply factors) if changes to the local provision of GP services were planned (Exworthy 1994b: 11). Additionally, questions have been raised about the way in which a geographical approach supports a policy to equalise the distribution of GPs; Butler (1973) raised the following questions about its *modus operandi*:

- Do list sizes ensure a fair distribution of GPs? As the average list size is now below 2500, this question is less applicable now;
- Is a list size of 2500 the maximum number for whom a GP can provide reasonable care? The figure of 2500 was set in 1952 but is irrespective of need of supply and ignores the contribution of other primary care professionals;
- Is average list size an adequate measure of GP workload? Need, supply and deprivation (among other factors) might suggest that list size is not a good measure;
- Is the MPC area the most suitable unit to base the administration of GP staffing? The MPC area consists of about 20–30 GPs but this varies widely. Large areas are less susceptible to an additional GP changing the average list size significantly.

In the wake of the NHS (Primary Care) Act 1997 and the NHS Act 1998, the MPC recognised the need for modernisation. As its 1998/99 Annual Report (3) stated:

> For the Committee the most significant change [owing to legislation] has been the shift towards assessment of the locality rather than individual practices, and to see responsibility for the definition of locality placed solely in the hands of health authorities.

The MPC reconsidered the value of its fourfold classification because the 'numeric parameters are no longer valid' and 'the health authority … determines the boundaries of the area to be assessed' (MPC annual report, 1998/99: 13). Hence, a range of factors were considered which 'will override the influence of a simple, average list size assessment' (12). The impact of salaried GPs and other PMS initiatives had called into question the value of the MPC's centralised structure.

In 2000, the NHS Plan noted that there were '50 per cent more GPs in Kingston and Richmond or Oxfordshire than in Barnsley or Sunderland' even after adjustments for age and need (DoH 2000: para. 13.10). It proposed, therefore, that the MPC should be abolished and replaced with a 'single resource allocation formula' including GMS non-cash-limited expenditure.

A Medical Education Standards Board would track the 'number and distribution of doctors in primary care' whilst 200 new PMS schemes would be introduced by 2004. This took effect from April 2002 (MPC 2002).

Special Area Payments

Two other mechanisms have been introduced which are designed to recognise the needs of GPs in particular areas. These are financial measures which are paid to GPs practising in these 'deprived' and 'rural' areas. As such, they partly met the criticism of the MPC's statutory inflexibility.

Deprivation payments were introduced to compensate GPs for working in 'deprived' areas. GPs received per capita payments according to the level of deprivation that their patients face. Currently, there are three levels of deprivation payments (electoral ward-based)(in England and Wales) ranging from £3.81 to £2.20 per patient. A scheme based on enumeration districts and attracting per capita payments ranging from £26.22 to £7.79 has yet (as of autumn 2001) to be introduced. (Deprivation payments in Scotland and Northern Ireland range from £33.70 to £9.99: *Medeconomics*, 'Your Pay', May 2001, 22(5), p.69.)

Three criticisms have been levelled against deprivation payments. First, the measures of 'deprivation' have been based on the Jarman scores (Jarman 1983) which are an index of GPs' workload, not deprivation (Senior 1991). Though the Jarman index is generally seen as a reasonable representation of factors affecting GP workload, it was based on a survey of London GPs (thereby ignoring rural areas) and so it may not correspond well to those factors that influence deprivation. Second, the payment is not conditional upon GPs responding to the apparent deprivation in their area. They receive these payments irrespective of whether or not they adapt services to meet the local needs. Third, the discrete divisions between the three categories make significant financial differences for an apparently minor change in the level of deprivation.

Rural area payments were introduced to recognise the additional costs of practising in rural areas such as the additional travel costs and the difficulty of attracting staff. Similar criticisms to deprivation payments are also levelled against rural area payments: they are conditional payments, they do not guarantee improved services and the definition of 'rural' is problematic.

International Comparisons

Traditionally, the UK health care system has spent relatively little on health care compared to other comparable countries. The UK spent 6.7 per cent of its gross domestic product (GDP) on health, equivalent to 12.8 per cent of its public expenditure (in 1997) (EOHCS 1999). Figures for other comparable countries are presented in Table 5.6.

Table 5.6   International Comparisons of Health Care Expenditure*

	UK	France	Germany	Sweden	EU average
Total expenditure on health care as % of GDP	6.7	9.9	10.4	8.6	8.5
Public (government) health care expenditure as % of total health care expenditure	85	78	77	83	n/a
Total expenditure on health care in US dollars per capita (purchasing power parity)	1347	2103	2339	1728	1743

Note: * All figures 1997.

Table 5.7   International Comparison of Health Status

	UK	USA	France	Germany	Sweden
Life expectancy at birth, male, 1990 (unless stated)	73.0	72.0	72.7	72.6 (in 1989)	74.8
Life expectancy at birth, female, 1990 (unless stated)	78.5	78.8	80.9	79.0 (in 1989)	80.4

Sources: Robinson *et al*. (1994).

There is some debate as to whether the UK's lower spending on health care generally is associated with relatively 'good' health outcomes. Table 5.7 shows that, at least in terms of life expectancy, there is evidence to suggest that the UK has reasonable outcomes in return for its health expenditure. However, life expectancy may not be the most suitable measure; health inequalities between social groups and areas temper the judgement about the UK (Acheson 1998). Moreover, the UK spends much less than other countries on administrative and transaction costs (despite the rise in costs associated with the internal market). Starfield (1998) among others has argued that those countries with well-developed primary care systems such as Sweden and the UK are able to control overall health care costs because of primary care's gatekeeping role.

Programmatic Level: the Health Authority/Health Board

Frenk's (1994) programmatic level involves the specific priorities of the system by, for example, defining a universal package of health care interventions. Although it might apply to the NHS as a whole, it is applied here to the Health Authority (or Health Board) level. It is seen here as an intermediate level between the macro decisions on the overall direction of (primary care) policy, and the micro decisions taken by individual practitioners in their own practices (Hunter 1980; Exworthy 1993b). It is axiomatic of primary care that, until recently, the Health Authority level was noticeably absent from primary care policy. However, in the light of managerialisation and integration, the programmatic level at which HAs (combined with FHSA functions) are located has become a potentially significant player in primary care policy. The changing focus of HAs is briefly summarised below.

In 1994, FPCs were transformed into Family Health Services' Authorities (FHSAs). Reflecting the managerial spirit of the time, these agencies had greater managerial powers; for example, for improving the quality and quantity of primary care services provided. Whilst they administered the former 'pay and rations' functions of the FPCs, they also managed the reimbursements of practice staff and conditional payments related to health promotion targets (Allsop and May 1986).

By 1996, FHSAs were merged with HAs. By combining responsibility for the management of HCHS budgets with those of FHS, the new combined HAs were supposed to take a more integrated approach to primary care. Nonetheless, there were limits as to how far HAs could intervene in primary care given GPs' independent contractor status.

However, the development of GP fundholding in particular from 1991 onwards had begun to affect the internal organisation of HAs. Many created primary care departments with the departmental head often having executive director status. This post became closely linked to the FHSA medical adviser and pharmaceutical adviser. Strategies to encourage teamwork and appropriate prescribing behaviour were examples of primary care strategies that were adopted at the programmatic level. However, historical commitments prevented a radical shift in direction towards primary care policy at this level.

PCGs were created in England in 1999 as subcommittees of the HA and, in time, they were expected to become free-standing PCTs. The 1997 reforms suggested that the role of the HA in local primary care policy was to become more detached, affording greater (managerial) scope to the PCT itself. Thus, it is debatable whether the potential of HAs in shaping local primary care since the mid-1990s had been fully translated into actual power and influence.

The 28 Strategic HAs (StHA) in England cover populations of about 1.5 million (DoH 2001c); they were designed to be coterminous with 'an aggregate of Local Authorities' and their boundaries 'should not cut across Government Office boundaries' (DoH 2001c: 18). StHAs will replace the 95 HAs and 'step back from service planning and commissioning to lead the strategic development of the local health service and performance manage PCTs and NHS Trusts' (DoH 2001b). StHAs will provide an overarching structure for all NHS organisations within its area; they will play a pivotal role in steering local networks of organisations, holding them to account and developing their capacity to deliver (DoH 2002a). Some of these roles might be seen as incompatible, such as accountability and development. The StHAs took on their responsibilities in October 2002 (DoH 2002a).

Thus, StHAs have become removed from any specific role in primary care policy, that task having been delegated to PCTs. Given StHAs' role in setting a strategic framework and performance management, it is unlikely that such organisations can ever play a detailed role in local primary care policy development. However, the effect of their decisions will filter through to PCOs and practitioners. Discussion of the equivalents in Scotland, Wales and Northern Ireland are included in the next section.

Organisational Level: PCOs

According to Frenk's (1994) classification, the organisational level involves the actual production of services through a focus on issues such as quality assurance and technical efficiency. The 'production' of services is somewhat blurred in primary care since the delivery of services is normally associated with practitioners. However, here it is taken to imply the organisational decision-making related to the patterns and content of such services. Thus, it is taken to be distinct from service delivery – the instrumental level.

Until the advent of GP fundholding generally and its derivatives specifically (such as fundholding consortia), the organisational level was noticeably absent from UK primary care. It could be argued that neither the health authority (programmatic level) nor the general practice (instrumental level) accurately described the organisational structures and processes related to quality assurance and technical efficiency, among others. Indeed, this was the lacuna of primary care. However, the current waves of reforms which instituted PCOs such as PCGs, PCTs and LHGs, mark a distinctive phase whereby primary care has become an organisational entity.

Describing, explaining and understanding such changes are the purposes of this book. Inevitably, therefore, this section of the chapter is detailed to take account of the recent reforms and to document the territorial variations within the UK.

'Organisation Level' Policy Reforms

The direction of health policy in the UK since 1997 raises questions about the degree of geographical variation in each of the four home nations. One of the most significant differences apparent between nations was the proposals for the replacement of the GP fundholding scheme. This shows clearly the centrality of primary care *organisations* in current health policy and the potential for greater diversity within the UK.

i. England

Primary care groups (PCGs) were proposed to replace the fundholding and locality commissioning schemes by being contiguous with each other and thereby covering defined geographical areas. The PCGs were designed to cover 'natural communities' of about 100 000 population, or the equivalent of about 50 GPs, or about 15–20 practices. In practice, the 481 PCGs contained populations of between 46 000 and 255 000 and from one per health authority (Isle of Wight) to 12 (Avon) (*Health Service Journal*, 12 November 1998, p. 3). PCGs were not voluntary schemes (like fundholding or locality commissioning); all GPs belonged to a PCG. PCGs had three main roles:

1. improving health;
2. commissioning (secondary) care; and
3. developing primary care.

Nonetheless, some similarities with fundholding remained. For example, PCGs operated at four levels from an advisory function to a 'free-standing' Primary Care Trust. The first wave of 17 PCTs was introduced in April 2000 (see Chapter 6); by April 2001, 124 had been created. GPs are, like fundholding, in the vanguard of PCGs (as PCG Board chair, for example) although PCGs also formally consisted of nurses and social services representatives. GPs were, however, numerically dominant. PCGs were intended to evolve into PCTs though the organisational structures and processes were somewhat different given its independent status (as a Trust).

ii. Scotland

The Scottish health reforms proposed 'greater flexibility ... over the pace and detail of primary care changes' than hitherto (Hunter 1998: 11). Add to the Scottish Parliament's ability to raise or lower income tax for Scottish residents by 3 per cent and to vire between budgets, the package of reforms could signal a dramatic shift in primary care; for example, adding greater democratic input into the commissioning process or abolishing the independent contractor status of GPs could be possible under these reforms.

In contrast to England, Scottish reforms involved the creation of Primary Care Trusts from the outset. These covered all primary care, community hospitals and mental health services. The Scottish PCTs incorporated networks of GPs in Local Health Care Co-operatives. These LHCCs were the replacement for fundholding but the White Paper referred to their function being one of 'budget-holding'. Also they were to be a 'voluntary organisation of GPs' (Secretary of State for Scotland 1997: para. 80). The Trusts cover populations of between 25 000 and 150 000. The three Island Health Boards retain a remit for strategic and operational management through directly managed units.

iii. Wales

Unlike Scotland, the Welsh Assembly has no law-making powers despite being able to make structural or organisational changes (Hazell and Jervis 1998: 34).

(In April 1999, before the Assembly started, the number of Trusts in Wales was reduced from 26 to 16 [Garside, 1999]). At the outset, health authorities were accountable to the Welsh Assembly who would monitor the population's health and identify/promote good practice. This latter function has been a hallmark of health policy in Wales for some time. Policy was clarified in 2001 by the publication of *Improving health in Wales: Structural Changes in the NHS*. It proposed the abolition of Welsh HAs and the development of LHGs into Local Health Boards. These Boards would 'include representation from Local Authority members and the local population' (NHS Wales, press release, 18 July 2001).

Although LHGs were coterminous with local authorities, they had similar functions to PCGs in England. However, there are no parallel 'levels' to English PCGs but the Welsh White Paper promised legislation to provide for the creation of Primary Care Trusts (para. 4.33). Their development into Local Health Boards has more in common with policy in Scotland than England.

iv. Northern Ireland

Given the political processes occurring in Northern Ireland in 1997 and 1998 and the opportunities opened by the Good Friday Agreement (10 April 1998), the reforms were proposed in April 1998 as a consultation exercise. The consultation exercises invited views on two 'primary care-centred' models which would both have a local commissioning system based upon GPs (and other primary care staff) and not disrupt the integration of health and social services (see Box 5.1 below). The abolition of fundholding in NI was proposed for April 2000, a year later than the rest of the UK. The proposed NI Assembly would have responsibility for health and social services.

Model A
- similar to developments elsewhere in UK;
- relatively little change to existing structures;
- incorporate HSS Boards, NHS Trusts and new 'primary care-centred commissioning bodies';
- the 'PCGs' would cover populations of between 50 000 and 100 000;
- stages of development (PCG levels) similar to England.

Model B
- involve greater change but still retain primary care in a pivotal role;
- Local Care Agencies to commission and provide services;
- LCAs to replace HSSBs and some/all NHS trusts;
- LCAs to have 'operational elements' (Primary Care Partnerships and provider bodies);

- 6 to 8 LCAs to cover between 200 000 and 300 000 population;
- Primary Care Partnership to cover between 25 000 and 30 000 population.

The results of the consultation, *Fit for the Future: a New Approach*, were published in March 1999, indicating the government's preferred direction of change and stressing that final decisions would belong to the NI Assembly. One of the 'six key themes' which informed the government's 'vision' was 'giving primary care professionals control over how services are planned, delivered and funded'. Another was to make the most of the integrated structure of health and social care, which would be retained at each organisational level. The paper set out a 'new role for primary care' in which 'health and social care partnerships' would be managed by boards of primary care professionals. Each Partnership would consist of 'primary care co-operatives at a more community level'. About five Partnerships were envisaged across Northern Ireland, with each containing co-operatives of between 50 000 and 100 000 population. The functions of the co-operatives would be akin to PCGs in England, namely to commission services, to improve health and to develop primary care. The Partnerships would play roles similar to health authorities/ boards, that is, assess needs, translate objectives into plans, commission specialised services, provide technical skills and provide public health functions. The Partnerships would devise and implement 'health and well-being improvement programmes', similar to HImPs elsewhere.

The Assembly is responsible for determining the final configuration of health and social services. The government's response (in March 1999) to the consultation sketched the policy direction, which favoured 'giving primary-care professionals control over how services are planned, funded and delivered' (Jervis and Plowden 2000: 24). It envisaged primary care co-operatives (PCCs) which would hold budgets to commission services. The boards would, in time, be replaced by PCCs which would be health and social care partnerships. In late 1998, ministers received advice regarding policy priorities which discussed 'organisational arrangements, including the development of new primary care-centred local commissioning arrangements following the abolition of GP fundholding from April 2000' (*ibid.*: 29).

In April 1999, five Primary Care Commissioning Group pilots were created to examine different ways of commissioning health and social services and to widen participation by professionals in commissioning. The pilots included 53 practices and 153 GPs. The pilots were supposed to end on 31 March 2001 but were extended in February 2001 for another six months. This extension reflected the Assembly's decision (30 January 2001) to delay the end of fundholding until April 2002 (which had been planned for 31 March 2001). The minister published a consultation paper (*Building the Way Forward in Primary Care*, December 2000) which sought views on new arrangements. The Assembly's decision has complicated the search for and resolution of an organisational structure for primary care in Northern Ireland.

Instrumental Level: the Practice

The instrumental level is the level that generates institutional intelligence for improving system performance through information research, technological innovation and human resource development. In primary care, the 'practice' is the focus of such activities. Here, we interpret the practice in various ways – as premises, as a managerial unit and as a site of service delivery.

The practice has been and remains the building block of the UK organisation of primary care, a managerial unit and the predominant focus of policy. Here, the term practice refers not only to the building – the physical premises of the health centre or 'surgery' – but also the collection of practitioners. General medical practitioners comprise the core of these practitioners since they, as independent contractors, have a financial stake in the practice partnership and employ other staff in the practice. Other staff such as health visitors, district nurses and social workers are 'attached' to the practice since their managerial and professional accountability have traditionally resided outside the practice with other agencies. Practice nurses are employed by the practice. The practice level has been the most significant organisational unit in primary care in recent years (Green and Britten 1999). Though its significance is changing with the advent of PCGs and PCTs, the practice remains the foundation of service delivery in primary care.

i. Practice as Premises

There are multifarious schemes which have supported the physical fabric of primary care. Although some primary care is delivered from health authority-owned premises and from NHS Trust premises, Bailey *et al.* (1997) describe the three main schemes which were operating in the 1990s.

a. Cost-rent schemes

These were 'administered by health authorities to reimburse GPs who wished to improve surgery premises, either by building new premises, acquiring premises for substantial modification or substantially modifying existing premises, for the provision of GMS' (15). Costs were based upon prescribed interest rates subject to certain limits. The total expenditure for cost-rent schemes was cash-limited at the HA level.

b. Notional rent reimbursement

These were 'reimbursed to all GPs not receiving cost rent, who financed their surgery premises' (16). The rent was based on a valuation according to the current market rent that would be paid for the premises. The rent was reviewed every three years. The notional rent was not cash-limited and so the health authority had the incentive to reallocate premises under the notional rent scheme but the decision was 'irrevocable'.

c. Actual rent reimbursement

These payments reimbursed GPs who rent their premises. Reimbursement was at the level of the lease rent or current market rent according to a valuation. The scheme was not cash-limited.

Bailey *et al.* (1999: 16) cite an NHS Executive/Valuation Office survey which showed that, in 1995/96, '63 per cent of premises are owned by GPs and reimbursed by either cost rent (30 per cent) or notional rent (33 per cent); 16 per cent are owned by trusts or HAs; and 21 per cent are owned by private landlords and reimbursed by actual rent'.

Practice premises have become significant components of any primary care policy especially in the last decade when the capacity of primary care has been stretched by new initiatives. However, the premises issue also reflects the tension between independent contractors and a publicly funded health service. This was perhaps most evident in the case of GP fundholding. 'Unplanned savings' from the fundholding scheme were allowed to be 'reinvested' in patient care. Some GPs reinvested these savings into premises. Whilst this investment is laudable, it also enhanced the value of the premises. When owned by the partnership, the sale of a partner's share of the premises was to the advantage of GP's personal finances. As such, it is similar to other partnerships such as law or accountancy.

The issue of practice premises has re-emerged under the Labour Government's modernisation plans for the NHS. The NHS Plan proposed to link premises modernisation with private sector involvement through a 'new equity stake company – the NHS Local Improvement Finance Trust (LIFT)' (DoH 2000: 45). Focusing on mainly deprived areas, the NHS Plan anticipated 'up to £1 billion' investment in primary care facilities and 'up to 3000 family doctors' premises will be substantially refurbished or replaced by 2004' (45). Thus, a new configuration of general practice premises (especially in some inner-city areas) needs to be viewed alongside other primary care service developments (such as walk-in centres and co-location of several services under one roof – the so-called 'one-stop shops').

ii. Practice as a Managerial Unit

A professional unit such as the practice may not initially appear to be a managerial unit but it should be remembered that GPs act as managers, employers and commissioners (or purchasers) as well as practitioners and primary care team members. Whilst these immediately create a conflicting set of demands, accountabilities and loyalties (Evans and Exworthy 1996), it does highlight GPs' managerial roles. These dual or hybrid roles of professional *and* manager are known as 'managerial professionals' (Causer and Exworthy 1999). It is significant, for example, that the GP fundholding scheme was directed not only at GPs (as opposed to, say, nurses) but also to the practice (rather than a new organisational form). Even the advent of PCGs recognises the role that the individual practice will play within the new structure.

Apart from practice nurses, health visitors and district nurses have been professionally and managerially accountable to their employers, NHS Trusts. Though also primary care team members, these nurses' dual role creates tensions regarding the direction and supervision of service delivery. These tensions have tended to result in nurses being seen as GPs' 'handmaidens'; the GP is able to direct much of their work by controlling the flow of patients and access to practice facilities. It is unclear how far PCT strategies will overcome this traditional division between GPs and community nursing.

The practice as the managerial unit has seen a large growth in the number of group practices and the concomitant decline in single-handed practices. For example, practices with six or more partners only accounted for 7.7 per cent of practices in England in 1973 but this had risen to 26 per cent by 1995 (Boaden 1997: 50). By contrast, in 1973, nearly one-fifth (18.6 per cent) of practices were run by single-handed GPs, whereas by 1995 this figure had fallen to one-tenth (10.6 per cent). Over the same period, the number of GPs had risen by about one third. The numbers of practice nurses and practice managers have also risen sharply. Between 1983 and 1994, the number of practice nurses rose from 3284 to 17 000 (Witz 1994: 36) and the number of practice managers by 35 per cent (1990–94) (Boaden 1997: 52).

iii. Practice as Site of Service Delivery

The practice is perhaps most readily recognised by patients and other non-primary care practitioners as a unit of service delivery. (Other sites include the pharmacy, dental surgery or accident and emergency). It is the place at which patients usually enter the health care system by seeing their GP, primary care nurse or another profession allied to medicine (such as a physiotherapist). The geographical distribution of practices (and practitioners) makes this point of entry readily accessible to most patients.

GPs

The practice as a site of service delivery is the location where GPs mostly deliver care to registered patients. Patients are free to choose their GP and the GP is able to accept on to or reject that patient from their list. (Most practices operate a catchment area so that new patients are only accepted if they live within this area. They may, however, move home and still remain registered with that GP/practice); hence the difference between resident and registered populations. Patient registration in the UK is about 99 per cent (EOHCS 1999: 53) but this varies according to social groups. The homeless, marginalised groups and students tend to have lower rates of registration. Inner-city areas (where populations tend to be more transitory) also have low rates of registration. Delays in updating patients' records and the nature of the population in these areas create problems of 'ghost patients' and list inflation. This inflation can be as high as 30 per cent in inner cities (Exworthy 1994b), a significant proportion especially when GPs' income is partly determined by capitation.

GPs' list sizes have been reduced to about 1804, a fall of 10 per cent in the 12 years to 1997 (RCGP 1999b). This is an average since many practices do not operate individual lists where patients can see the same GP whenever they visit. Of nearly 300 million initial doctor contacts in the UK each year, 95 per cent are with GPs (Kennedy 1999: 145). Of these GP–patient contacts in the surgery, about 12 per cent will be referred by the GP to hospital for tests, X-rays or further treatment whilst nearly 90 per cent will be treated from start to finish within primary care settings. As each patient contacts their GP, on average, about five times per year, the 'average' GP will hold about 9000 consultations per annum. About one-eighth (12.6 per cent) takes place in the patient's home, the rest being in the surgery.

The individual GP–patient relationship and the continuity of care have been further affected by the development of out-of-hours schemes (Boaden 1997: 42). Such schemes operate a deputising service which replaces the normal GP cover during the night and at weekends (Lattimer *et al.* 2000). Over 20 years ago, Acheson (1981, para. 3.62) found that 90 per cent of London GPs made use of deputising services. Lower patient registration, lower out-of-hours cover and the poor quality of some GP services has meant that accident and emergency departments and community pharmacies have often been used by some patients as the first contact with health care services (Acheson 1981: ch. 9). In essence, these constitute primary care also.

There are several types of GP. The main distinction is between principals and non-principals. Principals are those who have contracts with the health authority to take unsupervised responsibility for patients. They are divided into restricted and unrestricted principals according to whether the GP provides services to a limited group of patients or only provides specific services (RCGP 1999b: 6). Non-principals comprise assistants, associate, GP registrars and locums.

Primary care nurses

Primary care nurses provide services both within the practice premises, other service sites (such as schools or health promotion clinics) and within patients' homes. A broad distinction can be drawn between practice nurses on the one hand and district nurses, health visitors, Community Psychiatric Nurses (CPNs) and school nurses on the other.

Practice nurses (PNs) are employed by the GP working solely within the practice and for the registered patients. The PN's workload is largely controlled by the flow of patients referred (internally) by the GP and by the organisation of clinics and other services run by the practice. Chronic disease management, health promotion, immunisations and health assessments are usually undertaken by PNs.

Primary care nurses' caseloads vary depending on the population they serve, the staffing levels of their employer and local socio-demographic factors, among others. Indeed, caseloads have become an area of contention for many nurses (Atkin and Lunt 1996). Most operate on a referral basis, mainly from the GP but also from other nursing staff, social services or hospitals. The particular nature of health visiting has meant that some of their work is not determined by referral alone but rather by legal requirements. A common feature of the services delivered by primary care nurses is the continuity of care. Rather than just one-off discrete interventions, these nurses are involved in the care of patients often over extended periods of time often related to chronic conditions.

Unlike the GP and the PN, district nurses and health visitors work on a geographical basis. Though usually attached to a practice, they take referrals for patients living within particular geographical areas such as a village, town, housing estate or district within a city. In 1993–4, roughly 6 million patient contacts were made by district nurses, health visitors, CPNs and community mental health nurses. Most of these were undertaken by the 10 190 (wte) HVs and the 10 730 (wte) DNs (DoH 2002a).

Conclusions

The description of the history and current organisation of primary care in the UK presented in Chapter 4 and in this chapter illustrate many of the issues which permeate the rest of the book. Indeed, many of the reforms introduced in the late 1990s have challenged the taken-for-granted assumptions and values which had underpinned primary care for many years. Whilst the outcome of these reforms may not be known for some time and may be confounded by many other factors, three issues are especially relevant: the boundaries of primary care, the diversity of primary care and the integration of primary care (see Chapter 1).

Changing Boundaries

The boundaries of primary care apply not just to the organisational structures of primary care groups or general practice but also to the geographical and professional borders of primary care. The legacy of earlier policy reforms and professional and service developments have created the current boundaries of primary care. They are now much more fluid and permeable than ever before, to the extent that questions are being raised as to what actually constitutes primary care (see Chapter 3).

Organisationally, the boundaries of primary care have become malleable as they are subjected to closer policy scrutiny by government and subject to structural transformation locally. Resources flow in and out of primary care in ways that were unimaginable even ten or so years ago. New PCOs are likely to emerge from the current round of reform but the precise boundaries will be different in each area and nation according to local pressures and policies.

Geographically, primary care is becoming aligned like other NHS agencies. PCOs now have defined boundaries (in ways that practices never had) and they are contiguous with each other. Their coterminosity with local authority agencies remains, however, problematic (Exworthy and Peckham, 1998). The benefits of a population-based approach in primary care have been known for some time (despite the advantages that patient lists bring to general practice) but the co-ordination of commissioning and provision will be hampered so long as geographical boundaries prevent closer integration.

The professional boundaries of primary care are being redefined. Not simply are new relations within primary care being forged but external interests are becoming established. GPs' work, for example, is being reshaped by primary care nurses, PAMs and hospital consultants, *inter alia*. This process is one of the main ways in which medical autonomy is being altered. Combined with the managerialisation of primary care, the boundaries of GPs' work in primary care are fundamentally being redrawn. However, it would be premature to interpret all these 'boundary' changes as being inimical to medical autonomy in primary care. Besides, there is also evidence of re-professionalisation, a process whereby (some) GPs are enhancing their control over 'core' tasks and activities.

Diversity

The diversity of UK primary care has been a hallmark for many years, not just since the inception of the NHS. Many point to this being a distinct advantage in providing services that are appropriate to local needs and draw on the skills and experience of primary care practitioners. Indeed, this was one of the reasons why general practice was given the task of commissioning via fundholding.

However, whilst some may see diversity as an advantage, others see it as evidence of inequality. Since 1997, the Labour Government has highlighted the importance of tackling health inequalities. Whilst many see such a policy of health inequalities as applying simply to health status, it could also be seen as relevant to health care inequalities. Such inequalities apply to the usual aspects of primary care such as the quality, volume and type of services provided in primary care as well as the more latent aspects such as expenditure, resource allocation, access and usage (Rogers *et al.* 1999). The government has termed these inequalities 'unacceptable variations' (DoH 1997).

Medical practice variations may be considered as forms of inequality but variations are expected in medical practice where there is uncertainty, indeterminacy and a lack of agreement about the implications of research evidence (Anderson and Mooney 1990; Klein 1995). Research on variations in clinical practice has shown that 'the greatest variation in service occurs when there is a lack of consensus on the best approach' (Bindman 2001: 29). Developments such as clinical audit and evidence-based medicine are reducing the degree of variation but government has also introduced measures to accelerate this, including performance indicators and agencies such as NICE (in England) and the Clinical Standards Board (in Scotland).

Further diversity in the UK may be apparent following devolution to Scotland, Wales and Northern Ireland. A regional agenda for primary care in England is not yet apparent but could, in theory, emerge. Whilst many of the variations described above relate to individual practices or even particular areas (such as inner cities), devolution could introduce national differences in primary care policy, organisation and management. As this stage, only tentative conclusions are possible. Devolution could call into question the notion of the *national* health service itself (Mohan 1995; Powell 1999); devolution could thus institutionalise diversity.

Integration

Primary care, with general practice at its core, has, since the inception of the NHS, been semi-detached from the NHS. The current reforms can be seen as the culmination of a policy to integrate primary care into the mainstream of the NHS. Whilst the independent contractor status of GPs has not yet been abolished, GPs are being brought into the main body of NHS policy-making and decision-making structures. Managerialisation is the main process by which this is being achieved. It also includes greater accountability for their clinical and managerial decisions. PCOs, performance indicators and clinical governance are fostering this process. Such reforms may not necessarily reduce the power of GPs *vis-à-vis* other practitioners since GPs may colonise managerial tasks and/or remain in positions of power (such as chair of the PCG or PCT executive committee chair).

However, this integration is also creating problems in the sense that the number of actors and interests in primary care increased significantly in the 1990s alone. Although these actors and interests may improve the range and quality of primary care services, the difficulty of co-ordination may hamper the implementation of policy.

The first part of this book has sought to set the context in which primary care policy, organisation and management in the UK may be understood. In the second part, specific functions in and activities of primary care are examined.

PART II

Primary Care in Action

In the first five chapters of this book, attention was focused on describing and defining the context and parameters of primary care from a policy perspective. The chapters in this second part explore specific activities and tasks of primary care in action. The chapters on managing, commissioning, inter-professional working, interagency working, public involvement and public health examine the ways in which primary care addresses its roles and responsibilities, especially in terms of dealing with the environment beyond its own organisational and professional boundaries.

Part II

Primary Care in Action

CHAPTER 6

Managing Primary Care

If a book had been written on primary care in, say, the 1960s or 1970s, it is highly likely that there would have been no chapter on 'management' or about 'managers.' Whilst the absence of 'management' may apply to health care generally, it is notable that primary care has witnessed a period of managerialisation, associated with new ways of working and a dramatic rise in the numbers and types of manager since the 1980s. The process of managerialisation has tended to take place in primary care somewhat after the developments in secondary care. This chapter explains this development in six sections. The first outlines the nature of managerialism as applied to the public sector and the NHS. The second charts the emergence of managerialism within primary care. The third section deals with the contentious issue of the interface between managers and clinical professionals, whilst the fourth explores the nature of the managerial cadre itself. The fifth section examines 'management in practice' with reference to some of the specific mechanisms it uses to manage the performance of primary care and its staff. The final section draws conclusions about the implications of the development of managerialism in primary care in conceptual and policy terms.

Managerialism, Management and Managers in Primary Care

The management of primary care has become so crucial that it is important, first of all, to clarify the terms being used. Management, managerialisation and managerialism are certainly interconnected but, as will be shown later, there are critical differences between them.

The term 'management' has spawned many different definitions, perhaps as many as the number of management textbooks! This diversity highlights the lack of a commonly agreed term and has led some to define management as 'what managers do' (Walby and Greenwell 1994: 58). This is unhelpful though amusing; a more useful indicator might be the roles that they play (Dargie 1998). A basic definition might be:

> Management is the direction and supervision of human, material and financial resources.

Reed (1989) defines management as a set of activities and mechanisms for assembling and regulating productive activity. These definitions assume that management incorporates a set of beliefs and practices. Hence, management can be studied as a system of authority, a set of skills/practice, a social class or a sectional interest group (Reed 1989; Flynn 1999). These definitions imply that management operates within an institutional framework. For primary care, the 'institution' has been the general practice but, as shown later, this has not traditionally been an area considered a 'territory' for management or managers. All definitions imply that managers are primarily geared towards survival and success of the organisation.

Management developed as a separate function during the development of mass production in industrial capitalism in the nineteenth and twentieth centuries. It arose from the need for planning, co-ordination and control of the growing scale of production processes (Flynn 1999). The associated division of labour meant that subordinate workers had to comply with the direction from the newly emerged cadre of managers. Foremost among managers' tasks was monitoring work and its quality, an issue explored later.

Managerialisation is the process of change by which organisations and individuals become oriented towards and socialised in the routines and practices of managerialism. As a result, managers are appointed. This is important in considering the process and change over time in which primary care has been transformed. This has been mainly evident in the last 10–15 years.

Managerialism can be seen as a derivative of management in the sense that it still refers to direction, supervision and control. However, it has come to mean more in recent years with the introduction of specific policies in the UK public sector. In particular, this development has been termed the 'new public management' (NPM) (Clarke *et al.* 1994; Ferlie *et al.* 1997; Exworthy and Halford 1999). NPM refers to the specific principles and practice associated with the policies introduced in the UK during the 1980s and early 1990s (see Box 6.1).

NPM policies were, at least, inspired by the desire among governments in the UK and elsewhere to reduce or constrain the rise in public expenditure (Harrison and Pollitt 1994). Economies were subject to technological innovation, global economic shifts and declining rates in economic growth (especially following the 1972 oil crisis). The response precipitated the rise of service industries (replacing the dominance of manufacturing), decentralised organisations and flexible labour markets. The impact upon the welfare state included decentralisation, flexibility and the shift away from universal service provision to more market-oriented services delivered by different agencies (Flynn 1999: 20).

Harrison and Pollitt (1994) argue that NPM was pursued in fields in which privatisation was not possible or feasible. However, NPM did draw upon the private sector practices and applied them (with modifications) to the public sector. In particular, NPM introduced new measures of financial accounting and effectiveness. In short, the focus of NPM was on the 'three Es': economy, efficiency and effectiveness. The specific components of NPM included:

Box 6.1 'The Rise of New Public Management'

The emergence of NPM was facilitated by this new and emerging context in the public sector and wider economy. It drew on a variant of management called 'new wave management' which is closely associated with 'excellence stream' of the 1980s (Ferlie *et al.* 1996: 13) in which much emphasis is placed upon organisational culture and values. As such, it rejects rationalistic models such as Taylorism (see below). Texts such as *In Search of Excellence* by Peters and Waterman (1982) argued that the successful organisations were those which placed emphasis on shaping the culture of the organisation to promote innovation, learning and experimentation. New wave management thus fostered decentralisation, empowerment and a focus upon customers/users. Osbourne and Gaebler (1992) were among the first proponents of this in the public sector. Though applied to the USA, their approach has resonances with UK approaches:

> entrepreneurial governments *promote* competition between service providers. They *empower* citizens by pushing control out of the bureaucracy into the community. They *measure* the performance of their agencies, *focusing* not on inputs but outcomes. They are *driven* by their goals – their missions – not by their rules and regulations. (19–20; emphasis added)

Government (and in turn, managers) became more active agents (as opposed to the passive role of administration).

The most common distinction with new wave management has been with the Taylorist form of management. Based upon the ideas of the American, Frederick Taylor (1856–1915), Taylorism is founded on a tight control of the working environment including the regulation and supervision of workers by managers. This 'scientific management' aims for increases in productivity through the rationalistic techniques including a finely grained division of labour and mass production. Clark *et al.* (1994) see the role of managers in Taylorism as applying direct and continuous control (4).

New wave management and Taylorism clearly differ in their principles and practice, and are based on differing assumptions about human behaviour. For example, Taylorism sees managers as agents of control whilst new wave management sees them enabling creativity and fulfilling the organisation's mission. However, no organisation pursues a single form of management; rather there are multiple forms which co-exist within organisations and the public sector. Some are invoked at specific times or for different groups. Hence, in managing primary care, it is possible that Taylorist *and* new wave management styles are adopted in specific contexts and at certain times.

- 'more active and accountable management;
- explicit standards;
- targets and measures of performance;
- a stress on results, quality and outcomes;
- the break-up of large units into smaller decentralised units;
- more competition and a contract culture (known as marketisation);
- more flexibility in terms and conditions of employment;
- increased managerial control over the workforce; and
- efficiency in resource allocation'. (Flynn 1999: 28; see also Clarke *et al.* 1994: 2)

The saliency of these components clearly varied over time but many had a cumulative effect. For example, decentralisation was a prerequisite for the introduction of competition between units, within or outside the public sector. Ferlie *et al.* (1996: 11–15) expand on these NPM features by describing four forms of the basic NPM 'model.' These are:

a. 'the efficiency drive';
b. 'downsizing and decentralisation';
c. 'in search of excellence' (see above); and
d. 'public service orientation'.

In brief, during the 1980s and 1990s governments and public sector agencies invested great store in managers as a group of workers and in the language, techniques and values of managerialism (Exworthy and Halford 1999: 6). This set the context in which changes were effected within primary care such as the managerialisation of family practitioner agencies, the introduction of GP fundholding and later PCOs, and the development of organisational and clinical performance indicators.

Separate Developments in the 1980s; Convergent Developments in the 1990s

For the first 35 to 40 years of the NHS, management was not considered a discrete function; it was not a term widely used. Rather administration was the term to describe the way in which the service was 'run'. Although there had been calls for a generic management in parts of the public sector since as early as the 1920s, these were not implemented because of the continuing dominance of the professional autonomy and control (Exworthy and Halford 1999: 5).

The Under-managed NHS

From the inception of the NHS, hospitals were 'run' at the local level by consensus teams consisting of a doctor, a nurse, a finance officer and an *administrator*. Such a system allowed health professions a veto on change. This was an effective brake on major reform in the NHS. For administrators, they played a relatively passive role in initiating and implementing change. Harrison *et al.* (1992) described this role as one of diplomacy, in which 'administrators' were required to reach consensus between groups, a middle course between parties. In primary care, GPs dominated the management of the practice. Administrators (cf. managers) met the needs of GPs rather than instigating change themselves.

The Conservative governments from 1979 onwards were committed to major reform of the public sector including the NHS. Management was seen as the agents by which the public sector would be brought under control. Managers would 'do the right thing' (Clarke *et al.* 1994). This period coincided with the rise of management across all sectors; managers were gaining authority by offering solutions to organisational problems.

The 1983 NHS Management Inquiry (chaired by Roy Griffiths from the Sainsbury supermarket chain) was commissioned by the government to rectify what was seen as the 'problem': the NHS was under-managed. As the report graphically argued, 'If Florence Nightingale were alive today she would be wandering the *hospital* corridors trying to find out who was in charge' (Griffiths 1983: 22; emphasis added). The solution was the introduction of a cadre of general managers who would be installed at all levels in the NHS and have the power to overcome the 'institutional stalemate' generated by the multidisciplinary consensus teams. Managers would thus be able to override professional objections (Day and Klein 1983); they would no longer be diplomats (Harrison *et al.* 1992).

Despite the high profile appointment of these general managers, their impact has been questioned at various times. Their overall impact has been somewhat limited. Harrison (1999: 52) sums up the impact of general managers thus.

> Rather than conforming to the 'textbook' managerial stereotype of an authoritative individual, rationally pursuing organizational objectives by means of proactively generated change, the NHS manager possessed little influence relative to doctors, was very much focused on responding to the demands of internal organizational actors, and procured only incremental change.

Clearly, managers had some impact but this tended to be marginal or incremental change. By responding to internal issues, managers continued to act as diplomats and so were often likely to collude with health professionals rather than challenge them (Hunter 1992).

These managerial developments were focused on the hospital and community health service sector rather than primary care. It is notable that the Griffiths Report (1983) used the metaphor of Florence Nightingale wandering in hospital corridors rather than general practices or health centres. The 'problem' identified by Griffiths and pursued by the government did not apply to the entirety of primary care. General practice was seen as outside the remit of general managers. GPs were seen as the 'managers' of general practice and hence, at that time, did not fall under the remit of the Griffiths prescription. However, Griffiths' managers were appointed to the agencies responsible for 'administering' general practice and other primary care practitioners (such as opticians and dentists). General managers were appointed to head the Family Practitioner Committees (FPCs) but the general management structure did not permeate far in these organisations (Allsop and May 1986) Their role was to act as the agency administering the 'pay and rations' of GPs rather than instigating new initiatives and implementing change in the managerial fashion elsewhere in the NHS. (This reflects the impact of clinical power upon policy. Government avoided an overt challenge with the medical profession.) The transition from FPC to FHSA and then to a merger with HAs did instil a more managerial focus to family practitioner agencies. Within practices, however, management had been introduced through the post of practice manager, although these posts were often developed internally in relation to practices as small businesses. Health policy towards primary care had thus not focused its attention in such ways on primary care in the 1980s. Hence, the manage-rialisation (as it existed) in hospital and community health services on the one hand and primary care on the other can be seen as separate developments in this period soon after the inception of NHS general managers.

Griffiths' general managers were also appointed to community health services at the same time as hospitals. Ottewill and Wall (1990) argue that the distinctiveness of community health services was recognised in the Griffiths Report (267) in terms of its integration with hospital services. The same could have been argued for general practice although it fell outside Griffiths' remit. Ottewill and Wall (1990) show that the background of managers of community health services (the 'unit general managers', equivalent to chief executives) was similar to other services but medicine and nursing was more represented in community health services and administrative backgrounds less so (269).

GP Fundholding and Locality Purchasing: the Managerial Implications

The reforms introduced in April 1991 included the creation of the purchaser–provider system, the establishment of NHS Trusts and GP fundholding (GPFH). (For a more detailed description of the 1991 reforms, see Robinson and Le Grand 1994 or Le Grand et al. 1998; Mays et al. 2001). As shown earlier, decentralisation was a prerequisite for marketisation and similarly general managers facilitated both. Decentralised units such as NHS Trusts became the province of general managers, headed by a chief executive with a management hierarchy beneath. Market relations between purchasers and providers required managers to negotiate and monitor contracts.

Significantly, the purchaser–provider system incorporated primary care into a managerial framework through GP fundholding. Although GPs were the apparent focus of the scheme (hence its title), it had profound consequences for the managerialisation of primary care generally. The model of GPFH was only eligible for large practices initially and many of these were the more organised managerially anyway. Many had dedicated or part-time fundholding managers whose role was to manage the fundholding scheme with/for the GPs. Over time, smaller practices were allowed to join the scheme and practices began to amalgamate into multi-funds and consortia (mainly for economies of scale). These required greater managerial input given the co-ordination between practices and the increasing sophistication of the fundholding scheme and the contracting process. Moreover, some GPs were willing to oversee their practice's fundholding activities without becoming too embroiled in its minutiae. Such activities were therefore left to the growing number of 'fundholding managers'. Perhaps in part because of the way in which GPFH was conceived (Timmins 1996: 464), the scheme did not have a pre-existing managerial structure which was in any way similar to those in NHS Trusts or even Health Authorities. The analogy of GPFH and HAs to speedboats and supertankers was initially applied to their 'manoeuvrability' in the NHS internal market but it applies equally to the managerial structures. Speedboats have fewer crew and are leaner organisations compared to supertankers.

The implications of the 1991 reforms upon primary care was perhaps more profound in the way that it introduced managerial concepts. Markets, contracts and competition were notions generally alien to primary care. GPs and other health professionals were becoming inculcated into managerialism through the practice of GPFH. This happened in ways which were probably more pervasive than in NHS Trusts. GPs had, by virtue of their independent contractor status, *always* been managers of the practice and practice staff (Causer and Exworthy 1999). No doubt, GPFH extended this managerial role of GPs in a radically different direction. The internal market was thus having the effect of 'converting' professionals into managers (Hoggett 1996) but this process was patchy. Nonetheless, some GPs within GPFH practices could remain aloof from the details of the GPFH scheme (Mays *et al.* 2001). The size of Trusts meant that many clinicians could remain largely unaffected by the contracting process of the internal market. Primary care professionals (such as community nurses) in NHS Trusts were, however, forced to consider the implications of contracting upon their relations with GPs who were, from 1993, able to commission their services.

The internal market had far-reaching effects in primary care beyond the GPFH practices in three main ways. First, non-GPFH practices exerted their influence upon the HA decision-making process through a variety of locality and/or commissioning fora, some of which were in conjunction with fundholders (Exworthy 1993b). Whilst managers did not necessarily run these fora, locality purchasing did pull in many practices and GPs who did not want or were ineligible to participate in GPFH. As such, the managerial discourse of purchasing and commissioning was spread widely through primary care. These parallel developments of GPFH and locality purchasing/commissioning were infusing primary care with managerialism and laid the ground for subsequent PCOs after 1997.

Second, FPCs were renamed Family Health Services Authorities (FHSAs) in 1991 and, with it, were given a greater managerial role in shaping the direction and form of local primary care. They were, for example, allowed greater use of financial mechanisms to alter the type and nature of local primary health care services. The managerialisation of the FPC was further extended by the introduction of the 'new' Health Authorities in 1996. These combined the functions of the FHSA and the District Health Authority so as to promote the integration of primary and secondary care. Some saw this creation as a takeover of FHSAs by DHAs although the 'official' policy was that it was a merger. The new HA had new accountabilities which affected the new breed of primary care managers; they were now accountable either directly to the HA or to the Region.

Third, the managerial arrangements of GPFH combined with professional networks attempted to secure greater leverage over secondary care services. Whilst primary care was seen (at least in part) as a solution to the problem of unresponsive secondary care services, a managerial framework was required to effect this. Hence, fundholding was the managerial discourse adopted and fundholding managers were the individuals to implement such policies.

The period of the 1990s thus saw the slow convergence of primary care management into the mainstream routines and practices of the NHS. The internal market and its associated developments were the principal causes of this development. However, the process was ongoing, as the events of the late 1990s demonstrated. (Commissioning is discussed in Chapter 7.)

Fundholding is Dead, Long Live Commissioning!

The Labour Government, elected in May 1997, sought to end what was perceived as the 'unfairness' and 'two-tierism' of GPFH by abolishing it. In its place, the Government introduced PCOs; these organisations included all practices within an area. Despite variations within the UK (see Chapter 5), most forms had many of the functions previously included within GPFH (such as purchasing/commissioning) but with responsibilities for health improvement of the population in a defined geographical area and the broader development of primary care. There were thus many continuities with GPFH (Mays *et al.* 2001). In England, for example, all PCGs were expected to become free-standing PCTs by April 2004. In particular, PCTs have greater responsibility in commissioning. Given their ongoing provider responsibilities (of primary care and community health services), PCTs thus represent the partial return to an integrated system but (unlike previous systems) one to which all GPs are now subject.

Notably, PCOs have continued the managerialisation of primary care, although in a somewhat different fashion from past practice. Whilst the managerial structure of primary care under GPFH was oriented around the practices (or artificial amalgamations of practices), PCOs had a more defined managerial structure, albeit embryonic at the outset. They were headed by a chief officer, the first time this post had been widespread at such a level and with such a wide remit in primary care. Beneath, a nascent managerial structure of business and contracts managers were put in place but with strong ties to the HA. The English PCG remained a subcommittee of the HA. Policies such as clinical governance and risk management generated a review of the ways in which the managerial and clinical components of the PCG interrelated.

The managerial structure was much more advanced in those English PCGs that were allowed to become Primary Care Trusts from April 2000 (17 out of 481 PCGs became Trusts in the first wave and a further 23 in the second wave, from October 2000). These PCTs needed to have more clearly defined structures and processes given their independence from the HA. For example, the PCT has an executive and a trust board. The Executive Committee chair is predominantly a GP whilst the Trust chair is a lay person. Unlike PCGs, which were accountable initially to the HA, PCTs (and all other local NHS organisations) were accountable to the HA (or Strategic Health Authority, from 2002). PCTs represent a compromise between clinical and managerial interests because the CEO must work alongside the Trust chair (and board) and Executive Committee chair (and committee). This triumvirate has been termed 'three at the top' (Robinson and Exworthy 2000) (see Figure 6.1).

Although newly formed PCOs represent the most significant extension of managerial structures within primary care, they also comprise managerial mechanisms which may not directly affect the daily activities of clinical practitioners. As the scale of these primary care organisations have grown, there is a tension between aspects of management which impinge upon professional/clinical practice and those which leave such practice untouched. For example, clinical governance or the unified budgets of PCGs/PCTs make managerial action more necessary in order to ensure a balance between its responsibilities. However, the managerial structure of PCGs/PCTs which include quasi-superordinate GPs (such as the PCG chair or chair of the clinical governance committee) might mean that the rank-and-file GPs remain largely oblivious to managerial decisions. The quasi-superordinate GPs may thus act as a buffer between 'external' managerial pressures and the rank-and-file of GPs (Ackroyd *et al.* 1989). Alternatively, these GPs may facilitate the speedier introduction of managerialism within primary care.

Even over the last 15 years, the management of primary care in the NHS has moved from a position of 'semi-detachment' to one of 'integration' and 'inclusion' (Harrison and Pollitt 1994). Whilst this inclusion process may not be complete (note, for example, the potential for integrated health and social Care Trusts), there are signs in which this process may be heading. These signs include:

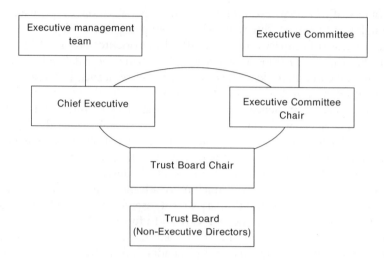

Figure 6.1   Governance of PCTs – Three at the Top

- a more extensive managerial structure within primary care, headed by a chief executive and a chair with a board of non-executive directors;
- the application (and somewhat reluctant acceptance) of managerialism and its processes by primary care practitioners; and
- the partial incorporation of primary care into other NHS managerial structures and systems (e.g. the potential for HCHS and primary care trusts merger and joint ventures).

Primary Care Professions and Management

It is evident from the two previous sections of this chapter that NPM was and remains a direct challenge to professional groups in the health care sector (Harrison and Pollitt 1994). Primary care has not remained immune. In order to make sense of the interrelationship between managerialism and professionalism (as competing discourses) and between managers and professionals (as individuals), this section explains the sources of tension, the nature of the challenge and the uneasy accommodation that has subsequently resulted. (For a more detailed analysis of professions in primary care, see Chapter 7.)

Since the formation of the NHS in 1948, GPs have retained 'semi-detached' from the NHS; they are an essential part of its functioning and yet remain independent contractors. This position has given them a managerial outlook in the sense that they are the principal referral agent to secondary care. As the referral process regulates the flow of work in secondary care, it means that GPs are gatekeepers to secondary care. Their decisions to refer, treat and prescribe effectively commit resources in terms of investigations, drugs and staff. The definition of management can thus see GPs *qua* managers. General practice also acts as a small business which invests and develops its premises and equipment. It also follows that GPs are employers of practice-based staff including practice nurses, receptionists and administrators. This involves the supervision and direction of such staff. GPs thus play managerial roles in the following areas:

- employment of practice-based staff;
- direction and supervision of staff (such as district nurses) as *de facto* leader of primary health care team;
- commissioning / purchasing of health care services;
- patient referral to secondary care; and
- committal of expenditure (through, for example, prescribing and treatment).

Using this definition, other clinical staff (such as community nurses and PAMs) can be seen to have similar but less developed managerial roles. Management in community health services has traditionally been profession-based (Ottewill and Wall 1990). Whilst Trusts did provide an overarching structure, the introduction of PCTs might presage a more integrated management of services across general practice and community health services. It can be seen, therefore, that professionals undertake managerial roles albeit implicitly and not described as such. This means that the distinction between managers and professionals is a somewhat false opposition (Exworthy and Halford 1999).

Whilst recognising that GPs and other clinical staff in primary care play various managerial roles, the challenge of NPM to such staff should not be underestimated. NPM represented a different form and level of managerial activity than was previously experienced. Managerialism and general managers challenged the position of GPs as semi-detached members of the NHS and with little overt (external) control. The perception of rising health care costs and the need to curtail autonomous professionals lay behind such developments. Primary care's relation with secondary care and the exercise of pressure through the referral system underpinned such strategies. NPM facilitated the introduction of commissioning, performance indicators and cost-containment measures. The move from Executive Councils to FPCs and FHSAs and later to new HAs represents one dimension of this process. A more recent example is where PCTs provide managerial structures across general practice and community health services. The managerial challenge to professionals (especially doctors) was evident in various strategies in the 1980s and early 1990s. In Table 6.1 below it is assumed that managers 'manage' clinicians and, as shown later, many of these have become superseded because overt managerial control has become less apparent. However, some strategies still remain in place.

The NPM challenge precipitated a clash of approaches between professionalism and managerialism (see Chapter 8). A key hallmark of professions is their autonomy which can be defined as the right to be 'unmanaged' (Harrison

Table 6.1 Strategies for Managing Clinical Activity

Continuum of management intervention		
< Minimal		*Maximal >*
Raising professional standards	*Involving clinicians in management*	*External management of clinicians*
medical/clinical audit	budgets for doctors (e.g. GP fundholding)	managing clinical work
standards and guidelines	resource management initiative	changing clinical contracts (e.g. consultants)
accreditation (e.g. Royal College or King's Fund)	managerial professionals (clinicians-as-managers)	extending provider competition
research and development (e.g. Primary Care Research Networks)	clinical involvement in contracting negotiations	Private Finance Initiative (PFI) commissioning

Source: Adapted from Ham and Hunter (1988).

1999: 50; see also Chapter 1). It entails the profession determining their own standards, caseloads and organisation of services. The self-employed status and (until recently) right to refer to whomever they chose illustrates GPs' autonomy (Harrison 1999). (Clearly, the medical profession has had greater success than nursing and PAMs in achieving such autonomy). Whilst autonomy is perhaps the most visible distinction between professionalism and managerialism, the clash between values can be stylised. Clearly managers and professionals do not simply fall into either category. Managers can, for example, be interested in effectiveness but the ideal type of managerialism tends to emphasise efficiency. This is illustrated in Table 6.2.

Professionals have traditionally coped with external pressures such as managerialism by means of a 'custodial strategy' (Ackroyd *et al.* 1989). This strategy is designed to 'preserve and perpetuate the customary [i.e. professional] kinds and standards of service provision' (603). This strategy takes the form of 'senior' professionals acting as a buffer between the external environment (including health authorities and the government) and rank-and-file practitioners. This strategy is evident across various dimensions of general practice such as GP principals acting as senior 'managers' in the practice and in the area of work performance where, until recently, only peers could assess the performance of fellow GPs.

These 'senior' professionals have often taken on more overt managerial roles and can be described as managerial professionals or hybrid professionals (Causer and Exworthy 1999). (In the USA, managerial professionals are often

Table 6.2 A Clash of Values?

Distinguishing features	Professionalism	Managerialism
Objectives	Effectiveness	Efficiency
Control	Trust/dependency	Rules/compliance
Client	Individuals (patients)	Corporate (organisations)
Reference group	Peers	Superordinate/superiors
Regulation	Collegial (self-regulation)	Hierarchical
Legitimacy	Clinical expertise	Hierarchical authority

Source: Adapted from Flynn (1999: 25).

termed physician executives). Such individuals are professionally qualified but have specific managerial roles. GP fundholder, Trust medical director and director of nursing and others have come to play central roles in primary care and other organisations as the effects on NPM have been apparent. Whilst the custodial strategy emphasises professional ownership, many commentators (such as Hoggett 1996) argue that NPM policies have sought to modify this strategy. The intent has not, therefore, necessarily been to usurp professionals *with* managers but to turn professionals *into* managers. In other words, professionals remain as professionals but a managerialist discourse is added. (The importance of distinguishing individuals from the discourse is thus underlined.) The key question, therefore, becomes 'who is taking over whom' (Harrison *et al.* 1992; Exworthy and Halford 1999)? Are professionals incorporating managerialism as they seek to protect their interests and as managerial skills become an essential part of a doctor's or nurse's expertise? Alternatively, are professionals becoming subject to greater managerial control and scrutiny?

A critical distinction among managerial professionals is the extent to which they retain their professional practice (such as a clinical caseload). Traditionally, doctors who have become managerial professionals have also retained some practice whilst nurses and paramedical professions have not. (This reflects their relative professional power.) The impact of their position rests upon their identity with their professional colleagues and their authority over them (Causer and Exworthy 1999). Indeed, such identity and authority of a professional is assumed to be more effective in managing clinical staff than general managers. However, as managerial professionals become more remote from clinical practice (either by specialty (general practice as opposed to surgery) or by the time since they last practised), such identity and authority becomes diminished. This strategy has been pursued much less successfully in non-medical professions. Nursing and PAMs have generally created their own managerial hierarchies, implying that promotion is associated with less clinical practice (Harrison and Pollitt 1994).

The Managerial Cadre in Primary Care

As much of this chapter has explored the nature of management and managerialism, it is useful to consider the manager as an individual, or rather their corresponding discipline or discourse. Who are the individuals who are the managers in primary care? What are their backgrounds? How has the changing policy towards management and primary care altered their roles and positions?

The number of managers in the NHS has risen substantially in recent years and whilst this is clearly due to some re-classification as administrators 'became' general managers, it indicates a 'very significant expansion of managerial posts' (Ferlie *et al.* 1996: 7).

Allsop (1995) estimates that the number of managerial staff in the NHS rose by 260 per cent between 1989 and 1992 (see also Timmins 1995: 510). Although the rise of 'general and senior managers' shown in Table 6.3. does not distinguish between primary care and HCHS, it is reasonable to assume that the vast majority of such managers would be found *outside* primary care.

The introduction of general managers in the NHS in the 1980s was expected to herald an influx of managers from the private sector with experience which had hitherto been lacking. However, in practice few private sector managers were recruited. Timmins (1995: 410) graphically describes the appointment of general managers within the NHS:

> As implementation [of general management] went ahead, it was chiefly [administrators] who became the managers, despite [Ken] Clarke and [Norman] Fowler ruffling feathers by insisting come hell or high water that at least some of the new appointments would be doctors and nurses and that some would come from outside the NHS.

Table 6.3   The Rise of Managers in the NHS

Directly employed staff (wte)	1982	1988	1992
Medical and dental	41 502	44 794	49 589
Nursing and midwifery	397 081	403 883	382 019
General and senior managers	na	1 235	16 692
Administrative and clerical	108 803	114 716	135 009
Total	547 386	564 628	583 309

Source: Data taken from Ferlie *et al.* (1997; table 1.3, p. 8).

Ottewill and Wall (1990) explain that about two-thirds of unit general managers (in hospital and community health services) came from 'administration/management' backgrounds whilst about one-sixth came from medicine and one-sixth from nursing (269). Some were appointed from military backgrounds but this was only 2.3 per cent of all Unit General Manager appointments (*ibid*: 270). Anecdotal evidence suggest that many of these general managers from 'outside' the NHS did not stay for extended periods, often owing to a culture clash of private/public values or because of the different managerial styles within the public sector.

Many general managers were not appointed to primary care in the 1980s since a managerial structure corresponding to HCHS did not exist. This changed as GPFH and associated commissioning structures established managerial positions but these were, however, much smaller in scale and size; hence, the numbers of managers were significantly smaller. However, the backgrounds of the managers coming into primary care appear to be different from those entering general management in the 1980s. Whilst the NHS has established the NHS Management Training Scheme (which is generating a [graduate-based] management cadre, some of whom go into primary care), it is important to track the emergence of managerial functions in primary care in order to understand the source of primary care managers.

In the 1990s, as GPFH began to take off and as FHSA functions were incorporated, many health authorities created departments of primary care which were often headed by managers with backgrounds in traditional general management or FHSA administration. Such departments tended to create locality management posts which had responsibility for primary care development across practices in the locality. (These localities became a useful foundation for subsequent PCGs). In contrast, GPFHs often attracted managers with non-NHS backgrounds, specifically because fundholding practices were trying to 'break the mould' and distance themselves from HAs. Hence, managers from industry and commerce were recruited. Some GPFHs recruited practice managers who had more grounding in primary care.

The emergence of PCGs and PCTs has generated the need for chief executives who have drawn on both strands of primary care management, that is, from the traditional HA/FHSA and external management traditions. A recent study of PCTs found that the backgrounds of the 17 first-wave PCT chief executives tended to come from a PCG background but had no experience as a Trust chief executive (see Table 6.4). Some felt that PCTs (evolving from PCGs) were perceived by mainly other Trusts as being 'minor' organisations. The comparatively lower pay that first-wave chief executives received (mainly because of the smaller populations within the PCT) reinforced this perception. The number of women chief executives in PCTs may augur an important balance of power within senior NHS management so long as primary care strengthens its position within networks of local agencies.

The impact of this is, as yet, uncertain. On the one hand, this may create a potent managerial mix, combining traditional public-sector values (of equity

Table 6.4 Chief Executives in the 17 First-Wave PCTs: Key Findings

Background	13 had been PCG chief officer
Experience	Most were a first-time Trust chief executive
Gender	6 are women
Age	5 were under 40

Source: Robinson and Exworthy (2000).

and probity) and the dynamism of external managerial experience. Alternatively, it could create an uneasy alliance between different and competing traditions.

Much will depend on the relations that these managers (of either background) establish with clinical colleagues and, in the case of PCTs, with their boards. These boards contain non-executive directors (NEDs) who will have a range of backgrounds. The election of the Labour Government in 1997 heralded a change in emphasis for board-member experience. Whereas the Conservatives had sought non-executive directors with private-sector (business) experience in the 1990s (to aid the functioning of the internal market), Labour now sought NEDs with community and representative links. This created claims of political bias which were largely refuted (OCPA 2000). This balance between PCT chief executives (and other managers) and their boards will be an important test of the blending of managerial styles and traditions.

Dargie's (1998) analysis of the work of chief executives in the public sector might be instructive for PCTs. As such, managers are never the main actor in public sector organisations; the roles that they play will be different. Dargie found that the roles of 'monitor, disseminator, spokesman, disturbance handler, resource allocator and negotiator were appropriate' whereas those of 'figurehead, leader, entrepreneur or liaison' were not (174). In primary care, these managerial roles no doubt will be more in demand.

In conclusion, it is evident that the managerialisation of primary care has involved the influx of 'new' managers and the transformation of 'existing' managers. Although the recent development of PCGs and PCTs marks a watershed for managers in primary care, the consequences are unclear. As primary care organisations become larger in scale, it will become increasingly important to identify and nurture future generations of management. Will they come from within primary care or from the HCHS sector (especially given the demise of CHS Trusts)? Will they be drawn from sectors outside the NHS? As PCTs become more significant in local health economies (as measured in financial terms), possibly by means of PCT mergers, it is likely that PCT managers will be considered more significant players by hospital Trusts. Hospital chief executives will no longer 'control' the local health economy's budget.

Management 'in Practice': Structures and Processes

A key managerial task involves the assessment of work performance. However, this is complicated by the professionalised nature of clinical services; managers cannot always know or understand the standards of clinical care and whether they have been achieved. However, in recent years, managerial developments have sought to gain greater leverage of clinical performance. Here, we briefly sketch some of these developments as examples of the mechanisms of managerialism in primary care.

Traditionally, assessment of clinical performance has been the preserve of clinicians, a reflection of their professional autonomy (Causer and Exworthy 1999). This has been described as a custodial strategy (Ackroyd *et al.* 1989) and might involve senior clinicians acting as mentors to juniors and restricting information about performance to others (Power 1999). These practices have been based on two assumptions. First, only fellow professionals (peers) have been deemed eligible to assess and take action on performance of other clinicians, although which groups are considered 'peers' is debatable. Second, professional etiquette has stifled open criticism of others, a custom known as the notion of equality of competence (Freidson 1994). In short, assessment of performance by the profession *or* management was cursory or non-existent. If it did take place, results were hidden from external scrutiny (Rosenthal 1995). However, the rise of a more aggressive managerialism, public concern about professional performance (e.g. Bristol RI Inquiry; DoH 2001d), the rise of evidence-based practice and the growth of information technology have challenged traditional forms of assessment.

Earlier schemes such as medical/clinical audit and accreditation did help shape the climate in which professions were *encouraged* to consider their own performance and act upon it. However, these schemes were rarely integrated into managerial structures and processes (Exworthy 1998b) and were largely voluntary. Clinicians thus not only set the standards of 'good' performance but also measured their colleagues' performance against these. Since the mid-1990s, developments have moved apace. The term clinical governance now captures a range of initiatives in which clinical performance and managerial decision-making are much more closely integrated. This is perhaps most advanced in secondary care, partly because of the semi-detached and independent nature of primary care and especially general practice. Clinical governance has been defined (in short-hand!) as 'the management *of* professionals, *by* professionals.' Assessing their performance is central to this strategy which draws heavily on US managed care schemes (Robinson and Steiner 1998).

One of the main ways in which their performance is assessed is via performance indicators (PIs). These have been closely linked to NPM (Hood 1991) as the latter introduced new parameters of what constituted 'success' and 'acceptable' performance (Exworthy and Halford 1999). PIs were, however, initially focused on financial and organisational aspects (Harrison and Pollitt

1994). They also became a means of remote control over decentralised units – or, more graphically, back-seat driving (Carter *et al.* 1992). As with other forms of assessment, a clinical dimension has been added to PIs in the mid/late 1990s. Though attention was invariably focused on the 'hard' quantitative information generated by PIs, Goddard *et al.* (1999) have demonstrated that assessing performance involved a combination of hard and soft (qualitative, interpersonal) information.

Clinical PIs in general practice are a recent phenomenon and are linked to NSFs and clinical governance. However, clinical PIs have often been resisted because they only capture one dimension of clinical work, namely activities which can be measured, usually by a computer. They fail to capture aspects of general practice such as the doctor–patient relationship, continuity of care and the emphasis on undefined need. Unless backed by strong sanctions, PIs may also lack sufficient authority to change clinicians' prescribing or referral behaviour. Wilkinson *et al.* (2000) found that GPs welcomed the clinical dimension of PIs, especially as they were based on strong research evidence (see also McColl *et al.* 1998; 2000). GPs also recognised that they would increasingly need to demonstrate their own performance for external audiences. However, some raised concerns that the use of research evidence conflicted with their experiential knowledge. They also feared the ulterior motives behind the introduction of PIs in general practice and made direct association with government/external inspections as in education (i.e. OFSTED, Office for Standards in Education). These new forms of assessment of their clinical performance were thus shaping their perceptions of their own autonomy (Exworthy *et al.*, 2000b). The sharing of clinical data is more likely in future for, Wilkin *et al.* (2001: 4) found, 'half [of the survey respondents] were sharing or planning to share identifiable information on the quality of care between practices and 41 per cent were planning to share anonymised quality information with the general public'.

The Managerialisation of Primary Care: Managers and Managerialism

The process of managerialisation is arguably the most significant development in primary care in the 1990s and early 2000s. Twenty or so years ago, management in primary care did not exist in any formal sense. Now it exists in multiple forms at various levels ranging from the 'practice manager' to the PCO chief executive. However, what has the process of managerialisation meant for primary care? What does it signify? This section attempts an evaluation of the impact and future direction of primary care management. Perhaps the greatest significance is for the way in which managerialisation has integrated primary care (traditionally a semi-detached member) more firmly into the organisation of the NHS. As Geoff Meads argues in the Foreword, primary care is no longer a 'small business outfit' but a multimillion pound organisation. Not only are the links between primary care and other sectors more explicit, but managerialism has spread into areas (via marketisation, performance indicators and audit) which were immune to management. This spread (the process of manage-rialisation) has been aided by three sequential policy developments: the intro-duction of general managers (in the 1980s), the decentralisation of responsibil-ity to smaller organisational units (via GPFH in the 1990s) and the placement of primary care at the centre of policy (from the 1990s onwards).

The impact of managerialisation is being felt in three main areas: the rise of a corporate identity in primary care, the changing relations between primary care professions and management, and the development of PCOs.

The Corporate Identity of Primary Care

Even within the last ten years, primary care has been gaining a corporate identity, more than simply the practice, which was unimaginable previously. This identity is being facilitated by managerialisation. General management, which had previously been installed in the HCHS sector, has now reached primary care. Indeed, many NHS managers (and clinicians) have only ever known general management or management in an era of GPFH, multi-funds and PCGs. One consequence is that managers have, in many ways, become part of NHS tribalism, which Griffiths (and the Conservative Government) tried to overcome. Professionals (especially doctors) still retain a strong voice (albeit not necessarily a veto) in decision-making and policy-making. The allocation of PCG chair to a GP and the creation of an executive board in PCTs illustrate this vividly.

Whilst some may bemoan the rise of 'corporate primary care', it represents a new set of challenges to primary care managers as they learn to apply managerial skills to areas which have traditionally been devoid of management *qua* management. As this identity is, by no means, well established, managers will need to create a sense of a single organisation working towards specific goals. They will need to co-ordinate the disparate groups, including practices, community nurses and other practitioners, into a coherent organisation. This is likely to be fraught with difficulty, especially when practices have tradition-ally not collaborated with each other at the local level (for example, in sharing data about clinical performance). Managers will thus require different skills. In particular, new forms of governance will be sought (see Box 6.2).

PCOs will have a relatively small management structure; Wilkin *et al.* (2001) found that 'the average number of managerial, financial and administrative staff employed by PCGs was 6.8 compared with an average for PCTs of 15.8' (2). However, the PCTs' influence will extend widely through governance net-works. For example, the PCT has responsibility for the 'management' of GPs and yet their independent contractor status remains. Perhaps more than other public sector managers, those in primary care have 'theoretical power' (Dargie, 1998). Hence, managers will need to be skilled in persuasion, negotiation,

---

Box 6.2   Governance

Markets, hierarchies and networks are alternative forms of organisation. The NHS has traditionally seen the shift from hierarchy (command and control), through to the (internal) market, towards an emphasis on networks (Exworthy *et al.* 1999). Although all three forms may coexist, the shift to network forms of management is illustrative of governance. Governance thus refers to the new organisational relations that exists with and outwith the public sector (Rhodes 1997). In an era of NPM, contracting out and commissioning, agencies must collaborate *and* compete with each other; their relations must be reciprocal and mutual.

Thus, primary care organisations engage with NHS Trusts, health authorities, social services and the independent sector in a variety of ways. As relations are conducted over the long term, relationship must develop trust and understanding whilst also being able to demonstrate accountability and value-for-money. It is this mixture of collaboration and competition, trust and accountability that distinguishes new forms of governance in the NHS generally and primary care specifically (Ferlie and Pettigrew 1996).

---

bargaining and conflict resolution (Hudson and Hardy, 2001). (These skills are a key justification for the managerial professionals; see below.) The PCO is and thus will be a 'virtual organisation' (Handy 1994).

One area in which NHS managers have traditionally been weak is account-ability, especially to the public and patients (see Chapter 9). Notwithstanding the difficulties of developing performance management measures for manage-rial and financial accountability to superordinate bodies (such as the Strategic HA), downwards accountability to the public may be facilitated by character-istics of primary care, namely its close and continual association with patients and communities, and its high level of patient registration.

Management of Professionals or Management by Professionals?

If, as argued above, primary care is no longer semi-detached from the rest of the NHS, it follows that neither are its professional staff. Whilst the independent contractor status has remained in place, many other initiatives have filtered managerialism into primary care. Whilst many such as GPFHs are high profile, others (such as the limited lists of prescriptions, medical/clinical audit and unified budgets) are less so. The introduction or existence of such initiatives are not in doubt; rather it is the impact of these that is less discernible. Will the organisational development of primary care be inimical to professions?

Clearly, the answer to this question will depend on each profession. A process of uneven re-professionalisation will benefit some professions and professionals to the detriment of others. In particular, this process of re-professionalisation will be demonstrated by the continued rise of managerial professionals. The type of integration strategy that they adopt will be crucial in determining the extent to which managerialism permeates primary care professions. If, as they have in the past, adopted the custodial strategy (Ackroyd *et al.* 1989) by acting as a buffer between their fellow professionals and external pressures, it is unlikely that initiatives such as clinical governance will affect the rank-and-file professional very much. This distance may be also enhanced by the growing organisational scale of PCTs. Nonetheless, managerial professionals will grow in number and power *vis-à-vis* their primary care colleagues; positions such as chair of the clinical governance committee and chair of the PCT executive committee will be occupied by clinicians. Whether this represents management *of* clinicians or management *by* clinicians depends on your point of view. It is indisputable that a shift has thus occurred but the scale and extent of this shift is debatable. Klein's (1989: 222–3) assertion that the NHS 'exercises least control over those who, in theory at least, exercise the greatest influence in determining the demand for health care' may no longer hold as true as it once did. However, indicative of new forms of governance, the nature of control has become complex as professionals have taken on managerial roles. An outstanding question in the area of managerial professionals is: can they 'become' *good* managers (or, at least, better than general managers)?

The Future Development of PCTs

PCGs (in England) were only formed in 1999 but have since been superseded by PCTs, which were introduced from 2000 onwards. Therefore, comments on managerial developments remain somewhat speculative at this stage. Indeed, the future structure of these PCOs is already under discussion. However, some indications have already emerged. *The 'New NHS'* (DoH 1997) instituted four levels to English PCGs/PCTs but, whilst a fifth level and more were not mentioned, they remain options for the future development of primary care organisations. In particular, Care Trusts were implemented in 2002 but the assimilation of NHS and local authority governance remains problematic (DoH 2001e). However, the integration with other NHS Trusts (which would require no further legislation) might be expected for 'level 5+'. PCT mergers would, no doubt, be required in order to achieve such new organisations because these would reduce management and transaction costs as well as provide a more robust financial structure. This merger process was already apparent in the first- and second-wave PCTs, as they effectively move into the 'organisational space' vacated by Health Authorities.

The reconfiguration of 95 English HAs into 28 Strategic Health Authorities (effectively through mergers wrought by 'Shifting the Balance of Power') in 2002 has been precipitated by these PCG/PCT changes, a development reminiscent of mergers in the early 1990s (Exworthy 1993a; DoH 2001b). (HA abolition has been planned in Wales for 2003: Exworthy 2001). Some argue that these changes make the transformation of primary care organisa-tions into American-style HMOs (Health Maintenance Organisations) more likely (Pollock 2001). Whether or not this happens, external (private-sector) management will increasingly be evident in primary care. The Private Finance Initiative (PFI) and Public–Private Partnerships (PPP) might be the most clear expression of this but others include the franchising of management teams for primary care organisations (which are awarded 'no stars' or 'red lights' in performance ratings) and the consequent imposition of external management upon 'failing' organisations. General managers still draw some authority/ legitimacy from government policy but this cannot be guaranteed in the long term; external management is being favoured more and more, though its presence in primary care is nascent.

Even though the government expects all PCGs to be PCTs by April 2004, it is undoubted that the trend towards greater managerial structures and processes will not abate in any PCO in the meantime. Managerialism is instrumental in shaping the future direction of primary care organisations irrespective of PCTs' individual contexts. It is unlikely that managerialism (in the form of NPM) is a short-term fad (Ferlie *et al.* 1996: 244; Marmor 2001) but surely the solutions which it offers to the problem of organising and directing primary care will change over time in accordance with prevailing policy imperatives and evolving managerial styles. Harrison and Wood (1999) and Ferlie *et al.* (1996) argue that governmental policy-making is less certain than previous administrations; there is no blueprint for primary care in a desk in Richmond House or Quarry Hill but rather a general direction in which the NHS is headed. In other words, the destination has not been clearly stated by government and managers have been given no road map. Managers will, therefore, have to survive off their skills and expertise in shaping the pace and mode of travel for primary care. The government is setting out the incentives for such pace and mode of travel but much will be left to local managers. It is unclear whether, for example, those further down the policy road (e.g. pilot and beacon sites) will necessarily provide a clear track for others to follow. Not all organisations will be able or want to follow this track. Diversity will be an outcome of this bottom-up approach which contains 'no blueprint'.

Managerialism involves a cultural shift in values that will take longer than a single policy paradigm such as marketisation; rather it is a generational shift. Seen in these terms, the management revolution in primary care is not yet over. Rather we may be on the verge of a step-change in the managerialisation of primary care.

CHAPTER 7

Primary Care Commissioning

Introduction

While management is a relatively new addition to the primary care world in the UK, commissioning must rank as an even more novel feature of the primary care landscape. Since its (formal) introduction in the UK in 1991, commissioning has spawned many different organisational structures which are variants of the 'official' model(s) (Smith and Barnes 2000). In short, commissioning may have had a brief life in primary care (and the NHS) but it has seen many changes in form and purpose. This chapter reviews this past decade by outlining the original purpose of commissioning, describing the conceptual contribution of different disciplines to its understanding, synthesising extant research evidence about commissioning, charting the emergence of PCTs and presenting some continuing dilemmas that will shape its future.

It is worth, first of all, reminding ourselves of the NHS system before 1991. District Health Authorities (DHAs) were responsible for determining the type and volume of services as well as being responsible for the management of (acute and community) units which delivered those services. In terms of the latter, line management involved functional heads of units (e.g. Finance and Personnel) being managed by functional equivalents in districts (James 1994: 5). FPCs (later to become FHSAs) were responsible for the 'pay and rations' of GPs and other primary care services. In line with administrative bureaucracies (see Chapter 5), both DHAs and FPCs were relatively hierarchical organisations, with a poorly developed strategic function of their own.

Two consequences of this 'unitary' system were apparent. First, organisations were subject to 'provider capture' in the sense that organisations were beholden upon those providing the services (clinicians in acute and community units). This led to examples of 'shroud waving' in which clinicians would use emotive cases as a way of securing additional resources. Second, units were subject to the efficiency trap. If units become successful, they would attract additional referrals of patients from GPs. Alternatively, if units could reduce their costs, more patients could be treated. In both cases, the units' revenue would not necessarily alter and hence there was no incentive to reward such 'success' of attracting more patients and/or reducing costs.

The Marketisation of the NHS

The White Paper *Working for Patients*, published in January 1989, proposed a reform of the unitary system on a scale unimaginable in the previous 40 years of the NHS (DoH 1989a). The reforms proposed by *Working for Patients* were implemented in April 1991, following the enactment of the 1990 NHS and Community Care Bill. (For an extensive review of the political and organisational context leading up the 1989 Prime Ministerial review, see Robinson and Le Grand 1994 or Timmins 1995). Central to the whole reform was the marketisation of the NHS; that is, it introduced market-style relations, the purchaser–provider split and hence the commissioning system. Attention focused on marketisation but the artificial nature of the market and the often heavy intervention by government meant that the NHS was a managed market (Klein 1995), internal market (Le Grand *et al.* 1998) or quasi-market (Bartlett and Le Grand 1993). (A similar purchaser–provider system was adopted elsewhere in the public sector: Bartlett *et al.* 1998.)

Purchasers (such as health authorities and certain GP practices [i.e. GP fundholders]) would commission health services from providers (such as acute and community health services units) by entering into contracts with providers (mainly NHS Trusts) which would deliver an agreed volume of services at a certain price. (The government strenuously avoided terms such as buying and selling since it had connotations of privatisation of the NHS, a policy which would have been political suicide at that time). GP fundholders (GPFHs) were responsible for their own elective acute purchasing (James 1994: 9) and so could contract with whomever they wanted and therefore refer to those providers *they* deemed most appropriate. At the outset, GPFHs were only responsible for about 20 per cent of their notional budget; HAs retained control of expenditure for the remaining amount and for particular services such as emergencies and specialist services. HAs also commissioned services on behalf of non-GPFHs who were thus required to refer patients to those providers with contracts with the HA. NHS providers could elect to become self-governing Trusts with greater managerial and financial freedom. Although the two approaches are not fully comparable, Mays and Dixon (1998: 175) saw HAs and GPFHs as 'seemingly incompatible models of purchasing' that coexisted. On the one hand, HAs had difficulty in understanding the needs of individual patients whilst, on the other, GPFHs had difficulty influencing providers to any great extent (given their relatively small budgets).

The purchaser–provider split has been likened to the distinction between steering and rowing (Osbourne and Gaebler 1992) or between strategic and operational responsibilities. Purchasers were supposed to operate a system which entailed an assessment of the health needs of their population, a process of setting priorities, specifying and negotiating contracts, and monitoring those contracts (Ovretveit 1995). As such, they become responsible for the health of the local population rather than simply the management of health services. This singular focus invariably broke down as the purchaser became embroiled in controversial rationing decisions and service issues. By contrast, providers would focus on the delivery of services. They would have greater freedom in running these services.

GP practices and acute/community units were granted Fundholding and Trust status respectively once they had satisfied Regional Health Authorities of their competence. They were thus created in waves. The first wave of GPFHs and 'self-governing Trusts' tended to be the more efficient and well-organised. (Smaller practices were permitted entry to Fundholding in subsequent waves). (This complicates evaluation [see below] as subsequent waves were qualitatively different from the first wave). For those who did not choose to become, or were ineligible to be, GPFHs or Trusts, the HAs retained responsibility. They would thus purchase on behalf of non-GPFHs. HAs oversaw the gradual delegation of responsibility from directly managed units (DMUs) to self-governing Trusts as the latter established self-sufficiency and reoriented themselves to commissioning (James 1994). Although initial policy stressed the voluntary nature of Fundholding and Trusts status, practices and DMUs experienced heavy pressure to become fundholders and self-governing bodies. The precise coverage of GPFH depends on whether the percentage of all practices, eligible practice or population is measured. In the first year (1991–92), 306 practices with a registered population of 3.4 million became fundholders; this extended to a further 280 practices and a further 3.2 million in the following year. Whilst all DMUs eventually became NHS Trusts, fundholding only reached 51 per cent by 1996 (Moon and North 2000: 57); this amounted to about 10 per cent of the hospital and community health services budget (Dixon 1998: 11). The entry size was reduced from an initial 11 000 patients to late versions with practices with list sizes of 3000 patients.

Defining Commissioning

The term 'commissioning' is often used interchangeably with purchasing in policy documents, by both practitioners and commentators. Also, the term 'contracting' is closely associated with commissioning as it is integral to the purchaser–provider split. There are distinctions between each definition, according to Ovretveit (1995: 18):

Commissioning	to maximise the health of a population and minimize illness, by purchasing health services and but influencing other organizations to create conditions which enhance people's health
Purchasing	buying the best value for money services to achieve the maximum health gain for those most in need
Contracting	involves selecting a provider and negotiating an agreement with them about the services they will provide in return for payment.

However, these differences in terminology need to be understood in the context of their usage. Commissioning, for example, has tended to have a wider application than purchasing as it has tended to include needs assessment and priority setting. Contracting has tended to be a rather narrow subset of purchasing and commissioning, referring only to the contract specification, negotiation and monitoring. However, such definitions are malleable; indeed those by Ovretveit are overlapping. Policy-makers, practitioners and commentators have often used these terms somewhat loosely. Here, we shall use the more encompassing term 'commissioning' to refer to the wider set of processes operating within the internal market.

Understanding Commissioning

The origins of the 1991 reforms did not lie in a rational assessment of the deficiencies and strengths of the NHS by the Conservative Government but rather a response to a developing financial crisis (Butler 1994). It is, therefore, somewhat surprising to find that the proposed solutions to this financial problem lay in organisational reform. Much of the reform programme proposed by *Working for Patients* (DoH 1989a) drew heavily on a monograph by Alain Enthoven, an American academic (see Box 7.1). While he was later to criticise the way in which his proposals were implemented (Newman 1995; Baggott 1998), his policy proposals found favour with the government as they appeared to resolve the perceived problems and corresponded to the general political climate.

Theories of commissioning have been most closely associated with models of marketisation and economic analysis. Whilst economic analysis does help to

---

Box. 7.1   Enthoven's Proposals for the NHS

'An internal market model for the NHS'

Description: 'A district would resemble a nationalized company. In itself, this change would not be privatization. It would be more a kind of 'market socialism.'

Advantages: Districts [DHAs] 'would use the possibility of buying outside as bargaining leverage to get better performance from their own providers ... [The change] would be almost invisible to most patients.'

Prerequisites: '1. incentives to make cost-effective decisions,
2. suitably trained managers who can analyze alternatives ...,
3. a culture of buying and selling health care services,
4. reasonable good cost information,
5. a supply of information on how to improve efficiency,
6. medical decision-making would need to be free of the conflict of interest that exists today' (Enthoven 1985: 41).

understand and explain commissioning, other disciplines can also provide compelling insights into the operation of commissioning and its impact. Disciplines such as sociology and geography can complement economics by identifying the limits to (quasi-)markets. The synthesis of these multi-disciplinary perspectives can illustrate the interaction between competing models of 'organisational co-ordination' (Thompson *et al*. 1991) or govern-ance structures (Rhodes 1997); these are markets, hierarchies and networks.

Markets, Hierarchies and Networks:

The NHS has been organised around each of the three governance structures throughout its history, the relative balance changing in line with policy. The competing models of organisational co-ordination are briefly described (below) before they are analysed in relation to the NHS. Markets are founded on exchange which creates (price) signals upon which buyers and sellers are sup-posed to act. The market's 'invisible hand' brings about equilibrium as supply and demand are balanced. Hierarchies are closely associated with bureaucracy, a high degree of centralised policy-making and resource allocation (Exworthy *et al*. 1999). Hierarchical organisations are vertically structured, based on authority and 'command-and-control'. Networks are characterised by informal, organisational forms and a common ethos (Thompson *et al*. 1991). Trust and co-operation are the network's co-ordinating mechanism whereas price and authority are the mechanisms for markets and hierarchies respectively.

Markets

Williamson (1975) addressed the principal–agent relationship in which 'agents act on behalf of principals to achieve some end' (Davies *et al*. 1999), a model with various manifestations in health care such as HAs and GPs acting on behalf of patients. Williamson argued that markets were the favourable model of co-ordination when three 'conditions' of the principal–agent relationship were satisfied. First, buyers and sellers needed to be knowledgeable about products and prices but *bounded rationality* places limits on such knowledge. In health care, it is impossible to know the precise details of each service or even its price/cost. Second, there needed to be no chance of *opportunism* for buyers or sellers. In health care, sellers/providers might inflate costs or activity since buyers/purchasers would be unable to monitor every clinical intervention to ensure it followed the correct guideline or protocol specified in the contract. Third, the (human and material) resources needed to have alternative uses, that is, the *asset specificity* of staff and equipment, must be low. In health care, assets cannot easily be put to alternative uses. Clinical staff can not readily change specialty and most equipment meets specific functions. These 'conditions' suggest that markets in health care are highly problematic, a finding supported by Titmuss (1974) who elaborated on Williamson's thesis by highlighting other limitations of markets in health care. Titmuss argues that health care is needed when the individual is most unable to afford it (such as being off work or under emotional strain) and the patient is unable to enter into a 'normal' contractual relationship with a provider (clinician) as they do not know what they *need* (*cf.* want or demand) (Stevens and Gabbay 1991; Bradshaw 1972). This explains why third parties (such as government or insurance companies rather than patients) are invariably responsible for health care funding.

Hirschmann (1970) argued that individuals have three forms of action in response to receiving a service: exit, voice and loyalty. Individuals can cease to purchase a service and go elsewhere (exit), can express their dissatisfaction in the hope of improvement (voice) or continue to support the service (loyalty). These strategies are problematic in health care because patients may have few if any alternative providers (and may be unable to distinguish between them in terms of service quality) and patients are often deferential to clinicians providing the service. Loyalty is the most common response of patients, given the importance of health and health care and their traditional deference to clinicians. In primary care, the GP may be seen as an advocate for the patient but, in commissioning terms, may be a poor proxy for their patients' needs (Lupton *et al.* 1998).

Hierarchies

Hierarchies are often equated with large, monolithic organisations in which policy is transmitted from the centre to the periphery by means of a command and control system – a conveyor belt. Decisions are taken centrally by politicians and civil servants and implemented at the local level. Many saw the NHS as a classical hierarchy from its inception in 1948 to the introduction of market-style reforms in 1991. Decisions about investment, staffing levels and pay awards had to be referred 'upwards' (A. Harrison 1993). Aneurin Bevan, the Minister of Health in 1945, famously explained the impact of the hierarchical system:

> When a bedpan is dropped on a hospital floor, its noise should resound in the Palace of Westminster. (quoted in Exworthy *et al.* 1999; see also Timmins (1995: 410))

Although the term bureaucracy has come to have negative connotations, its strict meaning implies impartiality and neutrality, attributes which help ensure fairness and equity of welfare provision.

There are doubts, however, as to whether the centre was ever able to command and control the entire NHS. For example, Holliday (1995: 95) argued that the planned system was a 'façade'. The 'weakness' of the centre is partly due to the lack of effective levers they had over the periphery. The notion that the centre emits orders which are faithfully carried out by managers and clinicians at the local level cannot be sustained. Lipsky (1980) argued that local practitioners enjoyed such a degree of discretion that their actions effectively become the policy of the organisations. For example, irrespective of the government's policy to contain costs, clinicians' autonomy to treat or refer patients may conflict with such a policy.

Networks

Networks operate differently from markets and hierarchies because they are characterised by informal organisational forms which create overlapping patterns of interaction between network members. Thus, some have argued that networks lie between market and hierarchy (Kickert *et al.* 1997). For example, the NHS has traditionally relied on professionalised networks between GPs and consultants to facilitate the exchange of patients between primary and secondary care; the quasi-market tried to transform these relations. (The exchange between GPs and consultants should not mask un-equal power relations between GPs and consultants, which have only begun to shift in recent years). The former was associated with high-trust relations which were replaced by low-trust relations during the era of the quasi-market (Harrison and Lachmann 1996). Whereas the NHS was based on trust, it became founded on contract after 1991.

The emphasis by the Labour Government (since 1997) on collaboration and co-operation stresses network-like features; hence it is valid to refer to Labour's commissioning strategies as akin to quasi-networks (Powell and Exworthy 2002). Whilst Labour claimed to have abolished the NHS quasi-market, they have instead transformed it into a more network-oriented organisation. However, since the purchaser–provider system has remained largely intact (albeit with a different language), a more relational system contracting with (initially) Health Improvement Programmes (HImPs), involving all local 'stakeholders' and longer-term service agreements, was introduced.

Closer inspection of the three models of co-ordination (markets, hierarchies and co-ordination) reveal that they are not necessarily competing alternatives but coexistent. Indeed, the NHS has witnessed the mix of models varying over time in response to its political administration (Exworthy *et al.* 1999; Rhodes 1997). Clearly, the period 1991–97 was an attempt to assert the market ahead of hierarchy and network but these persisted, albeit in different combinations. An example illustrates the coexistence of these models. The quasi-market (1991–97) was highly managed by the centre as a smooth introduction (steady state) was created at the outset (though later relaxed a little) and even several years into its operation continues to be highly managed. As the limits of competition were realised, contestability became policy (Ham, 1996). Contestability was the *threat* or sometimes the actual removal of contracts by purchasers away from providers to ensure that the latter remained competitive. Contestability might explain why 80–90 per cent of HA expenditure was directed towards providers located within the HA's borders (Exworthy 1998a). Moreover, this localism – a spatial market – also reveals a system of embedded relations between purchasers and providers, and also GPs and consultants (Granovetter 1992; Ferlie *et al.* 1996). For example, given the bounded rationality of purchasers in knowing information such as costs and clinical outcomes, the importance of networks based on trust between purchasers and providers increased. Ferlie *et al.* (1996: 59) argue that the quasi-market was relational as the relations were built around social exchanges which helped to reduce uncertainty on both sides. In short, localism and relational contracting illustrate the need to look beyond economic analyses, in this case, to geography and sociology, in order to understand and explain the linkages between markets, hierarchies and networks.

Commissioning in Practice

The chapter now examines commissioning in practice. What was the policy towards commissioning? What were the specific tasks and functions undertaken by commissioners? What did commissioning mean for the organisations and practitioners involved? What was the impact of commissioning? To review commissioning in practice is a mammoth task and it can, in no way, be adequately addressed here. More detailed assessments can be found in other texts; the most comprehensive are Robinson and Le Grand (1994), Le Grand *et al.* (1998), Mays *et al.* (2000) and Mays *et al.* (2001).

Contracting

First, it is important to clarify the nature of the contracting process as part of commissioning. As shown above, contracts were a new form of 'currency' in the NHS and were, *in theory*, the basis upon which purchasers and providers interacted. Contracts were documents that contained specifications about the volume and quality of services for which providers were to be paid by purchasers. Three basic types of contract were evident in the NHS.

Block	Funding independent of volume of activity
Cost and volume	Funding variable according to volume of activity
Cost per case	Funding for each individual case (patient). This tended to be for low-volume, high-costs cases.

Each created a different risk for purchasers and providers. Purchasers did not need to specify block contracts with any detail as providers would deliver services (until their funding ran out). However, there was no incentive for providers to increase activity since they were paid a 'flat rate'. Cost-and-volume contracts shared the risks more evenly, although difficulties related to the floors and ceilings specified in terms of the volume of activity. Defining activity was itself problematic. By contrast, cost-per-case contracts involved high transaction costs for both purchasers and providers even though purchasers only paid for each patient.

Patients who were treated as an emergency or in providers to whom their (non-fundholding) GP had referred (but with whom the HA had no contract), an extra-contractual referral (ECR) was created. Emergency ECRs were automatically charged to the host DHA but elective ECRs require prior approval. (GPFHs could refer on a cost-per-case basis.) ECRs accounted for about 1 per cent of patient activity (James 1994: 6) but created high transaction costs. ECRs were created to preserve clinical autonomy or, at least, give the appearance that the market did not threaten GP clinical freedom.

After 1997, ECRs were referred to as Out of Area Treatments (OATs) and, because of better information and service changes, they became less problematic than ECRs.

The first round of contracting in the quasi-market (1991–92) employed mainly a mix of block contracts and cost-and-volume contracts. The combination was designed so that contracts reflected traditional patterns of patient flows, hence the steady state. These contracts were inevitably rudimentary as the data were often inaccurate. James (1994: 6) cites one Trust whose activity was 20 per cent more than predicted because the quasi-market precipitated better recording systems and because some providers hoped that 'money would follow the patient', as the government has indicated. Contractual disputes were numerous. The emphasis of the second round of contracting shifted focus towards price (James 1994) as more GPFHs and Trusts became operational.

Contracts were often weighty documents which specified the volume/activity of services to be provided, the quality to which they should attain and their price. These documents did not always reveal a great deal because of the sensitivities of such a process in the NHS and of the substantial transaction costs involved in detailed contract negotiation and specification (Hughes and Griffiths 1999; Griffiths and Hughes 2000). Further concerns were identified in contract monitoring (Goddard *et al.* 1999).

Organisational Change Associated with Commissioning

Since 1991, the size and number of commissioners have proliferated owing, in part, to the changing pattern and purpose of commissioning. (Other factors such as service reconfiguration and IT have also been instrumental.) All commissioners (and other agencies such as providers and regional health authorities) have undergone radical reform and restructuring.

DHAs

In 1991, DHAs became the key commissioners within local health economies – their budget dominated GPFHs. As discussed before (Chapter 6),

DHAs were compared to supertankers whose size and power ensured manoeuvrability was poor. This position was weakened as more GPFHs were formed and as non-GPFHs demanded more. DHAs began to explore organisational options which would respond to this changing climate. They sought to prevent further disaffection of GPs (to fundholding) as this would decrease the DHA budget. They did so by seeking GPs' views about commissioning through fora and panels that were seen to respond to local needs (Graffy and Williams 1994; Exworthy 1993b). Some locality fora were strictly geographical (e.g. town), some were for all GPs, some for non-GPFHs only. DHAs were perceived as remote organisations (compared to GPFHs) and locality groups aided a more locally sensitive approach to commissioning. The government (and NHS Management Executive) also sought to streamline the commissioning arm by merging DHAs. Each DHA merger was expected to reduce management costs by between £1.3 million and £2.7 million (Exworthy 1993a: 281). DHAs increased their resident population from about 250 000 to around 500 000 as a result of merger. As DHAs became more (geographically) remote, locality purchasing/commissioning became a key strategy for DHAs in responding to the GPFH challenge (Balogh 1996). The variety of locality commissioning schemes defies simple conclusions but they can be seen as the forerunners of what became the Primary Care Groups after 1997.

GPFHs

Fundholding was founded on practices whose patient list size was over 11 000. This was later reduced as better information and risk management became available. However, at the same time as the 'formal' size of GPFH was diminishing, there was a trend towards agglomeration of GPFH practices. These formed a variety of structures called consortia and multi-funds. These ranged enormously in size depending on local circumstances such as the extent of fundholding or the power of the HA. GPFH's transaction costs were reduced by means of routine commissioning being managed by the consortium/multi-fund and more particular/niche commissioning by respective fundholding practices.

An extension of the fundholding scheme was made in 1993 when GPFHs were given all 'non-acute elements of community health services budget' (which included community nursing, paramedical services and specialist nursing), 'mental illness budget and the learning disability budget (Salter 1998: 87–8). The growing diversity of GPFH was further recognised in policy when, in 1994, GPFH was subdivided into three categories. This policy development marked the 'high point of political support for fundholding within central government' (Mays *et al.* 2001: 279). These divisions were community, standard and total purchasing. Their respective capabilities and responsibilities are shown in Table 7.1.

Table 7.1 Three Forms of Fundholding

Community fundholding	• practices with more than 3,000 patients • community nursing, drugs and practice staff
Standard fundholding	• original fundholding scheme and the 1993 extensions involving community nursing *et al.* • 'virtually all elective surgery and outpatient services'
Total purchasing	• introduced in 1995 through 25 schemes mainly through a consortium of fundholders • 'all hospital and community health services including emergency treatments'

Source: Salter 1998: 88.

Developments in both DHA and GPFH commissioning indicated the emergence of a system whereby some functions were most suited to 'higher' levels and others to 'lower' levels. When formalised, this process is known as *subsidiarity* (Exworthy 1998a). It also reflects a sense in which national commissioning policy was being overtaken by local developments. Commissioning had freed the innovative spirit and national policy could not anticipate the direction or speed of such change. Policy thus became emergent; it simply became the *de facto* developments by numerous commissioning agents (Harrison and Wood 1999). This perspective also reflects the formal change in the style of policy towards commissioning after the mid-1990s. Policy-making was much more consultative in the latter years of the Major administration (Baggott 1998: 163; see also Chapter 2). For example, in 1996, the Secretary of State (Stephen Dorrell) considered that locality commissioning and other schemes might be viewed as equivalent to fundholding (Mays and Dixon 1998: 180). This was associated with the 'rapid and unplanned development of a plurality of purchasers' (1998: 196).

NHS Trusts

Although not commissioners, NHS Trusts were heavily involved in the commissioning process. The extension of Trusts status proceeded faster and further than fundholding; there were over 150 Trusts created in the first two waves (1991–92 and 1992–93) (James 1994: 9). Whilst management clearly welcomed the opportunity that Trust status conferred, they had to find a balance between internal and external pressures. Internally, many doctors (and especially consultants) were against commissioning in particular (and the quasi-market generally) whilst externally, meeting the commissioners' specifications was problematic given internal resistance.

Solutions (which had echoes across the NHS and the public sector) included delegation and incorporation. Responsibility for managing the Trusts and meeting commissioners' requirements was delegated to clinical directorates. Whilst directorates preceded the quasi-market, their implementation was more rapid after 1991 as Trusts sought ways of managing clinical activity, monitoring services and controlling costs. (For a full description of clinical directorates, see, Packwood *et al.* 1991.) Providers were structured to reflect the major clinical specialties and each directorate was headed by a (part-time) clinician (a consultant) who worked alongside a (full-time) business manager. Clinicians were thus incorporated into Trust management. (Whether this incorporation was complete or partial depends on your point of view. It reflects the tension between managerial encroachment of clinicians and the clinical colonisation of management [Causer and Exworthy 1999]). James (1994: 5) concluded that organisational structures of directorates were straightforward but the requisite IT and finance systems were less developed initially. Equally less developed were the managerial skills of consultants but, as directorates have become established, this position is changing.

Commissioning: Reviewing the Evidence

Reviewing the evidence of commissioning is a daunting task given the number and scale of evaluations, research projects and programmes that have been conducted into the various different dimensions of commissioning. This task has been made somewhat more difficult by the lack of any formal evaluation at the outset of the commissioning initiative in 1991. Indeed, the notion of evaluation was specifically rejected by the government at the time. As Kenneth Clarke (health minister at the time) famously explained when asked whether there should be a trial of the reforms in one Region:

> If I do that, you buggers will sabotage it. (quoted in Timmins 1995: 468; see also Butler 1994)

This statement reflects the sense in which evaluation is contentious, its conclusions reflecting both the assumptions made at the outset and one's (political) point of view.

Further complications arose given the diversity of the reforms, the various different disciplinary communities within which the research has been published, the lack of clear aims which were set for the reforms, the voluntary nature of some components of the reforms (such as fundholding) and the changing resource base (Bartlett *et al.* 1998: 2). The lack of suitable comparative data either before the reforms were introduced or between suitable control sites also hampered some of the evaluation projects. Only a general outline of the reforms was proposed and details were determined during implementation (Harrison and Wood 1999; Wainwright 1998). This pragmatic, reactive approach to policy-making was reflected in Kenneth Clarke's claim that he was 'making it up as he went along' (quoted in Timmins 1995: 467).

This view contrasts with the argument of Bartlett *et al.* (1998) who claimed that 'the ideology [of quasi-markets] provided only the framework for a more pragmatic objective: to contain spiralling pressures' (2). Either way, the relative lack of evidence hampered the government's claims that the reforms were effective.

It should also be noted that, since then, the NHS has established its own research and development (R&D) programme and evaluations have become more firmly accepted as part of the policy-making process. Specifically, there has been a rise in evidence-based policy-making (Ham *et al.* 1995) which has been incorporated into government policy. This has been summarised by the Labour Government as 'what counts is what works' (DoH 1997; Davies *et al.* 2000).

Perhaps the most significant evaluation programme of commissioning (1991–1997) was initiated by the King's Fund, an independent health policy think-tank based in London. The evidence on commissioning draws on the King's Fund work; inevitably only a summary of this work can be presented here and readers are directed to Robinson and Le Grand (1994) and Le Grand *et al.* (1998).

The evaluative criteria adopted by Le Grand *et al.* (1998) capture the diversity of the reforms' aims and enable an appraisal of the likely compromises or trade-offs that have to be weighed in reaching a summative assessment of the reforms. The criteria are:

- efficiency
- equity
- quality
- choice/responsiveness, and
- accountability.

For each criterion, the evaluation is separated into health authority and GP fundholding, as distinct commissioning agents. These criteria broadly reflect those proposed by Maxwell (1984) in generic (health care) evaluations. His criteria are effectiveness, efficiency, accessibility, acceptability and relevance.

Efficiency

Efficiency is defined here as both the maximum output for a certain level of inputs (technical efficiency) and the best combination of outputs (allocative efficiency).

Health authority

In terms of technical efficiency, HAs appeared to do well by increasing activity (as defined by finished consultant episode [FCE]) by 29 per cent between 1991 and 1995 and also decreasing the average length of stay in hospital from 11 to 8 days (OHE 1995; Mulligan 1998: 22). These bare figures say nothing about the cost implications, the unit of measurement (FCE), and the effectiveness of the clinical intervention (during or after the hospital stay) or the impact of concurrent policy changes. In short, it is difficult to attribute such efficiency 'gains' solely to HA commissioning decisions.

In terms of allocative efficiency, HAs did not generally change the way in which they allocated their budgets but some shift is in evidence, especially out of London to more local providers. (In part, these decisions precipitated the crisis in London hospitals which prompted the creation of the Tomlinson Inquiry [1992]). For the most part, HAs have commissioned about 85 per cent of their budget from local (within their host HA) providers (Exworthy 1998a).

Fundholding

The technical efficiency of GPFHs can be gauged by considering, for example, prescribing, the impact of which has been extensively studied (Goodwin 1998: 45–6). Evidence points towards a lower rate of increase in prescribing costs among GPFHs than among non-GPFHs, at least in the first few years of the GPFH scheme. Whilst increases were evident in both groups, the Audit Commission (1995) concluded that differences were only statistically significant in first-wave GPFHs.

Allocative efficiency may be estimated by changes in the location of care wrought by GPFH. The shift of services from secondary to primary care (such as the introduction of consultant outreach clinics) is perhaps among the most visible changes in recent years (Godber *et al.* 1997). Clearly the burden of costs between patients and the NHS, and between sectors within the NHS, shifts as the location of service delivery does. Goodwin (1998) surmises that, in terms of the shift from secondary to primary care in both GPFHs and non-GPFHs, 'it is unclear to what extent this has occurred because of fundholding *per se*' (52).

Transaction costs are incurred by both HAs and GPFHs and hence there are costs of running two commissioning systems. The increased complexity and number of contracts, HA mergers and downward pressure on management costs makes transaction costs a poor proxy for efficiency.

Equity

Equity is often cited as a hallmark of the NHS and yet there are many examples of inequity in NHS expenditure, provision, access, use or outcome. Many of these *health care* inequalities pre-dated the NHS but have persisted since (Exworthy and Powell 2000).

Health authority

HAs were given the role of health needs assessment from 1991 and, whilst many claimed to consider equity issues, inequity persisted. The devolved nature of NHS decision-making (here, in terms of HA commissioning) meant that differences in what and how was commissioned were evident between and within HAs. This 'post-code rationing' became more evident from 1991 as the decision-making became more explicit. Reasons for not commissioning services included doubts about the clinical effectiveness, its relative priority and its costs. Hence, devolved decision-making is at odds with national equity (Boyne and Powell 2001). Few HAs made explicit contract exclusions partly because many feared the political consequences of making a decision explicit, that it would provoke claims that such rationing was the prelude to privatisation or a minimalist health service. Tattoo removal or cosmetic surgery were the most common exclusions but invariably traditional NHS ways of managing 'excess demand' were invoked – the Ds (i.e. delay, defer, deter, dissuade and decline).

Fundholding

GPFH generated particular concerns about equity in relation to the introduction of a two-tier system. Patients of GPFHs would, it was thought, benefit ahead of patients from non-GPFH (whose services were commissioned by the HA) because of the ways in which GPFH had, it was claimed, been more generously funded and because they were able to switch contracts more easily. Notably, GPFHs might be able to commission services from providers at the end of the financial year given their expected 'savings'. (HAs had usually spent their budget by this stage and hence placing patients on waiting lists was the only strategy.) This gave the appearance that GPFH patients were jumping the waiting list queue. Anecdotal evidence of such practices abounded and Goodwin (1998: 55) concludes that: 'there are strong reasons to believe that the practices of fundholding GPs have enjoyed better access to hospital treatment than other patients'. GPFH may be seen as a catalyst whereby providers improved their access arrangements for all patients, although initial benefits accrued to GPFH patients only.

A second equity concern about GPFH involved *cream-skimming*. This centred on concerns that fundholding would create incentives to select those patients who would make least demand upon the GPFH budget. Natural variations in the patterns of morbidity, it was thought, would make the allocation of budgets especially problematic. This risk management issue was addressed by policy which enabled individual treatments costing more than £5000 *per annum* to be transferred to the HA. Goodwin (1998) found little evidence of cream-skimming despite the potential for GPFHs to do so (Glennerster *et al.* 1994).

Quality

Health authority

Quality of services is difficult to define and hence it is particularly problematic in attributing changes in quality to commissioning. Specific difficulties relate to measures of quality, the availability of information about quality and the diffuse connection between inputs and outputs (or between cause and effect) of some clinical interventions. Linking commissioning decisions to the quality of services was rarely explicit in the NHS quasi-market even though mechanisms such as clinical audit might have facilitated this (Exworthy 1998b). However, penalising poor quality providers may hinder attempts to improve future services.

Fundholding

Many of the quality improvements attributed to GPFH relate to process and organisation rather than clinical care or outcomes. The lack of suitable control groups (such as non-GPFHs) complicates evaluations of GPFH commissioning and quality. Goodwin (1998: 63) argues that: 'it is unclear whether fundholding has been the catalyst to these [quality] improvements or whether it is a general effect of the purchaser/provider split'.

There was concern, especially at the outset of the reforms, that GPFHs lacked the suitable experience or expertise in commissioning. Whilst similar claims could be levelled against HAs, the involvement of clinicians (either GPs and public health doctors on the commisioner side or clinical directors on the provider side) in commissioning processes appeared to enhance the quality of such processes. Contracts thus became more sensitive to service delivery. In sum, the lack of adequate data makes claims about GPFH commissioning and quality difficult to substantiate.

Choice/responsiveness

Health authority

As commissioning operated in the 1990s, commissioning and other initiatives were being implemented in tandem. For example, local responsiveness was encouraged by the publication of *Local Voices* (NHS Management Executive 1992; Lupton *et al.* 1998). Hence it is difficult to isolate the effects of commissioning *per se* from parallel developments. However, there has been little evidence that HA commissioning has specifically been responsive to patients' choice (Mulligan 1998: 36). It should be noted, of course, that the HA commissioning adopted a strategic population approach and hence individual responsiveness was not part of its purpose (cf. fundholding). This does not mean that HAs did not try to be responsive. Many consulted the public through various means and many instituted locality commissioning schemes (Exworthy 1993a; Balogh 1996). However, these views had to be reconciled with financial constraints, a limited range of local providers and other competing priorities.

Fundholding

The analogy of HA commissioners as supertankers and GPFHs as speedboats conjures up the notion that the latter were more responsive commissioners. Indeed, their size, organisational structure and their *raison d'être* were meant to enhance flexibility, greater choice and responsiveness.

Patients' ability to change their GP was increased in the 1990s and some thought that, with fundholding, this may entail patients' seeking out GPs who would provide a 'better' service. The evidence for this is inconclusive (Petchey 1995). GPFHs were willing to refer patients further and to consider more than one hospital but patients were often indifferent to these choices (Mahon *et al.*, 1994). Indeed, Kind *et al.* (1993) found that 80 per cent of patients did not know if their GP was a fundholder or not.

Accountability

Health authority

Accountability can be defined as demonstrating and being held responsible for decisions and actions (Longley 1993; Lupton *et al.* 1998). HA accountability has traditionally been through performance management upwards to the Secretary of State but, as shown above, some HAs tried to respond to local views and demonstrate accountability for their decisions to local populations. The balance between upward and downward accountability has probably been towards to the former.

Fundholding

Accountability for GPFHs was complicated by their position in the NHS structure, reporting to HAs and Regional Offices. Concerns about fundholders' accountability were raised by the way in which GPFHs were able to use their 'unplanned savings', *inter alia*, for improvements to their premises which, by virtue of the partnership they held in the practice, would benefit them financially on retirement or when they sold the partnership. These and other concerns prompted the NHS Executive to publish the GPFH Accountability Framework in 1995. This assuaged many of those concerns.

In summary, the evidence on commissioning is mixed, its interpretation depending on the criteria adopted and 'political' perspectives taken. For example, increased activity may not be 'better' since evidence on outcomes or its opportunity costs is required for a fuller assessment. Furthermore, commissioning changed in nature and scale over time and both went through various transformations. As the two systems coexisted from 1991 to 1997, it is possible that there was a dynamic effect whereby fundholding prompted changes on HA commissioning (and possibly vice versa). These factors make interpretation of the evidence highly problematic.

The nature of commissioning changed with the election of the Labour Government in 1997 and the introduction of the proposals contained in the New NHS (1997). Whilst some evaluations of these reforms (notably the PCG Tracker Survey, conducted by the King's Fund and the National Primary Care Research & Development Centre (NPCRDC) (based in Manchester)) have been initiated, there has, to date, been relatively little published evidence relating to these reforms. This is largely because reforms such as PCGs were only implemented in 1999 (and PCTs in 2000) and there is a time lag between data collection and publication in journals or books. However, it is possible to begin to identify the direction of commissioning from current policy trends. The evolution of commissioning is, therefore, the subject of the next section.

Evolution of Commissioning

By the mid-1990s, the limitations of the commissioning models (established in 1991) were becoming increasingly apparent through published research and the experience of policy-makers and practitioners. This recognition prompted a shift from explicit emphasis on competition towards contestability and collaboration. The claims that the two commissioning models introduced 'two-tierism' and other forms of inequality into the NHS were increasingly common. Also concerns were raised about the high transaction costs of the internal market for both commissioners and providers in negotiating, formulating and monitoring annual contracts. These concerns were compounded by the relative lack of alternative available providers.

Policy, through the experience of local commissioning practice, responded by emphasising contestability; that is, the notion that the threat to switch contracts between providers need not always be exercised by commissioners to prompt improvements (Ham 1996). In effect, contestability represented commissioning of the last resort. Likewise, collaboration between commissioners and providers represented a recognition that the 'local health economy' was comprised of organisations responsible for ensuring health improvement and service delivery to a local population. The finances available for that population were (largely) fixed and so collaboration could meet multiple objectives.

However, there is evidence that the impacts of the market were not as widespread as its supporters had hoped (Le Grand *et al.* 1998). Commissioning may have had the effect, however, of shifting the balance of power within the NHS and of 'unfreezing' entrenched organisational positions. Hence, commissioning can be seen as a catalyst to further change (Moon and North 2000) rather than being an ideal solution to NHS problems.

The Labour Government in May 1997 was elected on a mandate for the NHS of promoting 'fair access' to services and ending 'two-tierism', 'unacceptable variations' and the unfairness of the internal market (DoH 1997). However, the basic division between commissioners and providers was retained but the language was of 'integration' and collaboration rather than competition. Instead of contracts, Service and Financial Frameworks (SAFFs) were created between commissioners and providers which would operate over longer periods of time and accord closely with Health Improvement Programmes (HImPs). These documents required multi-agency support and proposed the strategic direction of local services. The most significant reform involved the abolition of fundholding (except initially in Northern Ireland; see Chapter 4) and the creation of Primary Care Groups.

Primary Care Groups

The prime new mechanism to replace fundholding was the Primary Care Group (PCG) in England. The PCGs had three main functions:

1. to develop primary and community care;
2. to improve health; and
3. to advise on or commission secondary care services.

Four levels of PCGs were proposed whereby each level would involve more autonomy from the HA and a greater range of functions (see Table 7.2). It is important to note that the division between commissioning and providing has become largely redundant because GPs and nurses were involved in commissioning and provision at all levels but especially at level 4.

Clearly, PCGs and PCTs had their antecedents in fundholding but probably the closest resemblance came at level 2: 'in many ways, TPPs represented a scaled-down dress rehearsal for the so-called level 2 PCGs' (Mays *et al.* 2001b: 280).

A total of 481 PCGs were created in England in April 1999 and, although their average population size was meant to be about 100,000 based on 'natural communities', this ranged from 43,618 (south-west Shropshire, equivalent to 29 GPs and 8 practices) to 277,160 (Brighton and Hove, equivalent to 140 GPs and 53 practices) (Bojke *et al.* 2001). The number of PCGs per HA ranged from 1 to 12.

Table 7.2 English PCGs and PCTs

Level 1	PCG: • advisory role as subcommittee of the HA • to support HA to commission care for locality
Level 2	PCG: • still formally part of the HA • devolved responsibility for managing budget for health care of locality
Level 3	PCT: • accountable to HA for commissioning • established as free-standing body
Level 4	PCT: • accountable to HA for commissioning • responsible for providing community health services • established as a free-standing body

Source: Kent and Kumar 1999; Hudson *et al*. 1999).

Unlike fundholding (which was a voluntary scheme), PCGs incorporated *all* GPs in a locality. Hence, some see PCGs as not so much the abolition of primary care commissioning as its extension. Moreover, all PCGs were expected to develop such that they are 'responsible for at least 85 per cent of the total hospital and community health services (HCHS) and general medical services (GMS) expenditure for the local population' (Hudson *et al*. 1999: 6–7). This equated to a higher proportion of the NHS budget than standard fundholding. The HA remained as a local strategic body with the remit to produce the HImP, undertake public health functions and commission (some) services.

The governance of PCGs was notable given the mix of professional and managerial groups. PCGs were governed by a board which was chaired by a GP. Moreover, GPs were entitled to a numerical majority on the board. Many saw these guaranteed positions as a concession to the medical profession to assuage their concerns about the loss of fundholding and as an attempt to incorporate them into organisational decision-making. GPs's experience in fundholding or locality commissioning schemes proved valuable in the transition to new forms of commissioning.

In ways reminiscent of the consensus teams pre-1985, nurses were also represented on PCG boards. The selection of medical and nursing representatives on the PCG boards proved contentious in some areas, especially where the PCG consists of fundholders and non-fundholders and/or a mix of different types of area. Ensuring balance between geographical and interest-group representation hampered collaborative working between the board and its constituents (Hudson *et al*. 1999). PCGs were 'managed' by a chief officer – a general manager. This person was involved in the day-to-day operation of the PCG.

Social services were entitled to a nominated place on the PCG board to promote interagency collaboration. Hudson *et al*. (1999) found that the seniority of the social services representative and the PCG chief executive was crucial in determining the quality of such collaboration. In particular, similar levels of (financial and decision-making) autonomy were important in being able to formulate and implement strategies and initiatives that were sensitive to the PCG's needs. PCG boards also were comprised of a lay member and an HA representative (usually a non-executive director).

Primary Care Trusts

The creation of English PCGs was accompanied by proposals for Primary Care Trusts (PCTs). The PCT marks an important watershed for primary care in a number of respects. PCTs were given three roles:

1. to improve the health of the community;
2. to secure (commission) the provision of services; and
3. to integrate health and social care.

Not only do they represent the confluence of commissioning and provision but also the establishment of fully fledged primary care organisations *within* the NHS structure. Whether the latter represents the integration of primary care (especially involving the management of GPs) or an innovative approach to contemporary health care delivery is a matter of opinion.

A high percentage of PCGs expressed an interest in becoming a PCT (in part, so that they could be eligible to received further information from the NHSE about PCTs) and the NHS Plan (DoH 2000). 'Shifting the balance of power' (DOH 2001b) proposed that all PCGs will become PCTs by April 2004. In the first wave, 17 PCTs were created in April 2000 with a further 23 in the second wave which began in October 2000 (see Table 7.3).

In April 2001, a further 124 PCGs became PCTs, thereby creating a total of 164 PCTs. However, 237 PCGs remain (DoH website www.doh.gov.uk/pricare/pcts.htm, December 2001).

PCTs have evolved from PCGs, key differences being the role of com-document missioning and the community health services. On the one hand, level 3 PCTs can commission services and employ a limited range of staff but are not involved in provision. On the other hand, level 4 PCTs combine commissioning and primary care development, and provide community health services. By 2004, the DOH claims that PCTs will be responsible for 75 per cent of the NHS budget. (This compares with about 15 per cent controlled by GPFH in 1997). Though PCG/Ts have been established, the National Tracker Survey (Wilkin *et al.* 2001) has found the infrastructure less well-developed. For example, half of the respondents 'were developing financial incentives related to clinical governance' (3) and 'only a third had made any changes to the service level agreements for community health services and 43 per cent for hospital services'.

Table 7.3   Primary Care Trusts

First wave	17 formed in April 2000	Central Derby, Daventry, Epping Forest, Fenland, Hillingdon, Lincolnshire (NE), Manchester (S), Mansfield, Nelson & W. Merton, Newark & Sherwood, Peterborough (N), Peterborough (S), Poole Bay, Poole Central/North, Southampton (E), Southend, Tendring
Second wave	23 formed in October 2000	Airedale, Bexley, Birmingham (NE), Blackburn, Bournemouth, Bradford (city), Bradford (N), Bradford (S&W), Carrick, Dartford, Doncaster, Greater Yardley, Herefordshire, Hertsmere, Manchester (central), Manchester (N), Milton Keynes, N. Dorset, S.Hams & W.Devon, Stoke (N), Torbay, Trafford (S), W. Norfolk

Another important distinction is their governance. A PCT board will be chaired by an (appointed) (lay) chair and will be comprised of non-executive directors. This effectively makes the PCT like any other NHS Trust. Most first-wave Trust chairs (15: out of 17) had been NHS non-executives before their PCT appointment, reflecting, to some extent, the emphasis placed on community links by Labour (Public Accounts Committee, 2000). In first-wave PCTs, for example, five chairs are or have been local authority councillors. Whilst most chairs were male (9: out of 17), female chairs tended to be younger than their male counterparts.

Chief executives have been appointed. Most first-wave chief executives (13: out of 17) had been the chief executive of the PCG (Robinson and Exworthy 2000); their careers had mainly been outside primary care but still in the NHS. Most chief executives were male (10: out of 17) and, similar to chairs, female chief executives tended to be younger.

PCTs are also comprised of an executive committee chaired by a (usually elected) clinician (invariably a GP) with representation of primary care professionals. Though not present in the same form in other NHS Trusts, the executive committee can be seen as a concession to professionals' groups to ensure their involvement and to mollify their concerns about being taken over. The formal role of the executive committee chair in the governance of the PCT may arguably be seen as a transitional arrangement given the time commitment required and the relative lack of volunteers (at the moment) for such posts. Moreover, with the appointment of a Director of Public Health to the PCT board, it is likely that the role of executive committee chair will change.

The Trust chair, chief executive and executive committee chair have been nicknamed the triumvirate, three at the top or even holy trinity (see Figure 6.1). This form of governance is currently unique in the NHS. Given the newness of PCTs, the joint working between the 'three at the top' (and their links with their respective constituents) will have a strong bearing on the effectiveness of the PCT as a whole.

A feature of commissioning between 1991 and 1997 was the combination of large-scale (HA) and small-scale commissioning (GPFH). In the light of PCTs and Strategic HAs, this distinction is redundant. One possible impact is the loss of local responsiveness. For example, first-wave PCTs' population ranges from 79 000 to 245 000 (the average being 125,000). The average size of second-wave PCTs increased to a 135 000 population. (This compares to an average TPP population of just 'under 30,000', Mays *et al.* 2001b: 290)). With the prospect of PCT mergers, it is likely that PCTs may come to resemble former DHAs in both size and, to a lesser extent, function. The NHS has seen the ebb and flow of organisational size and population coverage (Exworthy and Moon 1998c) and the PCT pattern is the latest expression of this. For example, policy had introduced a population size for PCGs on the assumption that scale economies could be achieved in transaction costs (Mays *et al.* 2001b: 284). Yet there is 'no evidence that increases in the population size of primary care groups or trust beyond 100,000 will generate important cost savings or improvement in overall performance' (Bojke *et al.* 2001). However, this creeping centralisation will be inimical to meeting the needs of local communities or neighbourhoods. To enhance their responsiveness, locality initiatives are already evident in some PCTs.

The announcement of further PCT levels might be expected in terms of joint primary–secondary care ventures or integration with social care. Indeed level 4 PCTs can already register to become a new Care Trust and effectively provide social care services. Care Trust policy exemplifies emergent strategy development (see Chapter 2): 'The policy [for Care Trusts] is being developed as the detailed issues emerge and are considered' (DoH website www.doh.gov.uk/caretrusts/briefing/htm Para 3, December 2001).

Despite this ambiguity, the government has stressed that Care Trusts are not a takeover by either the NHS or local government but rather 'a stable organisational framework for long-term service organisational continuity and the kind of joined-up personal contact needed to improve services' (DoH website, December 2001). Rather than commissioning *per se*, they allow for new approaches to strategic decision-making (including financial flexibility), to service delivery and to quality improvement. As such, no single model is envisaged.

Care Trusts may represent a step towards unification between health and social care organisations, possibly akin to the Northern Ireland model. The House of Commons Health Select Committee (1998) favoured such an option.

> We consider that the problems of collaboration between health and social services will not be properly resolved until there is an integrated health and social care system, whether this is within the NHS, within local government or within some new, separate organisations. (para. 68)

The government initially rejected this view but the potential still remains. For example, the search for coterminosity between PCGs and local authorities

(Exworthy and Peckham, 1999), and the realignment of the former as they evolve into PCTs, makes this unification a possibility.

Primary Care Commissioning: Dilemmas and Possible Futures

It is important to note the pervasiveness of commissioning. It is now ten years since marketisation was introduced in the NHS and, since then, there have been several incarnations. Indeed, those who had hoped that the Labour Government would herald an end to the purchaser–provider split welcomed the end of the internal market but, ironically, also found that commissioning had been extended to all GPs through PCGs. Hence, 'fundholding is dead, long live commissioning'.

These incarnations and its extension have involved commissioning both *in* and *by* primary care. Initially, the commissioning was undertaken by GPs with the aid of fundholding managers but, with the advent of a managerial cadre in primary care, the role of clinicians has changed. They act in concert with primary care managers. Whether this heralds a shift towards further managerialisation of commissioning and the possible retreat of GPs is uncertain. Those GPs who retain commissioning roles may act not so much as a conduit for commissioning but rather as a buffer (or, at least, a filter) between the rank-and-file GPs and the wider organisation.

Services commissioned by primary care initially focused on elective secondary care but, over time, this has been extended into commissioning of primary care services including salaried GPs. Although the more extensive model of GPFH (i.e. TPP) made 'almost no impact' on GMS provision by GPs (Mays *et al.* 2001b: 279), this shift has been accompanied by a wider perspective on the role of commissioning, one which sees its aims in terms of service developments and, increasingly, more strategic aims such as health improvement and tackling health inequalities.

Whilst the notion of commissioning may have become established, its distinction with provision is becoming increasingly blurred. The distinction is apparent in the 1991 reforms but is contrasted with the 1997 reforms which stressed integration. The changing balance from competition to co-operation, the introduction of PCTs, and the Personal Medical Services pilots have been the main catalysts for this. These changes also reflect the changing organisational structure of primary care commissioning. The increasing scale is perhaps the most notable feature of this development. Fundholding began with populations of several thousand patients and its evolution enabled practices with few patients. Now, PCTs cover much larger populations (often more than 200 000), enabling economies of scale and greater management costs. As strategic health authorities 'step back from commissioning' (DoH 2001b), PCTs do, for example, represent a more significant organisation in local health economies than fundholding managed to achieve. However, with such gains, there is a possible commensurate reduction in local responsiveness and difficulty in ensuring PCT benefits accrue to practices (rather than the organisation) (Mays *et al*. 2001b: 282).

It is possible to see (some of) these changes as a strategy of integration. Commissioning has been one of the strategies whereby primary care has become tied more firmly into the aims and *modus operandi* of the NHS. For example, PCTs must demonstrate their ability to improve the health of their population as well as commission services for them. Moreover, central government has greater control over primary care through a tighter rein on its expenditure. Whilst initiatives such as clinical governance will diminish clinical isolation in primary care, the independent contractor status of GPs remains problematic for this strategy but PMS pilots and some PCT initiatives are eroding this. More women GPs and fewer GPs wanting to commit themselves to partnerships, for example, will accelerate this trend. One of the clearest manifestations of the integration concept is the governance of primary care. PCTs are comprised of a lay chair, a board and non-executive directors. Primary care clinicians have retained crucial roles in PCTs, primarily through the Executive Committee, but these roles may wane as PCTs extend across commissioning and providing, and reach into social care.

The blurring of commissioning and providing, and the extension into social care points towards possible futures for primary care. Integrated care, combining an intermediate function between primary and secondary care, is ideally suited for the evolving PCTs. This may also presage new organisational forms such as inter-organisational directorates and management. It may also facilitate the extension of the Private Finance Initiative (PFI) / Public–Private Partnerships (PPP) into primary care in terms of new capital (such as buildings and equipment via LIFT) and possibly staff. Though some have seen the resemblance of PCTs to American-style Health Maintenance Organisations (HMOs) (Enthoven cited in Newman, 1995; Robinson and Steiner 1998), the political sensitivities and tax-funded nature of the NHS are likely to militate against this, in the short term (Wanless 2001).

In summary, commissioning *in* and *by* primary care has had a short and eventful life in the NHS. It is highly likely that current arrangements will not last long and instead more integrated structures will emerge; purchaser and provider functions have largely coalesced in primary care organisations. In that commissioning models have demonstrated the scope for 'better cost control, demand management, efficiency improvement and service innovation' (Mays *et al*. 2001: 291), modified vehicles (such as PCTs and Care Trusts) will be used to develop PCOs. Therefore, although substantial elements will remain in place, it may no longer be possible to speak of commissioning as a separate and distinct function in primary care. In this way, commissioning both reflects and contributes to the changing nature of primary care in the UK.

CHAPTER 8

Inter-professional Working in Primary Care

Introduction

This chapter explores the contributions of and interrelationships between professional workers in primary care. Given the nature of health care generally and primary care specifically, service delivery is necessarily characterised by 'professionals' and by a high degree of interaction between them. The management of, organisation of and policy towards such inter-professional working has changed radically over time, not least because of the changes to work undertaken and to the composition of professions themselves. The chapter examines the nature of professions, reviews the actual interactions between professionals in primary care and considers current and future challenges of inter-professional work.

Before we examine the substantive issues of the chapter, it is necessary first to outline the terms and concepts being used. Perhaps the most crucial term and concept used here is that of 'professional'. Whilst the next section explores this in detail, its use here refers to professionally trained and qualified clinical staff including doctors, nurses and paramedical staff. Managers are usually professionally trained with their own credentials and qualifications but they are not considered here since clinical responsibilities add a significant and specific dimension to inter-professional working. However, social workers would be considered within the definition of professional (for the purposes of this chapter). The focus on professional groups enables comparisons to be made with other professionals such as lawyers, engineers and accountants (Flynn 1999: 19).

Inter-professional working implies a division of labour. This division exists in the sense of the number/range of professionals working in primary care, such as doctors, nurses, paramedical and ancillary staff. It also applies in the sense of the combination of professional skills in order to deliver health care to patients. This is clearly seen in the operating theatre in a hospital but also applies in primary care settings such as in the care of an older person in their own home. These divisions are not immutable but shift over time in response to knowledged advances, technological changes and political or regulatory shifts. It is consequent upon such divisions that issues of power and conflict arise in inter-professional working. Roles, functions, decision-making and leadership are all affected by unequal power relations between and within professions. This has implications for the way in which roles are delegated or substituted. As such, inter-professional working illustrates the changing boundaries within primary care.

The division of labour is becoming more complex as the range and combination of (clinical) professionals work in primary care. Even within the definition of primary care used here (including general practice and community health services), GPs are arguably the central players in the current primary care division of labour. This reflects not only their medical power (*vis-à-vis* other professionals) but also their role in policy. In terms of the later, for example, it is notable that it was GPs who became fundholders rather than any other professional group. Sibbald (2000) notes that GPs are the dominant medical specialty in primary care whereas there are several different specialties of nursing. This affects the relations between GPs and other specialties (on the one hand) and between GPs and nurses (on the other). Further, both medicine and nursing have been affected in recent years by the introduction of new public management in the UK, notably in terms of professionals-as-managers and the management of (clinical) performance (see Chapter 6). Williams (2000) argues that the impact of such management has been to add to insecurity within the health care professions.

The organisational changes in primary care have also created a new context for professionals. The policy emphasis on developing partnerships and the institutionalisation of these in new forms of primary care organisation have placed a renewed emphasis on, and provided a new context for, inter-professional working (Hudson 2002). For example, the NHS Plan described improved partnership working as being about achieving 'a radical redesign of the whole care system', and it is claimed that a key test of the closer working relationships 'will be how well they provide older people with improved services' (DoH 2000). The Plan goes on to specify service developments which will require 'cross-agency and cross-disciplinary working across health and local government services, particularly social care' including unified services such as rapid response (DoH 2001f).

There are also important changes in relation to the nature of professions, with new professions emerging and the blurring of boundaries between lay people and professionals. These changes are particularly relevant to the area of primary care. Complementary therapists mainly operate within the context of primary care being direct access and community-based. Increasingly primary care is building relationships with therapists such as acupuncturists, osteopaths, chiropractors and homeopaths – although not without criticism in many quarters. The role of patients and carers is also increasingly important and challenges the notion of professional expertise.

In briefly clarifying terms and concepts, a number of the themes that we will explore in this chapter have already surfaced. These include the notions of what it means to be a (primary care) professional, the changing balance of power between professionals, tensions between professional groups and the organisational structure within which professionals work.

Professions and Professionalism

Concepts of the Profession

In order to determine how individual professionals work together in practice, it is important to understand the constitution and composition of professions (as a collective group) and professionalism (as a discourse or paradigm) (Exworthy and Halford 1999: 129). (Such individual, collective and discourse distinctions can similarly be applied to managers, management and managerialism. These distinctions become important when an individual professional [such as a nurse] may be operating within a managerial discourse or the managerial discourse affects the composition of the profession). Although the literature on professions is vast, this chapter presents one perspective by focusing here on the collectivity and discourse; the next section explores the individual dimension.

The study of professions used to be characterised by the enumeration of the hallmarks of professional groups, usually in ideal types (e.g. Greenwood 1957). Such distinguishing characteristics usually included some or all of the following:

- limited membership;
- membership by qualification;
- body of 'expert' knowledge;
- assessment of performance by peers; and
- a relatively high degree of autonomy.

Such studies were often marked by an approach which assumed a beneficent role of professionals. This approach began to be undermined as studies also revealed malign aspects relating to professional competence, self-regulation and the degree of professional altruism. As a result, some saw professional groups as self-serving monopolies whilst others saw the potential for the exploitation of clients or patients. Nonetheless, Sibbald (2000: 19) argues that 'to the extent that the "defining" attributes of a profession have clarity and meaning for its profession, they frame the potential future development'.

A common approach to conceptualising professions relates to the notion of social closure (Weber 1949; Flynn 1999). This concept refers to the ability of professions to exclude competing groups and thereby to secure resources, status and power. A profession's ability to regulate itself, the ability to assess its own performance or to maintain salary differentials might be seen as examples of the success of social closure strategies. Citing Freidson's (1970) work in theorising professions (and in particular, the medical profession), Green and Thorogood (1998: 128) summarise the social closure concept:

> Freidson argued that the status of doctors derived not from a core of specialised knowledge nor an orientation towards service, but from the strategies that had been

used to gain a monopoly over practice. Only the profession itself can determine what constitutes medical work, practice, who is legitimately able to do it and how it can be done.

As a result, professions are able to enjoy (varying degrees of) autonomy. Harrison (1999) argues that the achievement of such autonomy has been manifest through the official policy of successive governments, the formal organisation of the NHS and the practice of management.

Most theories of professions see them in an ongoing process to assert and reassert their position *vis-à-vis* other (professional) workers. As such, it is useful to view professionalisation as a continual process or activity. Professions thus need to redefine themselves continually in the light of changing organisational forms, new policies, changing expectations of patients and new clinical roles etc. One theory which recognises this process of readjustment is 'negotiated order'. In clinical settings, the aims of professional and non-professional staff are usually not disputed, i.e. high goal congruence. This is most clearly in emergency care (Walby and Greenwell 1994: 166). However, professionals thus often talk about 'doing what is best for the patient' even though there are clearly differing opinions about how to achieve this or even what the patient might think. The teamwork between professional staff (and also ancillary staff) in clinical service delivery complicates the ways such aims are achieved. 'Negotiated order' refers to the way in which order is achieved and maintained. This is the essence of inter-professional working. Negotiation between professionals is conditioned by mutual tacit expectations of behaviour [rather] than explicit formulas for decision-making (Green and Thorogood 1998: 129), the relative balance of power (say, between a GP and a practice nurse) and their socialisation (i.e. the process by which *normal* practice is inculcated into new staff members). These 'negotiative' processes thus go beyond the 'formal rules'.

Professions are marked by hierarchies of status and power within and between professional groups. Within medicine, it is often assumed that the relative balance of power rests with surgeons as opposed to general (medical) practitioners, reflecting a societal value which values high technology, curative and specialist care above (lower) technology, preventive and generalist care. This division of medical labour has recently been stylised by the Christmas card analogy. In needing to win favour with hospital consultants, GPs (at least, mythically) had to send the Christmas card. This shifted with the advent of fundholding in the 1990s when consultants needed to secure funding from GPFHs (Harrison 1999: 57). The status and power of the medical profession is usually seen to be predominant among different professions (Williams 2000). Nursing has generally found it hard to define for itself a separate and distinct identity from that of medicine (Parkin 1995), reflecting a distinction between doctors' role to *cure* and nurses' role to *care* (Witz 1994: 33). Such professionalisation strategies in nursing have included the shift towards a degree-based education. The degree to which professional groups (or subgroups) have achieved *and* maintain social closure helps to explain the hierarchy within and between professions. For example, surgeons have traditionally managed to avoid 'competition' with others groups whereas the role of the GP is being redefined in relation to nursing.

More recently there has been a movement among some complementary therapists to professionalise. Saks (1995) sees this as a response to increasing consumer demand and fears about greater regulation within the European Community. He suggests that there may be strategic advantage for therapies to gain a recognised status (by the state). The recent registration of osteopaths and chiropractors and the establishment of registers for homoeopaths suggest that registration and formal recognition are seen as relevant to what has historically been an unregulated area of health care activity.

Challenges to Professions

As shown throughout the book (but especially in Chapter 2), policy is often concerned with changing the balance of power between or within professions and other groups (e.g. DoH 2001a). This balance of power is never static since professionalisation and professional power are dynamic and fluid concepts. The challenges to professions' power and to the process of professionalisation derives (in the case of health care) from within the profession, from other professions, from managers and from patients or the public (Gabe *et al.* 1991; Exworthy *et al.* 1996). These changes are, some claim, leading to de-professionalisation and proletarianisation. First, de-professionalisation refers to the loss of cultural authority (such as prestige and trust) held by professions which is due to

> broad social changes including consumerism, increased general levels of education . . . public concern with the privilege accorded to professionals . . . and the expansion of expert computer systems. (Exworthy and Halford 1999: 15)

Patients, for example, are now much more willing to challenge doctors, having lost some of the deference that they previously held. Second, proletarianisation refers to the transformation in professional labour as it becomes increasingly dependent on employment in and subject to organisations. As a result, professions begin to lose their autonomy and independence and so become like any other group of workers. For example, professionals are becoming subject to more government-initiated schemes to measure and assess their performance (see Chapter 5). (Some [heteronomous] professions such as social work have benefited from state sponsorship, their professional development being regulated, funded and protected exclusively by the state. Unlike medicine, for example, a private social work service does not exist.) Elston (1991) and Freidson (1994) are not convinced by these theories which they consider as suffering from a lack of robust empirical evidence.

Freidson (1994) offers a third theory – the internal combustion of the profession. He argues that 'the coherence holding a profession together may be undermined or even disappear as members cease to share the same interests' (Exworthy and Halford 1999: 15). This process is aided by greater specialisation within the profession, increased separation between administrators and the rank-and-file within the profession, and the managerialisation of professional associations (often linked to moves for self-regulation). Freidson (1994) sees the effect of some clinicians with entrepreneurial or managerial responsibility as 'driving a wedge into the principle of collegiality, of a community of autonomous peers at the local level' (Elston 1991: 74). Clearly, not all professions are experiencing these trends in the same way or at the same time. However, the differential patterns within or between professions are likely to exacerbate this stratification and hence fuel the internal combustion.

An alternative view on the future of professions is that power between and within medicine has yet to be seriously dented. The many challenges faced by medicine have often been incorporated into the profession and subsumed within its ethos. Demise of this profession is thus a premature and an incautious conclusion. For example, rather than managers taking over or controlling doctors, some doctors have themselves become managers, encroaching into managerial territory. Similarly, whilst doctors have delegated some tasks to nurses, they have usually resisted substitution by nurses. Moreover, the 'evidence-based' movement might be seen as a challenge to doctors but this has been colonised by doctors (and, to a lesser extent, other professions) (Harrison 1998). Some argue that the medical profession has emerged stronger from these challenges, with its power enhanced (albeit redistributed within the profession) whilst nursing has, to a greater extent, become subject to managerialism and evidence-based movement. Harrison (1999) sees that the power of professions (mainly medicine) may thus be enhanced through a process of uneven *re*-professionalisation. Some branches within the profession and some professions more than others will benefit the profession's restructuring. The profession is thus re-modelled within a different balance of power. The research branch (knowledge elite: Freidson 1994), generating the evidence base, for example, and the managerial branch (administrative elite, incorporated into organisational structures) are able to exert more influence over rank-and-file professionals because of the declining coherence within the profession. One interpretation of this restructuring sees the profession try to 'preserve and perpetuate the customary [i.e. professional] kinds and standards of service provision' (Ackroyd *et al.* 1989: 603). This 'custodial strategy' sees the administrative branch of the profession acting as a buffer (rather than a conduit) between the rank and file and external pressures. This may have been evident in TPPs whereby 'the majority of GPs in TPPs remained marginal to, and often ambivalent about, TPP activity' (Goodwin *et al.* 2001: 52). TPP as a managerial concept had failed to engage them but it is unclear whether this was because of the managerial structure (allowing 'free riders') and/or the buffering by the 'administrative branch'. This strategy has also been a way in which external assessment of the profession has traditionally been resisted by the (medical) profession (see Chapter 5). However, in 'managing' the profession, the administrative branch needs to retain credibility and authority with peers whilst also gaining legitimacy from managerial and governmental interests.

A different perspective on challenges to professions was taken by Alford (1975) who proposed a structural interest theory in which dominant interests (professional monopolisers, mainly medicine) were challenged by the interests of corporate rationalisers (such as managers and planners) in the reform of health care services. Community interests (such as patients and the public) were repressed and excluded from the struggle for power. This is discussed more extensively in Chapter 2 and the relationship between professions, patients and the public is explored further at the end of this chapter and in Chapter 10.

Finally, an important area for health care is the role of the state in regulating professionals. In the UK medical professionals have been self-regulated and this structure has been protected by statute since 1858. The establishment of the General Council of Medical Education and Registration (now known as the General Medical Council [GMC] enshrined the right of the medical profession to control the registration of doctors and their conduct. By contrast nurses and professions allied to health care have developed regulatory structures which are rested upon statute. At the other extreme while social work training is regulated through a central body, there has not been a regulatory body for social workers. This regulatory framework is now changing and in 2001 the government set out proposals for substantive changes to the regulatory machinery for health care professionals in *Modernising Regulation in the Health Care Professions* (DoH 2001g), with specific consultation documents for a new Health Care Professions Regulatory Board and a new Nursing and Midwifery Council – subsequently incorporated in the Health Services Reform Bill 2001. These developments involved a complete overhaul of the regulatory bodies and should be set alongside changes to the General Medical Council and how complaints are dealt with. For nursing, the English National Board and UKCC were abolished and have been replaced by a New Nursing and Midwifery Council that incorporate separate arrangements for health visitors. In addition there is to be a new Health Professions Council for the regulation of health care professionals previously covered by the Council for Professions Supplementary to Medicine. The changes to the professional regulatory machinery will apply across the whole of the UK and represent both a more structured role for professional regulatory bodies and one in which the regulatory mechanisms themselves are more centrally regulated.

At the same time there have been changes to the General Medical Council to strengthen its powers through a scheme of regular revalidation of the fitness to practise of doctors on its register, and the government is consulting further on new governance arrangements, revalidation and improved fitness-to-practise procedures. Finally, the government is also establishing a new Council for the

Regulation of Healthcare Professionals to which all professional regulatory councils would be accountable. These changes represent a significant change to health care professional regulation with greater government involvement in establishing and prescribing the functions of regulatory bodies and by establishing clearer links between regulation, accreditation and continuing professional development and reaccreditation. The introduction of new regulatory frameworks and stronger reaccreditation will have significant impact in primary care as new relationships and roles develop over the next decade and need to be considered alongside other challenges to professional autonomy and practice such as the introduction of guidelines, standards of practice and clinical governance.

Inter-professional Working: Experience in Practice

Changing Pattern of Professional Work in Primary Care

The pattern of professional work in primary care has rarely been static, reflecting fluctuations in the balance between and within professions as well as the myriad of changes in the organisation and management of primary care. However, the medical profession has remained largely dominant in various incarnations of inter-professional working. Nonetheless, the degree of inter-professional working has grown in the latter part of the twentieth century such that it is now a well-established feature of primary care in the UK.

The Primary Health Care Team

The primary health care team (PHCT) is often thought to be the main form of organisation within primary care and is held to be the most effective form of inter-professional working. It is also the main interaction between the medical and nursing professions' cultures, notably one type of doctor but different groups of nurses (Sibbald 2000). The development of PHCTs was stimulated in the 1960s by the Doctors' Charter (1966) which contained 'changes to the GPs' terms of service [which] encouraged GPs to delegate work to appropriate staff and introduced a 70 per cent reimbursement for employing a nurse in the practice' (RCGP 1998). Further changes at that time allowed greater collaboration between PHCT members. However, it was the rise of larger practices, rising workloads and the 1990 GP Contract which served to cement the concept and practice of teamwork in primary care.

Definitions of PHCTs have invariably been problematic. The definition offered by Wiles and Robison (1994: 324) sums up the key characteristics: 'a group of people working at or from a primary care practice with common goals and objectives relating to patient care'.

This definition places emphasis on the co-location of professionals in premises and the goal congruence of such professionals. (See also Acheson 1981; RCGP 1998; Wilson 2000: 44.) Whilst some doubt the extent to which the PHCT has become established (Bond *et al.* 1987), others have questioned even the notion of a team in the first place (Pearson and Jones 1994). Such disputes raise a series of issues relating to the PHCT, including team identity, leadership, access to GPs, philosophies of care, and understanding of (and disagreement about) team members' roles and responsibilities (Wiles and Robison 1994). For example, Sibbald (2000) notes GPs' ambivalent roles in teams: whether they work in or with the team; whether they run it; or whether they are the team 'captain'. In short, the opportunities presented by the PHCT are also related to their difficulties: namely the (overlap between the) relative contribution of professionals to service delivery.

Wiles and Robison (1994) found that the notion of PHCT was widely understood though not always practised. For example, some practices did not hold regular PHCT meetings. Also, nurses' access to GPs was often constrained to communicating with them between appointments; nurses would 'pop in to see the GP between patients'. Their study found that midwives and health visitors emerged as the least integrated members of the PHCT.

Richards *et al.* (2000) also found that teamwork in primary care was problematic. They explained this in terms of unclear roles, difficulties in face-to-face communication (owing to rising workloads), GPs' status (with GPs being reluctant to relinquish power), different management structures and duplication of some roles (especially between nursing owing to historical patterns of provision). They also cite 'conflicting hierarchies [as] a further obstacle to effective teamworking' (191). They advocate measures to enhance primary care teamworking such as 'workshops', 'vision sharing' and 'multidisciplinary learning' (191). Their latter measure has, however, been identified as problematic by Elston and Holloway (2001: 27) who argue that 'it might take a new generation to bring about an inter-professional culture to the NHS that can only be achieved through inter-professional education at an early stage'.

Their argument emphasises that many of the difficulties in inter-professional working stem from the way(s) in which professions are socialised into patterns of work and expectations of teamwork during their education and training. This has profound implications for the (subsequent) organisation and management of primary care, as policy statements have recognised: 'Expansion of professionals working with GPs will have an impact on the organisation and division of labour within primary care' (DoH 1996a).

Such views support what Hudson (2002) has described as the pessimistic tradition of inter-professionality. He argues that proposals for inter-professionality currently being developed represent an ambitious and demanding agenda for professionals in health and social care. This is also likely to become more complex and difficult as 'new' professional groups develop.

The integration of 'new' professional groups (such as those associated with complementary therapies) into patterns of primary care teamworking may prove problematic in future. Adams and Tovey (2000: 169) believe that integration has been sporadic to date but that complementary therapy is making its most significant contribution in primary care. They present three forms of teamworking between complementary therapies and primary care. The first, called 'referrals', involves 'lay therapists or medical colleagues who practise a form of CM' [complementary medicine]. The second, 'multi-disciplinary integrative primary care teams', involve co-location of therapists in the practice, thereby fostering 'collaborative treatments'. Thirdly, 'direct integrative practice' requires 'no direct input from other practitioners'.

Contrasting (policy) prescriptions for improved teamworking are evident in the Acheson Report on primary care in inner London (1981) and the document 'Shifting the Balance of Power: Securing the Delivery' (DoH 2001b). The Acheson Report adopted a structural solution to poor teamwork. It claimed that PHCTs were poorly developed because of the inadequate premises and the conflict between geographical responsibility of community nurses and the list responsibility of GPs. Grouping GPs/patients into larger practices was seen as one solution. More recent policy initiatives have not sought to reach a resolution of contributions to PHCTs but to provide greater flexibility. For example, 'new approaches to tackle the traditional demarcations between different professional groups and services will pave the way for innovative care pathways which better meet patients' needs' (DoH 2001b: 11). The latter policy will not take a generation to produce new inter-professional relations.

Skill Mix in Primary Care

The nature and extent of teamwork in any primary care organisation is largely shaped by the skill mix of the PHCT. In 1995 the BMA has defined skill mix as: 'the balance between trained and untrained, qualified and unqualified, and supervisory and operative staff within a service as well as between staff groups' (1; quoted in Richards *et al.* 2000: 186).

The skill mix within a PHCT can thus be a source of contention since the balance is dependent upon role definition, professional hierarchies, expectations, knowledge bases, workloads and organisational structure.

Skill-mix reviews have often been undertaken locally to determine the 'most' appropriate balance between professional inputs in service provision but they have been criticised for failing to take account of professionals' experience and competency or the organisational context (Richards *et al.* 2000: 187). Nonetheless, skill-mix reviews remain a persistent theme in determining the relative contributions of professions. Richardson *et al.* (1998) found, mainly from studies in the USA, that 25–70 per cent of doctors' tasks could be performed by other professionals. In the UK, Jenkins-Clarke *et al.* (1998)

found that, in UK primary care, 39 per cent of GP consultations had elements which could have been delegated and 17 per cent could have been delegated totally. If such delegation were to take place, this would have profound implications for the list sizes which GPs could manage (Exworthy 1994b). Delegated tasks might include some home visits, travel advice, ECG, suturing, diabetic management, depression management and advice on common illnesses.

Skill mix and delegation are intimately bound up with notions of professionalism and the consequent fears of incompetence, of de-professionalisation and of a deterioration in the doctor–patient relationship. As such, resistance to skill-mix changes exemplifies the value placed on professional autonomy by retaining social closure of the profession. At the root of such issues lie 'unequal power relations' (Richards *et al.* 2000: 192; see also Exworthy *et al.* 1996; Williams 2000). Whilst the GP retains clinical and legal responsibility for patients, power relations persist and, hence, delegation is an inaccurate description. Richards *et al.* (2000) concluded that it is better to view inter-professional working in terms of complementary rather than subservient roles. Complementarity becomes an important consideration in teamwork in the sense that patients often view doctors in terms of tasks (and functions) whereas nurses are often seen in terms of their relationship with the patient, reflecting the traditional perception of cure and care by doctors and nurses (Robison and Exworthy 1995).

The definition of the PHCT offered by Wiles and Robison (1994) does not illuminate greatly the balance, contribution or skill mix of members of the PHCT. It appears as if their definition relates mainly to the co-location and the common purpose in terms of goals or objectives. However, as Walby and Greenwell (1994) show, common objectives reveal little about the 'negotiated order' within a multi-professional setting.

To understand the broader picture of inter-professional relations in primary care (and teamworking specifically), it is important to consider the trajectory of the constituent professions of these teams. Many of the tensions and difficulties within and of PHCTs stem from the historical development of these professions.

Nursing and Inter-professional Working in Primary Care

Nursing represents a significant and varied professional group within primary care. It can be divided into two main subgroups by virtue of their employment and/or independence from GPs: first, practice nurse and nurse practitioners and second, health visitors, district nurses, school nurses and community psychiatric nurses (Williams 2000). It has undergone the most distinctive and significant professionalisation in recent years, a process largely shaped by its relations with medicine. Perhaps the most significant demonstration of this concerns nurse training. Nursing's curriculum used to be prescribed by doctors (Parkin 1995); indeed, women were excluded from medicine in the nineteenth century (Green and Thorogood 1998: 141). For many, the interrelationship between medicine and nursing reflected the distinction between curing and caring (Witz 1994: 33; Wilson 2000: 50), a differentiation as much about gender as about professions. Parkin (1995) argues that nursing is seen as essentially a female occupation which carries social perceptions of it as low-status work, involving menial tasks, uninteresting/routinised work and domestic duties. Sibbald (2000: 18) blurs the distinction as 'both caring and curing are central to the provision of primary health care which is characterised by the prevalence of undifferentiated illness which owes as much to the social and psychological context of people's lives as to their biomedical state'.

Over the last 30 or so years, nursing has undertaken a strategy of professionalisation. This strategy has involved the development of a body of knowledge, the associated changes in nurse education (towards a more degree-based profession) and practice (in terms of new roles and responsibilities). Witz (1994: 23) summarises the strategy in terms of credentials and legislation. She cites (29) the UKCC's 1992 change in code of practice for nursing as an example. This change placed 'less emphasis on certification and more on general, professional competency and individual judgement in applying principles to practice'. The intent was that nursing would be more involved in patient care than in overseeing such care (which was dictated by doctors).

The professionalisation of nursing strategy has been problematic because it has sought to define its territory more precisely and, as a result, to challenge medicine. Increasingly, it is being seen as an alternative rather than complementary to medicine (Wilson 2000: 50). This strategy of 'dual closure' (Witz 1994: 23) seeks to define who can practise nursing and to seek autonomy from medicine relating to nurses' roles and responsibilities. This parallels what Green and Thorogood (1998: 138) have termed a 'double bind' in which nursing has sought greater professionalisation whilst, at the same time, not trying to lose its patient-centred approach. In short, 'can the nurse be both an expert decision maker and the "patient's friend"?' (Witz 1994: 39).

Role delegation and substitution between and within professional groups is changing the face of inter-professional relations in primary care. This has consequences for the co-ordination of patient care:

> It is this notion of balance between members of staff which is considered to be crucial in order to deliver good quality, cost-effective care in the general practice setting and at the interface between the hospital sector and social service provision. (Richards *et al.* 2000: 186)

Sibbald (2000) argues that, traditionally, scant attention has been paid to the boundaries between doctors and nurses but this has been changing with the professionalisation of nursing. The identity and ethos of general practice, she argues, has thus been challenged. Delegation of roles from GPs to nurses (mainly practice nurses) has been encouraged by GPs, not least because they still retain overall responsibility. Substitution of GPs' work by nurse practitioners, district nurses and others is, as Sibbald (2000: 20) argues, 'another matter', largely related to power and control. For GPs, there has often been a sense of loss as their traditional roles are substituted by nurses whereas the situation is more 'ambiguous' for nurses, as Williams (2000: 4) suggests.

The changing balance between professional groups affects not only nurses and therapy staff but also GPs, social workers, pharmacists and groups beyond primary care (such as secondary care). The delegation of tasks to nurses and in some cases substitution by nurses changes the nature of what it means to be a GP, a generalist in a primary care setting. Similar processes are evident in the balance in GPs' roles shifting from a bias towards individual patients to becoming public health doctors for their locality (Green and Thorogood 1998: 102; see also House of Commons 2001). However, delegation and substitution debates have not yet addressed the issue whether such processes result in better quality or more cost-effective services (Sibbald 2000).

One of the major changes to occur at about the same time as this process started was general management. Managerialism represented a challenge to the nursing profession because nursing, in common with other professions, had traditionally sought 'occupational control through the creation of their own management hierarchies' (Causer and Exworthy 1999: 91). However, promotion up the nursing hierarchy was marked by a move away from professional practice, unlike medicine. Moreover, with the advent of general managers in the 1980s, nursing lost its automatic right of representation on higher-level decision-making bodies. This process has been only partly ameliorated by their automatic representation on PCGs since the vast majority of PCG chairs were GPs. Nonetheless, managerialism (through budgetary and organisational decentralisation) has reached down into the daily practice of nursing, shaping the work of ward sisters and district nurse managers.

One of the most significant attempts in primary care to enhance nursing's professionalisation was the Cumberlege Report on neighbourhood nursing (DHSS 1986b) (Exworthy 1994a; Parkin 1995; Wilson 2000: 50). The Report proposed that community nursing should be based on neighbourhoods of 10 000–25 000 population and managed by a neighbourhood nurse manager, drawn from any nursing background and responsible for all community nurses in that patch. This Report advocated nurse practitioners who could work independently, run certain clinics, refer, diagnose and prescribe certain medications (Parkin 1995). It also made recommendations about the PHCT liaison and nurse training. The Report sought to redefine the role of community nursing within primary care but in ways that were complementary or parallel to general practice. This led to much criticism by doctors and pharmacists. The Report's almost exclusive focus on community nursing and its failure to integrate with the wider primary care helped to shape the Report's relatively small impact. Allsop (1986: 492) saw the Report as 'overtly partisan. GPs are given short shrift ... Its main aim is to carve out an independent territory for community nurses'. Although about 30 per cent of community health services had implemented Cumberlege's proposals after two years, the 1989 reforms (implemented in 1991) overtook the concept of neighbourhood nursing (Exworthy 1994a). The dominance of GPFH effectively put paid to this professionalisation strategy.

The 1990s was a period of huge change for primary care nursing (including community nursing) as a result of the rise in the number of practice nurses and the development of nurse practitioners. The growth in the number of practice nurses was aided by subsidies to practices which employed practice nurses. Their numbers rose spectacularly from 1920 in 1984 to 9100 in 1994 (Green and Thorogood 1998: 100). Though working with the practice population and for the practice, practice nurses also experienced a huge rise in their workload (associated with the 1990 GP Contract). Richards *et al.* estimate this rise to be 75 per cent (2000: 187) as practice nurse roles were extended, especially into chronic disease management (e.g. asthma), health promotion, smoking cessation, family planning and treatment of minor illnesses. This was despite some delegation of practice nurse tasks to health care assistants. Although the number of therapy staff such as osteopaths, counsellors and physiotherapists also rose in the early 1990s (Green and Thorogood 1998), the number of new entrants to health visiting declined (Richards *et al.* 2000: 186).

In the late 1990s, there was an equivocal reaction to the introduction of PCGs among primary care nursing. On the one hand, nursing was guaranteed a role in decision-making but, on the other, it was only one place on a committee dominated by GPs. Only 2 nurses were appointed chairs in 481 PCGs in April 1999 (Richards *et al.* 2000) and only one was chair of the Executive Committee in the first two waves of 40 PCTs (from April 2000) (Robinson and Exworthy 2000). The recruitment of nurses and their quasi-managerial position on PCGs have been part of recent attempts to revive health visiting in a wider public health role (Acheson 1998; DoH 2000; Taylor *et al.* 1998).

The rise in number of practice nurses was initially thought to be at the expense of Nurse Practitioners. Such practitioners are distinguished from their nurse colleagues by virtue of their additional knowledge and skills which facilitate first-level assessment and treatment. Nurse practitioners are those with 'a level of education, clinical activity and responsibility higher than that of other nurses, but different from that of a GP' (RCGP 1998). Their tasks involve diagnosis, prescribing, telephone advice and home visits. Some see the nurse practitioner as shifting nursing towards a medical orientation and, hence, a diminished nursing role, whereas others see them as an alternative or complementary rather than subservient to doctors. The growth of nurse development units, nurse-led units and minor injuries clinics (often led by nurses), often part of walk-in clinics and healthy-living centres, illustrate how nursing practitioners are extending nursing into new clinical and organisational areas. However, many such developments have coincided with nursing's professionalisation rather than having been initiated by nursing. These developments should be cautioned by wider policy changes in primary care in which GPs remain mostly in control of resources. Witz (1994: 37) argues that this 'points to the limited expansion of the nurse's role, as [she] simply takes on routine tasks performed by GPs, without necessarily expanding her decision-making or forging new partnerships with patients'. As a result, she argues, the localised power of doctors and managers will remain crucial in influencing the direction of nursing and the roles that nurses undertake.

Single-handed Doctors and Inter-professional Working in Primary Care

Single-handed practitioners have been a remarkable feature of UK general practice since before the start of the NHS. One example of the rise and rise of inter-professional working is the changing structure of general practice. As Green and Thorogood (1998: 97) note, in the 1950s most GPs worked alone, often from their own home rather than in a health centre or dedicated facility. However, the 1965 Family Doctor's Charter (see Chapter 4) encouraged the growth of group practice and the rise of the health centre as the facility/location for primary care service delivery. One consequence was the decline of single-handed GPs. In 1952, 43 per cent of GPs practised single-handedly but this figure had fallen to 17.5 per cent by 1975 and 10.5 per cent by 1995 (Green and Thorogood 1998: 97). Although the notion of teamwork was not new (for example, the Dawson Report (Dawson 1920) recommended a form of teamwork; Chapter 4), the approach in the 1960s set in train a number of consequences. This new approach provided a more structured pattern of primary care and inter-professional working through the primary health care team (PHCT).

Single-handed GPs, especially working in inner cities, have traditionally been associated with poor service provision because they often failed to integrate with other primary care professionals (e.g. Acheson 1981; Green and Thorogood 1998). This inter-professional working has been hampered by their poor premises and the lack of out-of-hours cover.

Single-handed GPs represent a policy dilemma because, on the one hand, they are associated with generally poorer standards of provision but, on the other, they have the ability to know patients better (Green and Thorogood 1998; Moon and North 2001). This is invariably appreciated by patients as, in group practices, the patient does not always see the same GP on each visit. These GPs often have close ties with the local community and can also represent a resistance against what is often impersonal medicine (Green 1993). Moreover, given their occupational culture, socialisation and organisational position, GPs are generally not considered to be 'team players' and often see other professionals as a source of stress. Single-handed GPs make this aspect of general practice culture more transparent. This has wider implications for general practice and the implementation of reforms (such as PCTs) since it is unclear how far GPs will want to assume the new responsibilities such as Executive Committees and clinical governance. Traditionally they have 'strongly resisted attempts by previous governments to exercise greater control over the quality and content of their services' (Sibbald 2000: 25).

Clearly single-handed GPs have no other medical colleagues with which to engage within the practice but the structures and processes of clinical governance being established within PCGs and PCTs offer a chance for their continuation. By linking single-handed GPs into multi-professional clinical networks for education, peer review and audit, there is the opportunity for them to raise their standards of practice whilst also retaining the focus on personal aspects of care. Whilst single-handed GPs may be tolerated in the short term, it is debatable whether they will last as a distinct group. This is in part because they are a cohort who will, in the not too distant future, retire and won't be replaced in that setting. As such, the only future seems to be one of inter-professional working within larger practices.

Primary Care Pharmacy and Inter-professional Relations

It is only within the last decade or so that the contribution of primary care pharmacy (also known as community pharmacy) has been recognised. However, as it expands its roles, it is inevitably coming into tension with other established primary care professions. Primary care pharmacy fulfils various roles including 'services to GPs, over-the-counter advisory role, health promotion . . . services to special needs groups' and, more recently, medicines management (especially repeat prescribing) (Bond 2001: 251).

Primary care pharmacy is not usually seen as part of the PHCT and yet the vast majority of pharmacists want to be a member of it (Sutters and Nathan 1993). Pharmacists are most likely to be in contact with GPs. Differences have been noted about inter-professional working between these two groups. Sutters and Nathan (1993) found that 70 per cent of pharmacists thought that GPs did not want their input but only 17 per cent of GPs admitted this. Pharmacists also have close contact with district nurses; one survey found that 43 per cent had contact with PHCT members other than the GP (Smith 1990). However, communication was 'mostly initiated by the other profession, rather than the pharmacist' (Bond 2001: 256).

Primary care pharmacy, as a function separate from dispensing surgeries, is often professionally and geographically isolated from other PHCT members. However, pharmacy is a classic example of primary care in the sense that it is open access and does not involve patient registration (unlike general practice). As a result, many patients seek advice and medicines from pharmacists instead of and sometimes in addition to PHCT members. Primary care pharmacists are thus extending their roles, thereby encompassing tasks formerly undertaken by GPs The co-ordination of pharmacy with other strands of primary care has often focused on specific groups and/or specific needs (such as the homeless or drug misusers).

Primary Care–Social Work Relations

One of the most significant hallmarks of the policy, organisation and management of primary care in the last five years has been the emphasis placed upon inter-professional working. As the pitfalls of partnership have long been recognised (Callaghan *et al.* 2000: 19), the novelty has come from the degree of emphasis and, as Gillam and Irvine (2000: 5) argue, 'champions' of inter-professional working may question this novelty.

Organisational structures (such as PCGs and PCTs) and occupational cultures (of general practice, nursing and social work) have been overlaid on to an existing pattern of joint working between individual professionals in primary care and social services. Despite efforts to improve relations between primary care and social work professionals including those associated with the Community Care legislation in the early 1990s, the quality of inter-professional working between these sectors is still quite variable. Issues of language, meaning, management, governance and accountability are major differences which both facilitate and constrain opportunities for inter-professional working. More specifically, Gillam and Irvine (2000: 6) point towards the inexperience of primary care professionals as a limitation of inter-professional collaboration. They state that 'new forms of statutory partnership [are] unlikely to solve problems of joint working that have been present since inception of the welfare state'. They identify GPs' lack of strategic planning experience as a key deficiency to remedy.

Hudson (1999a) has identified four models of inter-professional collaboration between primary care and social services. These models are based on the ways in which individual professionals relate to each other and, although they can coexist, they represent an increasing level of sophistication in inter-professional relations (see Box 8.1).

Box 8.1   Models of Inter-professional Collaboration

i. Communication
Relating to the exchange of information:

- From GPs to SSD – this has been less well-documented and explored.
- From SSD to GPs – 'research has . . . shown that GPs prefer to work with a named contact from the SSD – something which requires a more structured form of communication' (15).

ii. Co-ordination
'Individuals remain in separate organisations and locations but develop formal ways of working across boundaries' (15). Hudson offers two forms:

- Shared assessments: GP assessments have tended to reflect a medical model and service-led approach with the result that they do not ask SSDs to conduct an assessment ... Hardy *et al.* (1996) found that, even in a project with co-located care managers in GP practice, there was only limited health input into assessment process' (16).
- Joint provision: such provision is often related to specific projects or initiatives.

iii. Co-location
Co-location involves members of different professions being physically located alongside each other and it is a widely used and preferred model. Somewhat like coterminosity between organisations, the benefits of co-location are 'deemed to flow from facilitation and promotion of greater understanding and trust, from co-ordinated approach to meeting individual needs and the provision of a single access point' (Hudson 1999a: 16–17). However, the inability to match the number of social workers to the number of practices (at least, on a full-time basis) and the lack of suitable accommodation in many GP practices frustrate such inter-professional collaboration. The internal organisation of social services into area teams or around client groups further limits the benefits of such collaboration.

iv. Commissioning
Commissioning can be divided into two types:

1. Practice: services commissioned by GP fundholders (and others) are at 'the margins of traditional health and social services responsibilities' (17). As a result, joint commissioning at practice level was a rarity and will be increasingly less so in the future.
2. Individual: such commissioning was unusual but changes proposed by *Partnership in Action* (DoH 1998b) and brought in by the 1999 Health Act has loosened the restrictions related to pooled budgets.

Fundholding and commissioning initiatives in the 1990s and the Labour Government's emphasis on interagency collaboration has spawned a number of models of inter-professional working. Many such models relate to the integration of services across professional boundaries. Mays *et al.* (2001a) cites a number of examples. In one example of community care co-ordination, an 'experienced social worker' liaised with the social services department and acted as a 'bridge' between the practice, social care managers and independent providers. Loosely defined, the role was to 'cover the grey areas' (108).

Hudson (1999a: 18) cites the work of Guzzo and Shea (1992) in recommending action for inter-professional working across the primary care–social services interface. No doubt, their advice is equally applicable to PHCTs:

- 'individuals should feel they are important to the success of the team';
- 'individual roles should be meaningful';
- 'individual contributions [to the team] should be identifiable'; and
- 'there should be clear team goals with built-in performance feedback'.

In more recent research Hudson (2002) has suggested that there is reason to be optimistic about health and social care inter-professional working. Inter-professional working is seen by many professionals to be a good thing, a way of coping with fragmentation and is an approach supported by policy and organisational changes (see Chapter 9). While Hudson did not find any significant positive developments, he argues that any movement towards better inter-professional working, even as limited as that identified in his research, provides grounds for such optimism in the future.

Current and Future Issues

> No one agency or group of staff is likely to be able to achieve all that is being asked of PCGs on their own. Successful PCGs will be those that harness the range of skills necessary to learn and work together for an effective partnership which will improve patient care. (NHS Executive 1998a: para. 8)

Delivering the NHS Plan will be about 'reform to break down the demarcations between different professional groups' (DoH 2001a: 5).

Inter-professional relations in primary care in the UK are not static but evolving. It is likely that the near future will involve significant reconfiguration of inter-professional relations. Since professionals only tend to collaborate when they are secure in their own professional identity, effective inter-professional working will arise when they can work from a position of confidence and competence. As primary care develops in an era of PCTs and Care Trusts, several themes emerge as likely to be significant influences in the coming years.

Recent reforms (such as the 1996 Primary Care Act and 2000 NHS Plan) are enabling professions (other than general practice) to adopt new roles in different organisational and occupational configurations. For example, nurse-led units, sometimes managed by a Trust, are providing new ways of delivering care that are distinct from the predominant patterns. These may not necessarily be opposed by GPs since, in some cases, it will free them from 'unwanted management responsibilities' (Sibbald 2000: 26). Hence it is possible, even likely, that the PCOs of the not too distant future will be organised and managed with little GP direction, supervision or even involvement.

The gender balance within primary care is changing and not simply because more women doctors become qualified. They have traditionally found general practice, primary care nursing and other professions attractive because of the flexibility they offer. Davies (1998) in particular has argued that gender is an important role in the transformation of professions and provides an analytical concept for understanding professions. This feminisation is likely to increase. It is also possible that doctors, nurses and PAMs will be split into 'core' and 'periphery' staff groups. This might involve name changes (such as associates) or different types of employment (e.g. temporary or conditional contracts). Such changes have been evident in teaching, for example. In short, professional stratification is unlikely to diminish in the near future.

Arising from and also shaped by role substitution, organisational reconfiguration will affect inter-professional relations, not least because primary care has traditionally been staffed by generalists, working in the community. The primary–secondary care interface is thus closely linked to changing inter-professional relations. Greater specialisation will be facilitated by the changing balance of general practice within PCTs. Some GPs, for example, are becoming specialist in certain clinical areas to the extent that patients might be referred from one GP to another *within* the PCT. Specialisation may precipitate further organisational change as the traditional boundary between hospital and primary care breaks down. Interagency directorates and clinical networks oriented around disease categories may result.

Changing inter-professional relations (and changes in organisational structures) may aid the integration of complementary therapies within primary care. Mostly, complementary therapies and primary care (especially general practice) have coexisted rather than intersected. Changing inter-professional relations may provide the opportunity for 'developing networks and communication between therapists and doctors' (Adams and Tovey 2000: 176).

However, inter-professional working is, in the future, likely to extend beyond 'inter-professional' by challenging the nature of professionalism itself. We argued in Chapter 1 that the shift of focus towards community-based care has been an important influence on developing primary care. Increasingly this has included a shift from hospital to home-based care and moving health care from hospitals to the community with more primary care, shorter hospital stays, more home-based care and involving, for example, parents in the care of their sick or disabled children is central to government policy (DoH 1989b; DoH 1991; DoH 1996b). Advances in medical technology and treatment now mean, for example, that there is an enhanced prognosis for children with chronic illnesses (Woodroffe *et al.* 1993). These changes mean that parents are often undertaking complex nursing care and highly technical procedures in a domestic setting (Kirk 1998a). Thus more children cared for at home are becoming technology-dependent – defined as those children who are dependent on a device or technology that is life-sustaining with a need for substantial and ongoing nursing care (Wagner *et al.* 1988). This includes children with disabilities, children with chronic illnesses, such as renal failure, and children with cancer. The increasing role of carers in these areas is challenging traditional concepts of the role of professionals as experts and the role of carers as lay people (Bloor 2001). More generally the concept of interdisciplinary working sees the patient and carer as part of the care team challenging notions of both professionalism and teamwork in health and social care. This blurring of distinctive roles is seen by some commentators as proof of a shift towards a postmodernist health care system where 'identity is no longer a stable phenomenon and ... pre-existing "modern" hierarchies, such as that between "senior" professions and professions related to them and between those who control the allocation of services and those who need or receive them, are in some way breaking down' (Biggs 1997: 371). Thus the blurring of patient and carer roles with those of the 'caring professions' is linked to wider issues where the government is placing an increasing emphasis on the involvement of patients and carers in health care services and individual care (see Chapter 10). Such views and policies present a challenge to health care and other professionals in terms of challenging both the nature of professionalism and traditional power structures between the patient and the professional.

CHAPTER 9

Health and Social Care Partnership at the Primary Care Level

This chapter examines the interface between health and social care in the context of primary and community care. Central to this chapter will be the coincidence of community care and primary care policy both of which emphasise the provision of care outside institutions and the importance of supporting people in their own homes. As in the last chapter, the changing organisational context of primary care will be examined in relation to collaborative working. It will, therefore, explore the different dimensions/ levels of horizontal government and current debates about 'joined-up government'. The discussion addresses wider issues of collaboration and partnership as these provide a developing context for future health and social care partnerships. The chapter will also discuss issues relating to decentralisation, integration and localisation drawing on current research in which the authors have been involved.

Difficulties in securing effective interagency and inter-professional partnership have been an apparently enduring feature of health and social care services in Britain. In particular, organisational differences have been compounded by differing professional cultures. The co-ordination of service delivery systems and staff was identified as a major problem by the Dawson Report as long ago as 1920 and the way in which the NHS was structured in 1948 only served to intensify the problems. Soon after the establishment of the NHS, criticisms were made of the fragmented health care system (separately administered hospital, community and primary care services), but also, and more importantly for the discussion in this chapter, criticism was made of the more important cleavage between hospital services and social care services provided by local authorities (Guillebaud 1956). Local authorities saw little incentive to support the expansion of community services as alternatives to hospitals which had been taken over by central government and were directly funded by the Treasury.

The eventual response to this was to create, from April 1974, two parallel structures based on coterminous boundaries and with a statutory duty to collaborate with each other through joint consultative committees (Wistow 1982). However, these arrangements were also seen to be deficient and, in 1976, joint care planning teams of senior officers from the NHS and Local Authorities were established (Wistow and Fuller 1983). At the same time, local authorities were provided with a tangible incentive to collaborate with the NHS through a joint finance programme which provided short-term funding for social services projects deemed to be of benefit to the health service. Although these formal arrangements were strengthened by the Care in the Community programme (DHSS 1983), the formal collaborative arrangements remained substantially unchanged until the 1990 NHS and Community Care Act. The 1980s also saw a shift in the location and organisation of community health services bringing closer collaborations with general practice and local authority services, especially social services (Ottewill and Wall 1990). Of particular importance to the discussion in this chapter was virtual lack of any involvement of general practitioners in these joint planning structures (Moon and North, 2000) which preceded more recent developments in PCOs and the new health and social care partnership arrangements developed from the late 1990s. More recently the Labour Government has placed an increasing emphasis on joined-up government and the need to find joined-up solutions to complex problems (Powell 1998).

This history of partnership has been covered in other texts (see for example Baggott 1998; Exworthy and Peckham 1998; Moon and North 2000) and, therefore, this chapter will mainly focus on the institutional and organisation of partnership in a primary care context from the 1990s onwards. In this chapter, therefore, the focus will be on the following two questions:

1. To what extent do PCOs represent a new dawn for improved partnership?
2. Will these organisations deliver a more integrated approach to health and care services – a goal which has eluded previous policy initiatives (Exworthy and Peckham 1998)?

Current health and social policies effectively encourage local authorities and health and social care organisations, including PCOs, to develop and make a commitment to more inclusive government through consultative and participative approaches to local policies and practices. In addition, there is a drive towards 'joined-up' thinking, generating 'joined-up' solutions to 'joined-up' problems (Clarence and Painter 1998; Powell and Exworthy 2001). In other words, the issues facing local communities – such as tackling health inequalities, promoting and tackling social exclusion, etc. – are multifaceted and require multi-agency and multidisciplinary attention. This new approach is embodied, for example, in the *NHS Plan* (DoH 2000) which stated that:

> The NHS will help develop Local Strategic Partnerships, into which, in the medium term, health action zones and other local action zones could be integrated to strengthen links between health, education, employment and other causes of social exclusion.

Collaboration and partnerships are the cornerstones of government policy in respect of achieving a joined-up approach to health and social care and to tackle wider problems such as health inequalities and social exclusion. PCOs are very much in the vanguard of local approaches to partnership through intra- and inter- organisational structures and processes. The shift from primary medical care to primary health care and the broadening of the organisation of primary care from general practice to primary care organisation provide a more appropriate context for partnerships to occur, and, as discussed in earlier chapters, partnership is an essential feature of a primary health care approach. In order to examine policy and practice in this area it is important to define what is meant by partnership and develop an analytical framework.

Primary Care and Social Care: a Framework for Partnership

The growing emphasis upon partnership arises in part from the acknowledged limits of organisational individualism. Huxham and Macdonald (1992), for example, identify four 'pitfalls of individualism':

1. *repetition:* where two or more organisations carry out an action or task which need only be done by one;
2. *omission:* where activities that are important to the objectives of more than one organisation are not carried out because they have not been identified as important, because they come into no organisation's remit, or because each organisation assumes the other is performing the activity;
3. *divergence:* the actions of the various organisations may become diluted across a range of activities, rather than used towards common goals;
4. *counterproduction:* organisations working in isolation may take actions that conflict with those taken by others.

Against such a background, Warren *et al.* (1974: 16) use the following definition of 'co-ordination':

> A structure or process of concerted decision-making wherein the decisions or action of two or more organisations are made simultaneously in part or in whole with some deliberate degree of adjustment to each other.

The Nuffield Institute developed a useful framework for analysing the collaborative dimension (Hudson *et al.* 1997) which distinguishes between isolation, encounter, communication, collaboration and integration (Hudson *et al.* 1998). Each of these represents points on a collaborative continuum ranging from weak to strong. In fact the first and last points are not strictly collaborative measures, since isolation involves *no* interagency activity, while integration is strictly an *alternative* to collaboration.

Isolation refers to the complete absence of joint activity in which members of different agencies never meet, talk or write to one another. *Encounter* exists where there is some interagency and inter-professional contact, but this is informal, ad hoc and marginal to the goals of the separate organisations. In those inter-organisational relationships characterised by isolation and encounter we would expect to find:

- loose-knit and lowly connected networks;
- infrequent and ad hoc interaction;
- divergently perceived organisational goals and interests;
- inter-professional rivalry and stereotyping.

Communication arises where separate organisations do engage in joint working of a formal and structured nature, but this still tends to be marginal to separate organisational goals, and needs to be able to demonstrate how such activity will help achieve these respective goals. In those inter-organisational relationships characterised by communication we would expect to find:

- more frequent interactions;
- a willingness to share information about mutual roles, responsibilities and availability;
- a willingness to share some information about patients/users whose needs cross organisational boundaries;
- some commitment to joint training;
- nominated persons who have some responsibility for liaison;
- relatively loose-knit and lowly connected networks;
- limited acceptance of the notion of membership of a team;
- prime loyalty to the employing organisation;
- a high degree of expectation of reciprocation.

Collaboration involves a recognition by separate agencies that joint working is central to their mainstream activities and implies a trusting relationship in which organisations are seen to be reliable partners. The following features might be expected to be present:

- a willingness to participate in some formal and structured pattern of joint working;
- acknowledgement of the value and existence of a team, and agreement on the membership;
- relatively close-knit and highly connected networks;
- a high degree of mutual trust and respect;
- a low degree of expectation of immediate reciprocation;
- a high degree of recognition of common interests, goals and interdependency;
- mutual secondments and other forms of cross-boundary deployment;
- clustering or co-location of personnel;
- joint assessments;
- joint planning;

- joint service delivery;
- joint commissioning.

Finally, *integration* represents a point on the continuum at which the degree of collaboration is so high that the separate organisations no longer see their separate identity as significant, and may be willing to contemplate the creation of a unitary organisation. Such arrangements would exhibit at least some of the following:

- very close-knit and highly connected networks;
- little regard for reciprocation in relationships;
- a mutual and diffuse sense of long-term obligation;
- very high degrees of trust and respect;
- joint arrangements which are mainstream rather than marginal;
- joint arrangements which encompass both strategic and operational issues;
- some shared or single management arrangements;
- joint commissioning at both macro and micro levels.

It would be wrong, however, to characterise the relationship between health and social care as being uni-dimensional – simply a linear continuum between isolation of primary care and integration with other agencies. This needs to be viewed both in the context of primary care partnership with social services and other agencies – other local authority departments, voluntary agencies and other primary care organisations. In practice, partnership occurs at a number of levels. In a study on joint commissioning Rummery and Glendinning (1997) identified three levels of partnership: locality/area-based commissioning; practice-based commissioning; and commissioning for individuals. It is not the intention of this chapter to examine only the commissioning context of the collaborative relationship but this does provide a useful model to examine the levels at which the relationship occurs.

Partnership can be seen to exist between individual workers in the context of inter-professional partnership (discussed in Chapter 8). There are important and ongoing relationships between social workers and primary care staff which continue within, but independently of, organisational and institutional arrangements – although it is presumably hoped that such arrangements support rather than hinder such joint working. In recent years there has been an increase in joint educational approaches with the training of social workers and health care students (e.g. University of the West of England). However, professional networks still tend to be uni-professional, although the Faculty of Public Health Medicine has begun to broaden itself into a more multi-disciplinary profession in line with government policy. Partnership can be contextualised in both formal and informal ways. Formal partnerships include organisational arrangements, such as cross-representation and joint budgets, and informal arrangements are those such as professionals working alongside each other and local networking. Generally formalisation occurs at all levels,

⇐ National ⇒	Joined-up Government
⇑ ⇑ ⇑ ⇑ Health Education Environment Transport ⇓ ⇓ ⇓ ⇓	⇑ Vertical partnership ⇓
⇐ Local ⇒	Local partnerships
⇐ Hoizontal partnerships ⇒	

Figure 9.1   Vertical and Horizontal Partnerships

with policy gradually increasing institutional and organisational structures to support this. Informal approaches have tended to be seen as less important but have also occurred predominantly at senior management levels and between professionals working in the community.

Traditionally government policy on health social care partnership has operated at these three main levels. However, it is also important to consider the context within which local partnerships can prosper. Since 1997 there has been an emphasis on the need for joined-up government – joined-up solutions to complex problems (Powell and Exworthy 2001). Powell and Exworthy argue that partnerships can be characterised both horizontally (within a national or local context) and vertically (between the national and local). This can be seen diagrammatically as in Figure 9.1.

National Partnerships: Joined-up Government

Since 1997 there has been an increasing concern to develop joined-up processes at a national and regional level, as well as increasing vertical partnership. Since 1997, the Labour Government has pursued a 'collaborative discourse' (Clarence and Painter, 1998) which has included 'joined-up government at the centre and joined-up governance at local levels' (Powell and Exworthy 2001: 21). Many attempts to promote greater collaboration (possibly including the current policy drive) have been 'largely rhetorical invocations of a vague ideal'. However, many argue that the collaboration has become the *zeitgeist* of the Labour Government (e.g. Hudson 1999b) as a result of its third-way philosophy (Powell 1998). As a response to the perceptions of fragmentation under the internal market (introduced by the Conservatives), various mechanisms have been introduced that cannot be considered simply rhetorical. These have been applied at both national and local levels and have been variously called joint working, partnership and collaboration.

At the national level, joined-up government has been promoted in policy-making and service delivery through cross-departmental programmes such as Sure Start, as well as initiatives (such as teenage pregnancy and rough sleepers) under the auspices of the Social Exclusion Unit (based in the Cabinet Office). These seek to overcome the long-recognised problem of departmentalism, i.e. the strong tradition and culture that civil servants and ministers seek to defend and, if possible, augment in their own sphere of responsibility (Kavanagh and Richards 2001). 'Turf wars' can ensue when one department appears to overstep its apparent role. Ministers thus become 'barons'. Issues that cut across more than one department (such as health inequalities or youth crime) might suffer from a lack of departmental ownership or sufficient accountability. Thus, Kavanagh and Richards (2001: 17) conclude that

> It is questionable to what extent joined-up government can be properly established when departments remain crucial holders of resources and continue to dominate policy-making and policy delivery.

Joined-up government can be interpreted as a rational solution to perceived fragmentation which matches the thrust of the Labour Government's emphasis on evidence-base approach to policy (Klein 2000). This has been summed up by Labour's dictum, 'what counts is what works'. This begs the question that priorities (what counts) are clear and unambiguous and that what works is unequivocal and uncontested (Exworthy *et al.* 2002).

Local Partnerships

At the local level, these new mechanisms include a statutory duty of partnership upon health and local authorities, with provisions for local strategic partnerships. Arrangements between health authorities, and Social Services Departments include the development of Joint Investment Plans and Community Care Plans. At this level there is also the focus on the Health Improvement Plan and Health Action Zones have also been developed – although these have a wider public health remit. In England at the level of the PCO there was an attempt to engage social services structurally by initially allocating one of the PCG board places and PCT Executive places to a social services representative. The development of Care Trusts takes these developments further with joint health and social care provision for adults (DoH 2000; DoH 2001b). PCG/PCTs have also been involved in developing partnership groups with a wide interagency representation and developing joint plans. In Wales these institutional and organisational arrangements are extended to include a further

Table 9.1 Horizontal Collaborative Arrangements

	Local authority	SSD	Voluntary organisations	NHS	Policy context
HA/LA	Strategic/ Planning	Strategic/ Planning	Strategic/ Planning	Strategic	Local Social Partnerships
PCO	Planning HImP	Organisational/ Commissioning	Organisational (in Wales)	Organisational/ Commissioning	HImPs, Community plans
Practice	–	Action on specific issues	Action on specific issues	Organisational/ commissioning	

local authority representative on Local Health Group boards along with voluntary agency representation. LHGs are also coterminous with local authorities. While these arrangements have focused on planning and strategy they have also included approaches to joint commissioning. Finally, at a practice level joint working has traditionally developed around specific issues or the need to meet individual patient/client needs but is supported through child protection measures under the Childrens' Act and community care developments in the 1990s (Glendinning *et al.* 1998; Moon and North 2000).

Local partnerships can, therefore, be seen to have a range of agencies involved, an organisational context and a range of purposes. These are shown in Table 9.1.

While much emphasis has been placed, both in policy and in practice, on health and social services partnerships, the widening health agenda means that for PCOs partnerships will also include: other local authority departments such as housing, education, leisure and environmental health; local voluntary agencies; and private organisations, and there will be an increased emphasis on partnership within the NHS: between practices; with hospitals; and potentially with other PCOs (see Chapter 10). This is a potentially complex set of relationships and shifts the focus to seeing partnerships as a network. Since 1997 the Labour Government has been trying to establish network co-ordination as the key organisational framework for the NHS and social care to take the place of the internal market arrangements introduced in the early 1990s – although the concept of the purchaser/provider split remains to varying degrees in the UK. In order to understand the current policy context for collaboration and partnership it is necessary to examine more clearly policy developments since 1990.

The Policy Background

The 1989 community care White Paper *Caring for People* (DoH, 1989b) provides a good starting-point from which to examine policy developments in the 1990s. This sets out the then Conservative Government's policies which were intended to provide a context within which interagency relationships could be revitalised. The White Paper provided a framework for partnership which had four elements:

1. Clarification of 'who does what' through the more explicit recognition of the distinction between health and social care as the basis for funding health and social services respectively.
2. Allocation of responsibility to social services departments for ensuring that assessment and care management processes take place within a multi-disciplinary context where appropriate.
3. Redefinition of joint planning through an emphasis on outcomes rather than the mechanics of joint planning and finance.
4. Strengthened financial incentives for joint working through the transfer of social security funds to SSDs and the creation of new specific grants.

Guidance on the development of joint community care plans, as part of the implementation of *Caring for People,* emphasised the need for joint agreement between health and social services agencies, and other agencies (particularly housing) about the needs of particular populations or client groups, and the development of jointly agreed strategies to meet these needs. The Department subsequently produced detailed guidance in the form of a workbook on joint commissioning (DoH 1995c), and the importance of joint working has consistently featured in the annual NHS Planning and Priorities Guidance. With respect to GP involvement in these processes, little had changed from the 1980s and on the whole GPs were not engaged with community care planning processes (Moon and North 2000). The purchaser/provider split also created problems in partnership with the voluntary sector where concerns have been raised about the role of voluntary agencies as both providers and advocates of service users. However, *Caring for People* provided a key framework for Social Services Departments to develop collaborative arrangements with the NHS.

As earlier chapters have discussed, the 1990s provided for rapid policy development in the area of primary care, with key organisational developments initially focused on commissioning arrangements – including fundholding, GP commissioning and Total Purchasing – but more latterly incorporating the development of primary and community services and public health. Partnership was mainly an implicit goal for general practice and primary care until *Primary Care: Delivering the Future* (DoH 1996a) placed a specific emphasis on partnership as a key element of delivering primary care. This view was later supported, and further developed, within Labour Government policy from 1997 that also sought to widen the notion of partnership beyond social care.

Despite these developments, research into the impact of these collaborative arrangements did not suggest that long-standing fragmentary forces were entirely overcome (Hudson *et al.* 1998), and the Labour Government elected in 1997, invested in a further and stronger push for effective joint working.

While devolution has meant some divergence between developments in England, Scotland and Wales, there also similarities. The key exception is in Northern Ireland where there have always been combined Health and Social Care Boards. The publication of *The New NHS* White Paper (DoH 1997) contained a firm commitment 'to get the NHS to work in partnership'. This emphasis was also reflected in *Designed to Care* (Scottish Office 1998). In part this involved strengthening relationships *within* the NHS, but it is also recognised that *inter*agency arrangements needed to be strengthened. This has been reflected in several measures:

- the portrayal of Health Improvement Programmes and Local Strategic Partnerships as vehicles for interagency partnership;
- the introduction of a new statutory duty of partnership 'to work together for the common good';
- a duty upon local authorities to promote the economic, social and environmental well-being of their areas;
- the establishment of 'programmes of care' between clinicians and social services to promote planning and resource management across organisational boundaries;
- the pursuit of coterminosity between health and social services boundaries in relation to Primary Care Organisations;
- joint monitoring of partnerships across health and social care by Regional Offices of the NHSE and the Regional Social Services Inspectorate;
- local authority/SSD membership on health authorities and PCOs;
- the creation of pilot Health Action Zones based upon local partnerships.

In addition to these developments, there was a promise to legalise the pooling of budgets between health and social services agencies, a commitment (from April 1999) to the pooling of hospital, community health and primary care budgets in a number of experimental pilot sites, and an anticipation that localities will be required to produce Joint Investment Plans, while professionals will work together better to improve the content and process of multi-disciplinary assessment of older people. As discussed in Chapter 3, the explicit aim of the government was to replace the internal market as the mechanism of co-ordination with a system of 'integrated care, based on partnership' (DoH 1997: Section 1.3). While the vision was broad, encompassing both vertical and horizontal perspectives, the key emphasis was on improving integration between health and social care.

The approach across the UK was not a unitary one as there are important territorial differences. In Wales, Local Health Groups are coterminous with District Councils to encourage closer partnership, and in Scotland, the Scottish Primary Care Trusts have limited commissioning responsibilities with Health Boards retaining the major commissioning role. In Northern Ireland the situation is somewhat interesting as the Health Boards have provided health and social care since the 1970s and there were concerns that developing PCOs would in reality fracture the existing partnership, although the favoured models of development keep a combined health and social care approach.

A number of these measures were central to NHS *Planning and Priorities* guidance (NHS Executive 1997) issued in the Autumn of 1997 which also set out the key principles for the NHS in England and Wales, placing a renewed emphasis on equity, effectiveness, partnership and accountability – issues which were further elaborated in *Partnership in Action* (DoH 1998b) a year later. In *Partnership in Action* the government outlined a number of proposals to remove legal boundaries on the pooling of budgets, for transferring funds between agencies to allow lead commissioning and the widening of powers of health and social care agencies to provide integrated health and social care services. These powers were formalised within the NHS Act 1999. The partnerships had to be focused on the needs of users and be justified by improvements in services to these users. Agencies also had to establish effective monitoring arrangements and demonstrate accountability. In particular, pooled funds had to be separately audited and agencies were required to have partnership agreements.

This emphasis on partnership was also echoed in the Social Services White Paper, *Modernising Social Services* (DoH 1998c). In 1999 the House of Commons Health Select Committee investigated partnership between health and social care and identified the need for an integrated approach. They saw the involvement of social services and community NHS trusts in PCGs and PCTs as 'providing an excellent opportunity for improved collaboration between health and social services, but falls well short of unifying the two agencies' (House of Commons 1999: para. 68).

These organisational developments clearly challenge traditional organisational and professional boundaries. They are also leading to greater integration between agencies and also of primary care and ultimately social care services into the NHS. At the same time we are seeing an increasingly diverse number of agencies and services. Before looking at some of these developments – particularly arising from the NHS Plan in England – it is worth reviewing the evidence on primary care partnerships with social care from the late 1990s. The following section, therefore, examines the development of primary care organisations during the 1990s and explores the extent to which these new forms of primary care have engaged in partnerships. Most of the evidence relates to England where there have been a number of studies examining the experience of PCGs in particular.

Reviewing the Evidence: Partnership in Practice

This section reviews the research on partnership between primary care and social care. The focus is predominantly on the post-1997 experience drawing on work by Hudson *et al.* (1998; 1999), the Audit Commission (1999; 2000),

Shapiro *et al.* (1999) and the National Tracker Survey of PCGs (2001). However, before examining this work in more detail it is worth briefly reviewing the experience of these early PCOs' partnership with social services leading up to the reforms post-1997.

Research on GP Fundholding found that their main focus was on commissioning for individual patients and that little joint working was undertaken with social services (Audit Commission 1995; Glennerster *et al.* 1994). The development of multi-funds offered more opportunities as these had a broader geographical base but again the approach was dominated by health care commissioning (Le Grand *et al.* 1998). It was the development of more locality-based approaches such as GP Commissioning and Total Purchasing that perhaps held most hope for developing joint working. However, again the evidence for this is limited although Total Purchasing Pilots (TPPs) did start to develop partnerships with social services (Hudson *et al.* 1998).

Mays *et al.* (1998) reported that TPPs mainly limited their initial purchasing intentions to service areas where they had a special interest and were related mainly to local issues. The evaluation of the pilot projects found that there was little awareness of national or local policies for community and continuing care (Myles *et al.* 1998). In terms of partnership, the main focus in the pilot projects has been on service developments in the sense that pilot status has seemed to act as a catalyst to developing joint approaches with social services and often included organisational approaches such as SSD representation within TPP executive boards.

In a report on the first two years of TPPs (Mays *et al.* 1998) a number of key lessons were identified:

- TPPs focused mainly on local health service issues at a practice level rather than strategic service changes;
- change was focused on developments in primary care rather than secondary care;
- changes in community care were often based on past experiences and previous initiatives rather than new innovations;
- boundary differences between TPPs and HAs, providers and social services created enormous problems in relation to budget-setting and making service changes.

The other major change that occurred alongside developments within primary care itself was a gradual shift by health authorities towards locality commissioning structures (Exworthy 1993b; Balogh 1996; Exworthy and Peckham 1998a; Exworthy and Peckham 1999). Locality approaches were in one sense a reaction by DHAs to changes in primary care but also provided structures for drawing together representatives from different NHS and LA organisations. These developments need to be seen in the context of decentralisation and localisation across the public sector generally (Hudson *et al.* 1998) and generated new debates about the importance of coterminosity as a precondition of greater partnership between local health and social care agencies (Exworthy and Peckham 1998a; Exworthy and Peckham 1999).

We will now turn to examine the research on PCGs and partnership. The first major study examining partnership and PCGs was undertaken by the authors with Hudson and Callaghan (Hudson *et al.* 1998; Hudson *et al.* 1999). This involved a survey of health authorities, social services and housing departments in the two Regions, Northern and Yorkshire and South and West Regions in 1998 and in-depth case studies of PCGs (two from each Region). Other early studies included another by Hudson for the Association of Directors of Social Services (Hudson 1999b) and a survey by the Social Services Inspectorate (SSI 1999). These surveys were all conducted during the run-up to and the first six-month period of PCGs (which were established in April 1998).

The survey in the Northern and Yorkshire and South and West Regions (Peckham and Exworthy 1998) found that, while all social services departments were represented on PCG boards, the level of representation varied. In this survey 2 respondents reported councillor representation (1 in each region), 10 reported director or assistant director representation (8 in Northern and Yorkshire and 2 in South and West) and 13 reported locality or area manager representation (6 and 7 respectively). It would appear that where PCGs were more coterminous with unitary authorities social services representation was more likely to be at director or assistant director level. Conversely, the larger the local authority area covering more than one primary care group the more likely the representation was at area manager level. These findings were similar to a survey undertaken for the Association of Directors of Social Services (ADSS) in the summer of 1999 (Hudson 1999c). This survey found that around 10 per cent of PCGs had director level representatives, 33 per cent assistant director and the remainder were third-tier managers. Interestingly, around 15 per cent of the boards had additional social services representation and nearly 20 per cent had an elected member presence (although not always a social services committee member).

This difference in levels of representation had important implications because the sort of partnership that was developed between PCGs and social services. Higher level representation suggested a more strategic approach – potentially ideal for commissioning roles and area manager role had a more operational approach better suited to local developmental and service provision roles (Hudson *et al.* 1999). The survey by Hudson for the ADSS found that most SSD representatives needed more time and support to undertake their PCG activities and that mechanisms for feedback were very patchy.

In the two-Region survey few (five) housing departments indicated that they would be represented on PCG boards. In the South and West Region one housing department indicated it would be represented at councillor level. While actual representation is low in the South and West Region, nearly half of the housing department respondents expressed a wish to be represented through co-option. The desire for representation may be related to the predominantly two-tier nature of local government in this region compared to

Northern and Yorkshire. Clearly there are compelling reasons for housing involvement in PCGs both on broad housing and public health grounds as well as in relation to community care issues. The ADSS survey in the summer of 1999 found that only about 10 per cent of all PCGs had local authority officers' representation from departments other than social services.

The findings suggest that there is a strong desire for collaboration and partnership and this has been noted elsewhere. However, the two-Region survey (Peckham and Exworthy 1999) also found that there were differences in how agencies viewed existing partnerships. Health authorities were more likely to report stronger partnerships than social services. Again, not surprisingly, housing departments reported poorer levels of partnership than social services. When asked about service integration all respondents thought services and organisations would become more integrated in the future.

The survey also asked respondents to indicate key factors that encourage or hinder partnership at a locality level. The majority of respondents emphasised the need for good-quality relationships in terms of personal relations, commitment and trust – which was seen to be best achieved through joint working. In particular, respondents cited joint priority-setting, developing joint structures and having joint responsibilities. One significant point that arose from the survey was that both social services and housing departments emphasised the importance of the national agenda for encouraging partnership. Lack of trust and debates about budgets were identified as the principle hindering factors. However, accountability issues were also highlighted – such as differing organisational and geographical boundaries, the lack of clear priorities and lack of time made available for collaborative working. When asked to identify measures of effectiveness of partnership the respondents provided a wide range of indicators with little consensus between organisations. There were, though, a number of indicators that were more frequently cited, such as user satisfaction as a measure of the effectiveness of joint working and joint services as a measure of service configuration. These findings have important lessons for primary care groups and other PCOs in developing collaborative and responsive locally based services.

Not surprisingly the focus on partnership in these studies remained at an organisational level. However, this organisational engagement provided, in some places, opportunities for more directed joint working on health improvement around Single Regeneration Bid funding and on service delivery (NHSE *et al.* 1999). Similar messages about organisational links were also identified in an SSI report on services for older people (SSI 1999). The SSI found that there was a broad range of small-scale partnerships between social services and primary health practitioners and professionals but few strategic partnerships. This may reflect the traditional general practice focus (Rummery and Glendinning 1998) and link with a lack of engagement by GPs, in particular, in joint working. The SSI identifies potential through joint investment plans for PCGs (and PCTs) to develop more integrated service plans with SSDs and it was optimistic about future partnerships. PCT status has provided the opportunity to reorganise community health services with, in England, community nursing and other community services being transferred from Community Health NHS Trusts to the new PCTs. This may provide a greater impetus for developing PCT/SSD, and even wider LA, partnerships, as traditionally, much of the service level partnership at a primary care level has occurred between community nursing and social services (Ottewill and Wall 1990). This development of horizontal partnerships has not been mirrored to the same extent by the integration of providing and commissioning functions in PCTs.

The optimism was also found by Hudson *et al.* (1999) in the case studies conducted in the two Regions. In the case studies PCG board members and other key stakeholders (NHS Trusts, housing, CHCs, etc.) were interviewed and it was found that that there was an enormous amount of goodwill towards the concept of the PCG and the potential of PCGs to develop good partnerships. It was also clear that while there was little experience of utilising the freedoms outlined in *Partnership in Action*, there was support for the principle of the freedoms promised therein. Such goodwill will be extremely important but it is not clear how far this can overcome other problems identified, such as the enormity of the task, low resourcing of PCGs, tensions between practices and GP board members, and unease about the current boundary arrangements and size of some PCGs and PCTs. These tensions are likely to increase as PCTs develop into larger, more complex, organisations and then as newer Care Trusts emerge. However, the research found that there was a will for PCGs to develop new ways of working and certainly there is some hope for improved working to develop primary care and community services based on experience from the TPP pilots and the intentions of PCGs. However, it was clear from this research that there are still considerable problems when it comes to working with local communities.

The key finding for Hudson *et al.* (1999) was that, in terms of the co-ordination continuum, there was some bunching around communication. Almost by definition, the formal representation of many of the relevant parties on the PCG board guaranteed that relationships had gone beyond the point of *isolation and encounter*. However, there was still relatively little that could be categorised as *collaboration*, and even less that could be seen as *integration* – in only one of the case study sites was there any speculation about Primary Care Trusts encompassing social services to create a new 'integrated' PCT. What was discernible was evidence of *communication*.

This description clearly did not fit all parts of each PCG, but it did contain the elements that appeared most frequently. At such an early stage of development this was interpreted as an acceptable level of attainment, for where more substantial developments had taken place there was normally a history of partnership working upon which PCGs could draw. However, given the low involvement of GPs in previous joint working initiatives few places had this basis to develop from.

By contrast, LHGs in Wales are more firmly established as partnership organisations. While there is a similar representation of social services on the board (as in England) there is a further local authority representative and a representative from local voluntary organisations. GPs do not form the majority on the Board. Unlike their PCG/PCT counterparts in England, LHGs are tending to focus more on broader partnership aims. In a survey of their first year the Audit Commission (2000) characterised the difference as LHGs making steadier progress on a broad front while PCGs were making faster progress on a narrower front.

More recent research on PCGs/PCTs in England has charted the development of health and social care partnership. The National Tracker Survey found that nearly half of the PCGs and PCTs surveyed do not routinely consult with social services when commissioning community health services and fewer consult when commissioning acute care (Glendinning *et al.* 2001). In contrast, the relationships between frontline social services staff and community-based and practice-based health professionals was improving (*ibid.*). The survey found that partnerships were slowly developing in joint commissioning, with the NHS Plan priorities most widely quoted as service goals particularly in relation to broader national priorities such as older people and mental health services. Incompatible boundaries continued to be seen as an important barrier to good partnership working, as did structural and organisational differences and a preoccupation in PCGs and PCTs with medical issues (*ibid.*).

The Current Context

Current developments in creating partnerships between primary care and social care are focused in the establishment of Local Strategic Partnerships and organisational changes to health and social care. The Health and Social Care Act 2001 placed a 'duty of partnership' on each agency. As part of this, Health Authorities and Primary Care Groups and Trusts are required to have representation on their Boards from the local authority. There are distinct differences in organisational developments in England, Scotland and Wales. However, the principles of partnership and the development of local strategic partnerships are characteristic of policy across the whole of the UK, although in different forms.

The Local Government Act 2000 placed on local authorities a requirement to prepare community strategies as part of their duty to promote the economic, social and environmental well-being of their areas. Each local area will be required to have a Local Strategic Partnership (LSP) that brings together the public, private, voluntary and community sectors in pursuit of the aims of the local community strategy. Such changes are located within the broader framework laid down by the Act relating to the modernisation of local government and democratic renewal. LSPs are a key strategic element of intersectoral partnerships in England (DETR 2000; DETR 2001) and have key roles in engaging communities in partnership arrangements and provide rationalisation of other strategic planning processes. There are fears that they are being dominated by local authorities with little community input (Biles *et al.* 2001) and that they may simply be another layer of bureaucracy. Certainly Health Improvement and Modernisation Plans remain separate from community plans, being developed by local authorities, and there does not appear, at present, to be any significant dovetailing of NHS planning with these new LSPs. Yet public health, in its broadest terms, is clearly expected to be a prominent issue for the LSPs to pick up; addressing health inequalities is an important consideration and, for example, Learning Disability Partnership Boards are to be located within the LSP framework (DoH 2002b). There is a similar scheme in Scotland where local authorities have to develop community planning to provide a strategic framework for joint planning, partnership working, and to address fragmented public policy and service provision (Fernie and McCarthy 2001). However, the main focus of these partnerships is on urban regeneration and it is too early to see what impact these approaches will have on a shared health and social care agenda or on public health. It is likely that such approaches will increasingly play an important role given the new duty on local authorities to promote the well-being of their populations and the increasing emphasis on health in regeneration strategies.

In 2000 the publication of the *NHS Plan* provided a further impetus to the development of partnership and provided for a potential next step in the form of Care Trusts (DoH 2000). The *NHS Plan*, which applies to England and Wales, highlights partnership aiming to develop the implementation of the Health Act 1999 flexibilities, invest in intermediate care and make specific organisational arrangements for improving local partnerships. In addition to Primary Care Organisations with social services representation on the board, the Plan proposed:

1. NHS community care trusts, which bring together providers of health and social care into one organisation;
2. Care Trusts, which integrate primary and community health and social care, and also fulfil a commissioning role.

Table 9.2 The Organisational Context of Partnership

	Community health services	Primary health care services	Social services	Commissioning
NHS community care trusts	✓		✓	
PCG/Ts	✓ in some cases	✓		✓
Care Trusts	✓	✓	✓	✓

Thus in England three forms of PCO will develop that include different responsibilities as shown in Table 9.2.

However, it was not just formal organisations that were highlighted in the Plan. There were also specific proposals to develop, for example:

- *rapid response teams:* made up of nurses, care workers, social workers, therapists and GPs working to provide emergency care for people at home and helping to prevent unnecessary hospital admissions;
- *arrangements at GP practice or social work level to ensure that older people receive a one-stop service:* this might involve employing or designating the sort of key workers or link workers used in Somerset or basing case managers in GP surgeries;
- *integrated home care teams:* so that people receive the care they need when they are discharged from hospital to help them live independently at home.

In Scotland the flexibilities have been integrated into three proposed organisational forms to take partnership working forward, although these lack the independent legal form of Care Trusts (CCD7/2001). These are:

1. Joint Management Structure – where health and social care budgets are aligned but which has no independent legal identity;
2. Partnership Body (Aligned budgets) – has a distinct identity but not a legal entity, cannot employ staff but offers streamlined organisation and management;
3. Partnership Body (Pooled budget) – has a host partner and distinct identity but no legal identity; however, host agency employs staff.

The *NHS Plan* also established specific performance measures for partnerships:

- To reduce the risk of loss of independence following unplanned and avoidable admissions for people over the age of 75;
- To improve the delivery of appropriate care and treatment to psychiatric patients discharged from hospital;
- To reduce the national percentage of delayed discharges of people aged over 75 years occupying acute hospital beds.

At the time of writing it is too early to identify whether such arrangements have stimulated partnership working. The first 9 English Care Trust demonstrator sites were announced in July 2001 with a further 29 expressions of interest registered with the Department of Health (see Box 9.1). However, most sites did not go live in April 2002 but most should be up and running within 2002 (Revans 2001). Some developments are seen as a natural progression (such as Wiltshire) whereas others are being developed across new partnership boundaries (such as Camden and Islington where two local authorities are involved). There may, however, also be schisms within social work itself as proposals for Care Trust pilots from 2002 have specific focii, as shown in Box 9.1.

Box 9.1   Care Trust Pilots

Area	*Client group*
Bexley	Older people
Birmingham	Mental health
	Learning difficulties
Brighton and Hove	Range of vulnerable client groups
Essex	Housing and older people
New Forest	Older people and physical disabilities
North Somerset	All services except mental health
Northumberland	Working age adults (except mental health)
Wiltshire	Older people, physical disabilities, learning difficulties and children's health

---

These new forms of organisation are based upon a horizontal and value-added metaphor (as compared with a vertical or command-and-control metaphor). Moves to joined-up agencies (such as Care Trusts or integrated services) will create new management concerns and challenges, not least that of how to achieve integration. In the main, most attempts to change organisational forms in order to attain integration have taken place within the existing bureaucracy of either the NHS or local government. One key, major shift can be characterised as a shift from vertical bureaucracies to horizontal corporation. Castells (1996) argues that this shift is characterised by a new emphasis on:

- organisation around process not task;
- a flat hierarchy;
- team management;
- performance management based upon customer satisfaction rewards and team performance;
- maximisation of contacts with suppliers and customers;
- information, training and retraining of employees at all levels.

Revans (2001) argues that despite widespread confusion and the lack of central guidance there is an underlying enthusiasm about the potential benefits of Care Trusts for service users. Research in an established combined Trust in Somerset post-1998 has suggested that there is room for optimism as professionals develop shared culture, which is seen as essential for developing integrated services (Peck *et al.* 2001). This finding is also supported by Hudson (2002) who also found room for optimism in developing inter-professional working between health and social care professionals.

Conclusion

Partnership is currently being institutionalised through organisational changes within both horizontal and vertical dimensions. The restructuring of the NHS in England has seen the development of two layers of operation – Strategic Health Authorities, and Primary Care and Secondary Care Trusts. In Wales the moves were to abolish health authorities, replacing them with Local Health Groups coterminous with local authorities, while Scotland retained its two-tier approach of Health Boards and Trusts. The proposals provide for differing levels of integration between commissioning and providing functions but all contain a strong focus on partnership through institutional and management arrangements. This reflects the Labour Government's political approach to developing public services and a clean break with the internal market approach of its Conservative predecessors.

From a policy perspective these moves are interesting as they suggest a centrally driven shift towards PCOs. Yet PCOs are supposed to find their own solutions to partnership issues while working within a very prescribed organisational format that prescribes who the partners are. For policy, therefore, a key question must be whether PCOs will be able to devise their own solutions to partnership issues or whether they are being forced towards integration at an unnatural pace. What is clear from surveys on health and social care partnership is that there is wide support for a partnership approach among frontline workers and management staff. Clearly the process flexibilities and new organisational forms provide ways to overcome what have been seen as often insurmountable barriers to joint working (Exworthy and Peckham 1998a). Yet the very organisational changes may possibly destroy many of the fledgling partnerships that have been established since 1997 (Glendinning *et al.* 2001). Constant organisational change has a tendency to shift the focus of attention towards internal organisational issues (an issue identified in research on new primary care organisations from TPPs onwards – see, for example, Mays *et al.* 2001d). In addition, changes in organisation have also often resulted in changes to geographical boundaries resulting in staff having to develop relationships with new people.

These challenges can be seen in England with the development of three alternative partnership arrangements – two based within PCT organisational formats and a third in a provider-only format. Already PCT has generated reconfigurations of PCG boundaries. The development of Care Trusts takes this a step further but also raises important questions about the nature of social care and its broader relationships within local authorities (such as with housing).

It is possible to discern two tensions, which are at the heart of the move towards partnership approaches between health and social care but also reflect the wider partnership agenda (see Chapters 10 and 11). The first is that between integration and fragmentation. Both these forces are apparent in policy objectives and organisational development. The integration of social care into primary care will tend to fragment its relationship with other organisations. There would also appear to be an increasing emphasis on placing PCOs at the front line replacing health authorities – thus creating a fragmentation of commissioning and established local partnerships built up over a long period. The second relates to the vertical dimension of partnership which sees a tension between decentralisation and centralisation. The government has continued to state that one of its key aims is to decentralise decision-making and responsibility in the NHS to PCOs. Yet at the same time it is also committed to a national health service with equal access and standards across the country. Thus PCOs see themselves constrained by an increasingly nationally imposed agenda through SAFFs, NSFs, NICE, CHI, etc. Even partnership is being driven centrally as part of the modernisation agenda. Care Trusts will be established from April 2002. While such moves are voluntary, the increasing emphasis being placed on Trust status (originally a voluntary development) may reflect a political impatience to establish mandatory partnerships at local levels.

CHAPTER 10

Patients, the Public and Primary Care

Introduction

In many ways the NHS in the UK has been built upon the relationships between health care providers in the community and their patients. In the past health care was predominantly undertaken by local doctors (general practitioners) and community nurses who would work both in the community and in local hospitals. Even today, in any one year most of the population will have contact with a primary care professional. It is the relationship between the doctor and patient that lies at the heart of the UK's primary medical care service (Gillam *et al.* 2001). Yet this focus on the patient's relationship with primary care hides a more complex relationship between local primary care providers and local communities. The development of community nursing was very much driven by a focus on local communities (Ottewill and Wall 1990) and the role of the general practitioner in the nineteenth century was also much more about his link with the community he worked in.

However, the increasing medicalisation of health care delivery during the twentieth century created a paradigm shift in health care, with doctors and nurses focusing more on the delivery of care to individual patients and their families. This paradigm shift was reinforced by organisational changes in the delivery of health care through the expansion of insurance schemes in the early part of the last century, the establishment of comprehensive general practice following the introduction of the NHS in 1949, the transfer of community nursing to the NHS in 1974 and contractual and financial changes in the 1980s and 1990s. However, this paradigm of the individual patient relationship did not remain unchallenged during this time, and organisational changes in the late 1990s and early into the current century have directly raised the need to explore the complex relationship between primary care and the local community. In addition, over the last 20 years there has been an increasing emphasis on involving patients and the public in health care and there are specific contexts at a primary care level for the relationships between:

- patients and primary care practitioners;
- patient/self-help groups and primary care organisations;

- the public and primary care organisations as commissioning groups;
- public health and primary care organisations.

Proposals which have developed from the NHS Plan (DoH 2000; DoH 2001b) are also radically reforming arrangements for patient and public involvement in the NHS. These changes have particular implications for primary care organisations as they develop to Trust status.

This chapter examines the relationship between primary care and the public. In particular, it explores key concepts of participation and involvement in general practice and primary care more generally examining the evidence for supporting such involvement and how far this occurs in practice. It also assesses the potential of primary care to develop this area of activity in the light of past experience. The discussion will focus on the dichotomy between the individual and the public and how this relates to consumerist and democratic models of involvement. It will also explore professional–lay relationships and the broader role of structural interests.

Establishing a Policy Framework

The policy framework for patient and public involvement is set at a number of levels within the health service. It is also true that it is not just those policies directly aimed at such relationships – as seen increasingly from the mid-1980s onwards – but also other policies on the organisation of general practice and the regulation and pursuance of professional practice. For example, the basis of the individual patient relationship and the GP is at the heart of primary care and the GP contract as well as being closely related to the concept of clinical autonomy. Shifting relationships brought about by changes to the GP contract and changes in the organisation of primary care, such as with fundholding and more recently primary care organisations, affect the way professionals relate to their patients and to the wider public in their locality (Moon and North 2000).

Policy on patient and public involvement has been developed across a combination of all of Frenk's (1994) four levels of policy. At the systemic level, while predominantly concerned with the health system overall (hence the emphasis on primary care) there have been debates about issues of accountability and patient involvement which have implications for the organisation and practice of primary care. Increasingly, at the programmatic level there has been some attempt to engage local populations in decision-making processes (Lupton *et al.* 1998). Similarly, at the organisational level there has been an emphasis on providing structures for involving patients and the public in the development of primary care, such as lay representatives on PCGs and PCTs (DoH 1997) and the establishment of patient and citizen fora (DoH 2000; DoH 2001h). At the instrumental level the concern has been how to ensure the implementation of these policies and primary care professionals have begun to explore their relationships with their patients and their local populations to increase communication and collaboration.

As has been demonstrated in the preceding chapters of this book, primary care is becoming an increasingly complex area of the NHS with patients seeing a range of health care practitioners within the practice setting and their own homes. In many practices patients can choose which GP to see at any time. What does this mean for the traditional idea of the doctor and his patient? There are also different views about the relationship between the patient and the GP. Clearly doctors such as David Widgery (1991) saw themselves as patient advocates in a health, social and political sense and for Julian Tudor-Hart (1998) the patient in the community has been the focus of his life work. For other GPs the lifelong relationship that has been established between themselves and their patient, may go little further than the consulting room. However, it is important not to focus solely on the GP–patient relationship as practice and community nurses and health visitors also build up close relationships with patients and also often with local community groups. Increasingly, a range of other practice and community-based staff are also providing primary care including counsellors, physiotherapists, specialist nurses (cancer, paediatric and mental health) and complementary therapists. More recently the development of Primary Care Walk-In Centres and NHS Direct have further changed the context of the patient's and public's relationship with primary care.

Such complex relationships mitigate against an easy understanding of the changing relationships between the public and primary care. The situation is further exacerbated by the context. In order to explore the relationship between policy and practice it is useful to draw on three conceptual frameworks that can be applied to the area of patient and public involvement. The first is that developed by Alford (1975) and described in more detail in Chapter 2. Alford's theory of structural interests in health care has been used as a heuristic device both in the USA and UK. Despite concerns about its explanatory power it is helpful in exposing the structural interests that underpin political processes in health systems and it provides a lucid analytical framework (Harrison *et al.* 1990; North 1995). To date, its application in the UK has been primarily in relation to an NHS dominated by health authorities and hospital providers, although recently it has been used more widely to analyse the role of patient associations (Wood 2000) and has been applied to primary care (North and Peckham 2001). It has, however, been helpful in focusing attention on embedded interests underpinning political processes within health services and in providing a lucid framework for analysis. Alford's three groups – the professional monopolisers (the medical profession), the corporate rationalisers (managers) and the community – reflecting in turn dominant, challenging and repressed interests in health care, have provided a succinct representation of the key stakeholders, visible or not, in health care politics. For Alford the professional groups are dominant but continually challenged by management with the community remaining 'unheard' because 'no social institution or political mechanisms ... insure that these interests are served' (Alford 1975: 15) and this meant that the community has to muster enormous political and organisational energies to overcome their institutionalised disadvantage.

The second framework explores the differences in consumerist and democratic approaches to involvement (Lupton *et al.* 1998). Consumerist approaches relate to a market model of organisation and focus on the individualistic nature of medical care – epitomised in general practice – with an emphasis on individual patient or user involvement. The emphasis of this approach is on the rights of consumers to information, access, choice and redress in relation to a specific service or product. This approach is often found at two levels – that of the clinical consultation and in relation to service issues. Democratic approaches are more generally concerned with issues of accountability and the wider engagement of the public with health care services. The democratic approach emphasises the importance of equity and empowerment with 'participation' a key concept. As Lupton *et al.* (1998: 45–6) argue:

> The two approaches have different implications for the extent and nature of public involvement. Whereas the consumerist model views involvement as a series of discrete episodes, the democratic model may encompass a more developmental and incremental process in which those participating broaden their perspectives and experiences through collective action.

The third framework, *patient-centred care*, is directly related to the practitioner–patient relationship – a conceptual framework increasingly being debated and discussed in relation to clinical practice (Stewart *et al.* 1995; Little *et al.* 2001; Stewart 2001). This conceptual framework provides a model for patient–practitioner encounters within a holistic approach to clinical practice. The framework is premised on involving the patient in all aspects of diagnosis and treatment, developing an equal partnership between patient and practitioner. This does not mean that the patient is always actively involved or makes treatment choices. The key concept is that the patient is engaged in making decisions about how s/he should be treated, including giving the responsibility for making choices to the practitioner – i.e. choosing not to be involved. However, to do this the patient has to be sufficiently empowered to make a conscious decision.

While neither of the first two frameworks has been specifically applied to a primary care context in the UK, they are useful in analysing policy development and are clearly reflected in primary care and broader health policy over the last 20–30 years. The third framework has been specifically reviewed within a primary care context (Little *et al.* 2001) and can be seen within the broader contexts provided by Alford and the consumerist/democratic framework. The other key concept central to the relationship between the patient–public and primary care is the concept of power. This debate is explicit within Alford's framework but is implicit in the remaining frameworks. The position of the patient and the relationship with the medical practitioner is widely discussed in the sociological and medical literature and the relationship has been viewed in both structuralist (Parsons 1951) and Foucauldian terms (Foucault 1993) (see Chapter 2). The power imbalance between general practitioners and patients can be viewed in four ways. Pendleton and Archer (1983) see doctors' power based on knowledge, moral authority and charismatic authority. Silverman (1987) has also added a further view which is based on the passing of responsibility for decision-making from the patient or carer to a health professional where difficult and risky medical procedures are being undertaken. It is also useful to draw on the power framework of structure and agency (see Chapter 2) to help understand the relationships described in this chapter where the biomedical model and authority of doctors are social structures limiting the agency of the patient.

The discussion of involvement is also commonly related to two broad concepts. The first was developed by Arnstein (1969) who envisaged a ladder of participation ranging from manipulation and therapy – where participation is an aim only as a 'feel-good' factor – to citizen control – where people are in control. Arnstein provides us with a way of thinking about participation process and the way that power is exercised within it. The other useful concept is that suggested by Hirschman (1970) who set out options for the public in terms of 'exit', 'voice' and 'loyalty'. These conceptual approaches are discussed fully elsewhere (see Lupton *et al.* 1998; Chapter 2). Here they may help to provide a useful backdrop to thinking about patient and public involvement alongside the three frameworks outlined above.

Patient and Public Involvement: a Brief History

The history of patient and public participation in primary care is a mixed one with weaknesses in general practice but some strengths in community nursing and wider primary health care services. In particular the focus has been on individual patient contacts and the wider concept of community or public participation is very underdeveloped. Yet the idea of community involvement in primary health is not new; as far back as the 1920s it provided the basis for the Peckham community health project in London. More recently the World Health Organisation focused attention on involvement by including it within its definition of primary health care developed at the 1978 Alma Ata conference:

> Primary health care is essential health care based on practical, scientifically sound and socially acceptable methods and technology made universally accessible to individuals and families in the community through *their full participation*. (emphasis added)

The emphasis on participation has since been reinterpreted by the WHO (1991) to define three sets of activity:

> a contribution by people to their own health and health care the development of organisational structures that are needed for *participation to be effective empowerment* of patients and their organisations and advocates, *so that their voice is heard not assumed*. (emphasis added)

Such a definition recognises both the individual and group perspectives related to involvement. Yet general practice in the UK is primarily driven on an individual demand basis and characterised by a dominant biomedical model. As we move towards developing primary care organisations, practitioners face a major new challenge to shift the focus from the patient and the practice list to the wider population. The idea of the Peckham Health Centre lives on and the development of new healthy living centres is part of the current government's strategy for public health (DoH 1998a) and the first centres, such as Bromley by Bow in London and those being developed in Bristol and Sandwell, are the forerunners of new community-oriented health centres or health parks.

How far these centres and PCOs will be able to manage the individual patient–practitioner partnership within a broader population perspective remains to be seen. Accountability to your patient and accountability to a population – or to the government for effectively using resources – will create tensions that will require careful management. Yet patient and public involvement are essential to the delivery of good health care and, while the relationships may be complex, the rewards for professionals and health care service users are clear. There is growing evidence to demonstrate that patient involvement is likely to lead to an improved clinical outcome (Coulter 1997) and clearly an informed user of services may gain more than simply improved health. There are also important issues in terms of addressing the health care needs of the community that require partnerships between local people and professionals (Lupton *et al.* 1998).

In the UK it was the increasing interest in primary care-led purchasing and commissioning in the 1990s that provided a focus for patient and public involvement in the UK. However, this sat within a broader context of an increasing interest in, and belief in the value of, patient and public involvement (NHSME 1992; DoH 1996c; NHS Executive 1998b; Lupton *et al.* 1998). Essentially this context was framed by the developing commissioning and quality agendas (Lupton *et al.* 1998; Pickard *et al.* 1995; Taylor and Lupton 1995). However, there was also a growing interest in public involvement in relation to public health and health promotion, although this remained some-what detached from other approaches to involvement by health authorities focusing on the commissioning and quality agendas (Taylor *et al.* 1998).

The introduction of fundholding and its derivatives (such as multi-funds and total purchasing) in the 1990s provided a new policy context for public involvement. The initial response to this was the Accountability Framework (NHS Executive 1995) which identified the need for fundholders to be accountable to their local populations (essentially the practice population). However, as with the wider NHS, the emphasis was on a consumerist approach focusing on patients and service users. With increasing emphasis on primary care in the late 1990s the emphasis shifts towards a population and/or geographical focus with the concept of community much more central in policy development (DoH 1997). However, primary care policy, general practice and policy on patient and public involvement have tended to emphasise the

Table 10.1 Matrix of Relationships

	Patient	Practice population	Community/public
Practitioner	Strong	Variable	Weak
Practice	Variable	Strong	Weak
Primary Care Organisation	Weak	Weak	Strong?

importance of individualistic, patient relationships with the NHS – a focus that underpins current developments (DoH, 2001h–j). This individualistic emphasis was not reflected in more localised approaches which sought to promote public involvement, such as community health development and patient consumer groups and movements (Lupton *et al.* 1998; Allsop *et al.* 2002). This is a point we shall return to later in the chapter and also in Chapter 11.

Thus, primary care encompasses a range of relationships (see Table 10.1) but retains a strong practitioner/patient element which at times is juxtaposed with more community/population oriented approaches to involvement.

This matrix can be overlaid on the framework for primary care shown in Figure 3.3 in Chapter 3. The dominant axis of the relationship is, however, that which links practitioners and patients, practices and their practice populations and, more recently, primary care organisations and their communities – perhaps this is more an aspiration as the extent to which this context has developed varies from area to area (Gillam and Brooks 2001). It is these relationships which are explored in the next sections of this chapter.

Practitioners and Patients

The history of the relationship between the public and primary care is a complex one that has been dominated by the context of the GP–patient relationship – which has been the focus of much research and debate. The wider context of primary care and the public has, for most GPs, come more recently, although other primary care practitioners, such as health visitors, have recognised this important context for many years.

If the patient was the 'ghost in the machinery' of the hospital (Klein 1995), for general practice the patient has always been something real and tangible, central to the work of the practitioner with whom he (or now, more increasingly, she) would develop a lifelong relationship (Balint, 1964). The predominant view of the GP is that of being the patient's advocate. The physical and professional closeness of the GP to his patients was central to the development of the profession. This view can also be seen as being instrumental in the development of current policies such as GP purchasing where the GP acts on the patient's behalf to secure secondary health care services. However, such policies are based on the premise that being close to the patient is the same as knowing what the patient wants and being able to advocate the 'needs' and 'wants' of the patient.

The patient remains central to the practice of primary care. However, there is a growing recognition that the role of the patient is changing from one of passive recipient to one of informed partner. This concept of partnership between practitioner and patient involves a whole patient focus, a high degree of knowledge of the patient, caring and empathy, trust, appropriately adapted care, *patient participation and shared decision-making* (Leopold *et al.* 1996). The increased availability of information for patients coupled with higher expectations is perhaps one of the biggest changes in recent years. It is likely that this trend will continue, encouraged by NHS policy, but also supported by the growth of new technologies such as access to the Internet, video consoles in GP surgeries and a growth in consumer health information services, such as Help for Health in Winchester, and helplines such as NHS Direct. Patients in the surgery are more likely to be able to obtain relevant information before consulting their general practitioner.

This contrasts with traditional views about the patient–doctor relationship which, while based on trust and knowledge of the patient, have been more focused on the patient presenting their illness to the professional doctor who diagnoses and validates the illness (Lupton 1994). This relationship has been seen as paternal in nature and also one in which the patient is passive (Parsons 1951) and is based on a biomedical model where the practitioner is expert (Florin and Coulter 2001). For nurses that patient–practitioner relationship has always been viewed as different. Just as the relationship between nurses and GPs is marked by a clear power differential, the relationship with patients is seen as less privileged and less powerful. In particular, nursing has always been characterised as patient-centred or -focused, taking a holistic approach to care. In practice, there have been concerns that nursing has been as much dominated by the medical care model as has general practice.

The wider context for much of the development of shared decision-making and patient involvement in general practice is the concept of *patient-centred care* (Stewart *et al.* 1995). The pressure for patient-centred care comes from both developments in clinical practice and patient pressure. In a study on patient preference for patient-centred care, Little *et al.* (2001) suggested that patients want patient-centred care which:

- explores the patients' main reason for the visit, their concerns and need for information;
- seeks an integrated understanding of the patients' world;
- finds common ground on what the problem is and mutually agrees on management;
- enhances prevention and health promotion;
- enhances the continuing relationship between the patient and doctor.

The approach places the patient at the centre of care where decision-making is undertaken in partnership. It does not mean that the patient will always want all the information or be responsible for taking a decision. The key point here is that the patient is involved in making the decision about how much information she or he may require at any time or passing responsibility to the practitioner (Elwyn *et al.* 1999; Gwyn and Elwyn 1999). The practice of shared decision-making, and the research literature, is growing. There have been a number of projects developing decision aids – including interactive videos, computer simulations, written material and group interviews – but on the whole the quality of such aids has been poor (Coulter *et al.* 1999). However, in more recent projects such as the King's Fund's PACE programme (Dunning *et al.* 1998) interactive videos are beginning to address such problems. Pursuing shared decision-making within a patient-centred approach will, however, require substantial changes in the role of the practitioner creating challenges for all primary care professionals, not just GPs. The need to make such changes is widely acknowledged not only from a policy perspective, with documents such as *Patient Partnership* (DoH 1996c) and White Papers *Primary Care: Delivering the Future* (DoH 1996a), *The New NHS: Modern, Dependable* (DoH 1997) and, more recently *The NHS Plan* (DoH 2000), but also by the medical profession itself (Toop 1998; Gillam and Pencheon, 1998; Florin and Coulter 2001).

However, it is not just in the context of the individual patient that changes are occurring as there is an increasing interest in viewing patients as a group. Recent emphasis on involving patients in their own care has brought the debate about the nature of the patient–practitioner relationship into central policy debates. The clear emphasis in *Patient Partnership* (DoH 1996c) and *The NHS Plan* (DoH 2000) underpins the increasing importance of ensuring that there are structures and processes giving patients access to information and organisations promoting and supporting their involvement. In addition, the expert patient programme has been promoted by the NHS (DoH 1999a; DoH 2000; DoH 2001i) to support and encourage user-led self-management programmes. This is not a new idea and is aimed at improving the self-esteem and quality of life of those with chronic illness (DoH 1999a). The rationale for the programme is based on the high prevalence of chronic disease and disability, and the self-management programme is being used as the basis for the programmes development in the UK (Lorig *et al.* 1996). In the UK a number of programmes have already been developed by health care charities such as 'Challenging Arthritis' run by Arthritis Care and others run by the Multiple Sclerosis Society and the Manic Depression Fellowship. While such approaches are supported by users and by government policy there are concerns that the lack of a strategy to challenge professionals assumptions about people with a chronic illness may undermine the expert patient programme (Wilson 2001). Such programmes would appear to be set within a consumerist framework and are open to being labelled as manipulative or therapeutic approaches as defined by Arnstein (1969). However, proponents of a patient-centred approach would argue that such approaches are based on ensuring real choices and a shift in the power relationship between patients and professionals.

Practices and their Populations

To date, most public involvement initiatives, and subsequently research on public involvement, have been focused on acute providers and Health Authorities as purchasers/commissioners of health care and the involvement of users in social care, in particular through Community Care Planning (Lupton *et al.* 1998). In primary care, the main focus has been on service provision issues such as involvement in practical matters relating to GP surgeries or for health promotion purposes (Pritchard 1994; Heritage 1994). Traditionally the population focus of the practice has been the practice list – the aggregate of individual patients. Involvement has, therefore, revolved around how patients can be involved in the practice beyond the patient–doctor relationship.

Developing patient participation groups has often been seen as the most effective method of participation in general practice but, as Pritchard comments, progress has been slow, with only some 3 per cent of all practices having such a group, although in the early 1990s this represented over 400 groups nationwide (Pritchard 1994). In addition, doubts have been expressed about who participates in such groups:

> The extent to which patient participation groups reflect the profile and needs of the practice population is unclear. It may be that the group provides a forum for the higher social classes in which to articulate their needs; the views of those patients in social classes 3 and 4 who may be less likely to attend meetings may therefore go unacknowledged though their needs may be greater (Agass *et al.* 1991).

Patient participation can, however, be very effective both in terms of benefits to the practice through the development of care and support schemes and for patient groups where they can articulate their concerns and in some cases input into practice decisions (Peckham *et al.* 1996). Recent developments flowing from the 1997 White Paper have seen increased support for Patient Participation Groups through direct financial support of the National Association of Patient Participation Groups. However, despite such funding, in October 2000 the National Association claimed membership of only 200 groups nationwide – a small number compared to the 11 000+ total number of practices in the country.

The development of GP Fundholding in the 1990s helped to develop the concept of the participation of the patient population with the exploration of the health needs of the practice populations (Harris 1995) and, at least an acknowledgement of, an input into service planning and priority setting. With the Accountability Framework (NHSE 1995) there was also a requirement to develop public accountability, although there is little evidence of this being achieved by primary care purchasers (Lupton *et al.* 1998). This focus on the practice population has been an important step but already there is a further shift taking place moving beyond individual practices to looking at whole populations in particular communities or areas.

Primary Care and the Public

This wider view of primary care is essential within the current context of developing primary care organisations and for improving public health (an issue explored in the next chapter). For some general practitioners there has always been a link between their practice and their community in respect, for example, of social conditions (David Widgery 1991) and public health (Julian Tudor Hart 1988). The shift towards primary care commissioning in the 1990s provided a significant impetus to the need to explore public involvement. However, most work on public involvement in health care commissioning has traditionally been undertaken by health authorities (Lupton *et al.* 1998) with little evidence of public involvement in primary care commissioning developing during the 1990s. In the West Midlands Smith *et al.* (1997) found a 'conspicuous absence of significant user involvement' (40) and the TPP evaluation (Myles *et al.* 1998) found no evidence that any of the TPPs had developed appropriate and specific initiatives. One explanation for this is the perception that GPs are themselves best placed to understand patient's needs because of their closeness to them and, therefore, a wider consultation process is unnecessary (Tranter and Sullivan 1996: Myles *et al.* 1998). Le Grand *et al.* (1998) suggested that the idea of the GP as the natural and obvious advocate of the patient was accepted uncritically in policy. Thus, until recently there has been less focus on issues of patient/public involvement in primary care and there is some reluctance among primary care practitioners to accept any challenges to their ability fully to represent the health needs of their patients. There is also evidence to suggest that GPs are neither effective collaborators with community groups nor supporters of participative activities (Taylor and Lupton 1997; Taylor *et al.* 1998).

The development of multi-practice arrangements such as GP commissioning, Total Purchasing, LHGs, PCGs and now PCTs has, however, shifted attention beyond the practice list to geographically defined populations. Within the UK the preoccupation with populations has traditionally been the role of the DHA, thus creating a distinction between the patient-centred approach of general practice and primary care and the population focus of the health authority (Ham 1996). This is new ground for many GPs and there is clearly a tension between these approaches which will need to be managed. However, not all primary care professionals within the practice will find this orientation new as health visitors have had a public health role with a focus on communities and populations for many years – a role which has become more widely recognised and seen to be increasingly important (DoH 1995a; Cowley 2002).

Moving to a population focus requires PCOs and the professionals within them to become more outward-looking, forming alliances with local community and voluntary groups, working with other statutory agencies and developing new skills such as needs assessment. Experience of these approaches is very limited in general practice and it is not clear that all GPs will want to go down this road (Peckham *et al.* 1998). One major issue was that despite policy intentions, PCGs were not, on the whole, constituted around natural communities and subsequent reorganisations to Trust status have been affected predominantly by existing District Council/Unitary Authority boundaries.

For PCGs the formal connection with their communities was through the board lay representative. The government envisaged that this representative would act as a conduit to the community (Milburn 1999) but this in itself raises complex questions of how such a conduit will work, what mechanisms exist to support individual lay representatives in their role, how representatives are selected, etc. Early evidence suggested that lay representatives were quite isolated but it is important to recognise that they did at least provide a public voice on PCG boards. One important link that requires further exploration is that between PCGs, and now PCTs, and local authorities, especially District Councils and Unitary Authorities. Developing these links, potentially around discussions on public health and HImPs, have provided significant opportunities to engage in wider discussions about public involvement and public accountability which owe more to the legacy of Health for All and Healthy City approaches than to the NHS.

It is around these issues of participation and public health that distinct differences have developed between England, Scotland and Wales. In the latter two countries the establishment of national assemblies and, in Wales the coterminosity between local health groups and local authorities, may have important consequences. The Scottish Parliament is likely to have a significant influence on health issues and may be in a stronger position to address public health across departmental boundaries. The two national assemblies are also closer than the House of Commons to services and the people – it is rather like each region in England having a local Parliament. Given the emphasis on the public health role and accountability in *The New NHS* it will be interesting to watch developments in Scotland and Wales to see if there are lessons for England. In Northern Ireland the debate about how PCGs are to function has been more complex given the pre-existing joint health and social services boards. Decentralisation to PCGs seemingly threatens existing joint arrangements rather than creating new ones.

Public Involvement in the New Primary Care Organisations

In England PCGs' boundaries as far as possible were to cover 'natural communities', although other, more bureaucratic considerations such as coterminosity with Social Services' boundaries and the preferences of some practices at the geographical margins of putative PCGs also merited serious consideration. As Hudson *et al.* (1999) suggest, PCGs could not avoid 'being shaped by, and having to fit into, existing inter-agency and inter-professional relationships' (133–4). The locality focus, as opposed to differently configured PCG popula-tions – for example, covering geographically overlapping populations thereby offering a choice of PCG membership for practices and ultimately patients – both simplifies the collection of area-level data and in theory reduces the number of service agreements with which a more diffusely populated PCG would otherwise have to engage. It shifts attention from practice-level concerns but may not succeed in subordinating practice-level interests within PCG debates. It is important to differentiate these from patient interests, responsi-bility for the promotion of which has traditionally been claimed by professional practitioners. However, practice interests may not necessarily be in harmony with patient interests. Furthermore, the promotion of the patient's perspective by GPs, which was institutionalised within fundholding and which has been offered as an appropriate mechanism for the representation of patients and synonymously the community on PCGs (Marks and Hunter 1998; North *et al.* 1999), is not an adequate substitute for genuine consultation and participation. It also conflates a number of different constituencies that PCGs need to reach.

However, the record of PCG performance is somewhat equivocal. There is evidence of engagement with the agenda of lay consultation and participation (K. Smith *et al.* 2000; Anderson and Florin 2000; Harrison *et al.* 2000) and of PCGs indulging in a variety of activities including public meetings, citizen juries and networking with local patient or health interest groups. Active consultation with the general public was less common and more frequently communication was one-way, for the purpose of only informing the public (J. Smith *et al.* 2000; Harrison *et al.* 2000). Only one study so far (Harrison *et al.* 2000) has asked respondents to identify the outcomes of the public involvement process: less than a third of respondents were able to offer satisfactory evidence of changes in service planning as a result of public or patient involvement. In addition, Anderson and Florin identified a certain reticence among the sampled PCG board members over the advancement of public involvement in health care planning – particularly so with GP members. The risk of tokenistic consultation is further compounded by the danger that the presence of the PCG lay-member may be regarded as obviating the need for more vigorous consultation with the community. The studies provided evi-dence of some conceptual ambivalence in the role, most problematic being that they were there to represent the local community and their views (Anderson and Florin 2000).

In Wales the context is somewhat different, with the development of Local Health Groups whose boundaries are coterminous with local authority boundaries and where the board includes a social services and one other local authority representative. In addition, the board includes a local voluntary organisation representative as well as the lay representative. These differences may have significant consequences for the approach taken to public involvement with a stronger link being established between primary care and local government. However, the Audit Commission (2000) study on the first year of LHGs found that there had been a major reliance on the Community Health Council (CHC) and with only a few developing other mechanisms for consulting or informing the public.

Williamson (1992), using the terminology of internal markets, identified three categories of consumer: patients and carers, consumer groups, and consumerists. Notwithstanding the change in emphasis following *The New NHS*, the relevance of these categories for consultative and participatory processes within PCOs remains. Patients have the right to direct representation of their views, rather than by the proxy of GPs' impressions. Williamson touches on the expressed concerns of some GPs in noting the limitations of individual patients' views, although she argues that their usefulness can be tested against consumerist principles. She also identifies practice-level patient groups and research as ways of channelling patients' views of their experiences. Since patients' perspectives may challenge professional ideologies, not all professional monopolisers will be accepting of practice-level mechanisms. However, the government has indicated the use of HA-level consumer satisfaction surveys covering primary care as well as secondary services (DoH 1997) and any emerging issues will require the attention of the primary care organisation corporate body, whatever the misgivings of the GP constituency.

Primary Care Organisations will need to consult specific client groups when planning dedicated services, a process which perhaps excites the greatest concerns over balancing the competing claims of well-organised groups against those more weakly articulated. Whatever difficulties might obtain in the mediation of differences, these should not discourage PCOs from involving groups in the planning process. In the same way that Health Authorities were required to consult with 'local people' when planning services, PCOs will need to solicit the views of the local community. GPs, concerned about being labelled as rationers of health care (Marks and Hunter, 1998; North *et al.* 1999) – something from which professional monopolisers recoil – have recognised the need to secure public support for PCG plans (North *et al.* 1999). PCG members in Hudson *et al.*'s (1999) study also accepted the need for public legitimation but there was uncertainty about how best to respond. However, the 'legitimation' of end-stage and selectively presented proposals is some distance from genuine consultation or participatory processes conceptualised within community development approaches. These, Hudson and colleagues suggest, are probably not widely replicated. The risk of tokenistic gestures is further compounded by the danger that the presence of the PCG lay-member may be regarded as obviating the need for more vigorous consultation with the community. Unlike either health authorities or GPs, however, Social Services Authorities have a well-established record of client consultation that can inform consultation processes on commissioning priorities as well as specific service developments.

For 'the community' in all its forms, a further danger, and one that Alford predicted, is the risk of exploitation by the more dominant professional practitioners (professional monopolisers) and NHS managers (Alford's corporate rationalisers). The role of professionals, particularly doctors, in patient organisations and voluntary agencies is widely recognised (Lupton *et al.* 1998; Wood 2000), with professionals exercising significant control through appointment as chairs and specialist advisers. Thus, while there may often be a synergy between professional and lay interests, this is often mediated in patient groups through the key role of medical professionals. Health managers have also sought to engage the public in debates about rationing and service priorities (Redmayne 1995; Hunter 1998). Of interest here is the managerial control of the consultation agenda and the manipulation of agendas as managers seek legitimation for their own actions through public consultation and support (Lupton *et al.*1998). Both may lay claims to championing the community's interests in pursuit of their own goals. Professional monopolisers, for example, might seek to challenge PCO policies by prescribing non-PCO formulary medication whilst corporate rationalisers insist that, for the greater good of all, some treatments are proscribed. In this way 'the community' risks being drawn into the agendas of the professional monopolisers and the corporate rationalisers. In addition, there is a further danger as, even where such exploitation is not explicitly pursued, local consumer health groups are unlikely to have the resources or perhaps the skills to negotiate demands successfully where these offend prevailing professional models of care, as Alford predicted. While such attempts may appear to be giving 'voice', real participation, as defined, for example, by Arnstein (1969), is limited to the lower rungs of the ladder.

Though evidence has suggested that lay representatives may have been marginalised within PCGs/LHGs it is important to recognise that they did at least provide a public voice on these organisations' boards. With the establishment of PCT lay boards in England there are different criteria for nomination – replacing the concept of a locally recruited lay representative with an appointed lay representative and one to be elected by the new Patient Forum.

These changes were introduced alongside a wider attempt to develop patient and public participation which was outlined in the NHS Plan (DoH 2000) and a consultation document a year later (DoH 2001h). The main thrust of these proposals were, in England and Wales, to replace CHCs who have traditionally played a limited role in primary care with a range of new organisations and structures. In Scotland it has been decided to retain Community Health Boards – the Scottish counterpart to CHCs. The role and position of Community Health Councils has always been an ambiguous one since their creation in 1974 (Moon and Lupton 1995). They have represented one important element of local accountability but have suffered from a number of structural and resource weaknesses, an expanding agenda, and also enormous variance in activity from area to area (Lupton *et al.* 1995).

In the place of CHCs the government proposes establishing four new elements for patient and public participation, Trust-based Patient 'Advisory Services' (PALS) and new scrutiny powers for local authorities (DoH 2001b; DoH 2001h; DoH 2001j). To support patient and public involvement the proposals include Patient Fora for each PCT and NHS Trust, with half their membership appointed from local health consumer/voluntary groups and half from recent or current patients of practices in the PCT area, and the National Commission for Patient and Public Involvement in Health (CPPIH – an independent statutory body) (DoH 2001j). Successive amendments to the NHS Reform and Health Care Professions Bill have now led to proposals to base local staff in the 300+ PCT patients' fora, which will have a wider role in their localities than patients' forums in NHS trusts. PCT patients' fora will:

- promote the involvement of the public in decisions and consultations on matters affecting their health
- provide independent complaints advocacy and commission specialist advocacy where necessary
- help fora work together.

Both the fora and CPPIH will have statutory powers and Patient Fora will elect one of their members to sit as a non-executive member of the Trust Board. The independent advocacy services will support the patient, replacing this important function currently undertaken by CHCs. While these certainly represent a strengthening of the public and patient role it is not yet clear what resources will be made available for supporting their work and thus truly rectifying some of the weaknesses of the CHC system.

Locally, these new arrangements for patient and public involvement will have to link into existing networks of voluntary organisations and arrangements at practice-level for patient participation. It is not clear how these relationships will develop. The link to PCOs is formalised by the nomination of a lay executive member on to the PCO board. How this person will be supported and linked into the wider networks in the community and among patient organisations is not clear and, whilst linking through the Fora and the CPPIH will provide some cohesion, there are complex and important relationships to be worked through.

Central to the changes is the establishment of the CPPIH to represent patient and public interests at a national level (Health and Social Care Bill 2001). Membership of the Council will be drawn from local Fora and the lay-members on Local Strategic Partnerships. The linking of such a body to the wider consumer health movement and local patient and public fora and councils represents a new dimension to accountability in the NHS. The role of the CPPIH will be to monitor and develop local arrangements providing expertise and advice to local fora, a scrutiny role and guidance to Ministers (DoH 2001j).

These proposals do represent a radical new challenge for primary care organisations. For the first time they will be statutorily accountable to lay bodies and will have to make formal arrangements for patient/public involvement and support. Current experience suggests that PCOs are finding this a difficult task. What is particularly interesting about the government's proposals is the blending of consumerist approaches through patient representation and lay executives alongside more democratic representation from community and voluntary organisations with a health focus. The proposals also blend individual advocacy with wider representation through fora and the local parts of the CPPIH.

Primary Care and the Community

Given the emphasis on the development of primary care organisations which have a specific population focus it is useful to consider the context of their relationships with the public. While the medicalisation of primary care has meant that the traditional focus has been on engaging the individual patient, patients and local communities have generally adopted group approaches to articulate their interests in relation to health.

Since the 1970s there has been a rapid development of the community health movement providing a different context for public involvement which focused on public health issues such as needs assessment, health outcomes and active involvement of local communities in promoting their own health. The first community health initiatives in the UK were developed in the late 1970s but these were short-lived and were thought to be insufficiently rooted in the local community (Scott-Samuel 1989). Following these early developments a wide range of initiatives grew up in the 1980s, numbering in their thousands and leading to the establishment of the National Community Health Resource in 1988.

The development of the user movement and voluntary sector from the 1960s onwards reflected a discontentment with state bureaucracies and a challenging of professional autonomy by service users (Lupton *et al.* 1998). The first organisations were predominantly national, such as the Association for Improvements in Maternity Services (AIMS) established in 1960, the National Association for the Welfare of Children in Hospital (NAWICH) established in 1961 and the Patient's Association, established in 1963. The Patient's Association originated from concerns over unsatisfactory individual treatment and, in particular, about research being undertaken on patients without their knowledge and consent. The main growth in patient and user groups occurred, however, in the 1970s and 80s with a particular emphasis on the development of local organisations. The development of local user groups and local voluntary groups in the health and social welfare field has constituted a significant part of the growth of the voluntary and community sector in the UK. Interestingly, this large reservoir of public action was largely ignored by the NHS and certainly by primary care organisations such as general practice (Lupton *et al.* 1998; Taylor *et al.* 1998). With the advent of geographical conglomerates of practices in the 1990s and with more recent developments, the relevance and need to collaborate with these groups has only just become recognised.

Clearly proposals for public involvement have taken this context on board with the inclusion of voluntary health group representatives within the new arrangements for public and patient involvement. However, in Wales such representation is directly to the board through the voluntary sector representative. There are, however, new paths to tread in relation to the way that communities are engaged as partners in health through involvement in the development of health policy such as through the HImP process and in the delivery of health services through Healthy Living Centres and Health Parks. Some of these issues are discussed in the next chapter. What is interesting is that proposals for public involvement and the establishment of an institutional framework for such involvement continue to focus predominantly on service delivery rather than on public health. There is an aspiration on behalf of the DoH that eventually public involvement will address all the determinants of health and not just health care (DoH 2001: 17). The Department's original proposals set out in the consultation document were that 'Local Voice' organisations would:

> work with StHAs ... [so that] ... they can pull together an overview of trends and themes, and take account of broader community issues and wider determinants of health. Armed with this information, Voices would make reports and recommendations to their StHA about the strategic planning of health services in their area, which the StHA would have a duty to take account of. (DoH 2001h: para. 5.19)

With the changes following the consultation process, proposals for Local Voices organisations have been scrapped, there will be local elements to the CPPIH and references to local public involvement on public health have disappeared (DoH 2001j). These wider issues of participation and public health are discussed further in Chapter 11.

Conclusion

There is no doubt that a significant shift has occurred in patient and public involvement over the last 20 years. There is an increasing professional acceptance of the efficacy of involving patients in their own care and in decision-making. The expert patient programme provides another approach to drawing on user expertise in self-management. However, these shifts are not without some resistance from health care professionals. While not specifically anti such approaches, there is a conservatism in professional practice which does not address the power differences between patients and professionals (Wilson 2001). There is a need for greater cultural change. To what extent such a change will occur in primary care is difficult to assess. Undoubtedly there is a shift in the boundary between patient and professional which challenges traditional clinical practice.

A similar shift is occurring in the planning and delivery of health care services. Primary care will increasingly come under the scrutiny of lay people through executive members on PCO boards and patient fora. Traditionally sheltered from the remit of CHCs, primary care organisations are only just beginning to encounter the need for more openness in their decision-making processes and in the provision of services. These moves create new accountability structures at a local level which, alongside proposals for Local Authority Scrutiny Committees (LASCs) and independent advocacy (DoH 2000; DoH 2001b; DoH 2001h), create a new framework for involvement, accountability and scrutiny at a primary care level. One outstanding question, however, is how this new structure is to be resourced. The approach is at once both a challenge to existing boundaries and creates a diverse structure of agencies, roles and responsibilities ranging from PALS, incorporated within Trusts, to independent scrutiny by LASCs and the CPPIH. There is also a sense of incorporation of patient and public involvement structures. Is this relevant to the way that user groups and the voluntary and community sector work? In fact we know little about health care user organisations and health sector voluntary groups. Few studies have explored the extent of their role and influence or their organisation and functions (Wood 2000; Allsop *et al.* 2002). In the new NHS such groups will play an increasingly important role with local and national nomination rights to the local and national voices.

However, the main challenge is for primary care to engage with the patient and public participation agenda. There is little history of active patient or public involvement in general practice or primary care more widely. Where there has been work developed it has focused very much on the medical agenda of the health care professionals – for example, providing support services to practices – rather than addressing patient concerns or providing opportunities for local people to shape local services. Such conclusions can be generally drawn for the NHS as a whole (Lupton *et al.* 1998) but it is more true within primary care. PCOs and the new participation agenda therefore create real challenges for primary care managers and professionals. The extent to which they are able to address these issues will, in part, be dependent on the priority afforded at a national level and how activity is measured. There are signs, however, that public participation has been drawn into PCO agendas through the actions of lay representatives and the new proposals can only serve to ensure that the issues remain on the agenda even if, in the near future, little activity is observable. More importantly, there may be the potential to move away from the predominant individualistic approaches of the past – through PPGs and market research type approaches to a more democratic model of participation that engages the public at a number of levels and over time.

CHAPTER 11

Primary Care and Public Health

This chapter explores the increasingly important connections between primary care and public health. As a focus of primary care services throughout the last half of the twentieth century general practice has, as we have discussed in earlier chapters, developed as a reactive medical service for individuals and their families. This contrasts strongly with the focus of public health which is on 'populations' and a concern with both cure and prevention. Thus there is an immediate tension. With the development of primary care organisations and reform of the NHS in the early twenty-first century the government has been shifting responsibility for public health in England to PCOs. Similar approaches have been developed in Scotland and Wales, although in these countries the devolved assemblies have taken a stronger political interest in public health.

As we have seen from earlier chapters, the development of PCOs and Primary Care Act Pilots projects (PCAPs) are substantially changing the face of primary care in the UK. Such changes provide new opportunities for examining the role and structure of primary care in relation to public health, which, particularly at a local level, has also been rapidly changing with a greater emphasis on local/community-based developments such as Healthy Living Centres, Health Action Zones, Health Parks and community-based regeneration projects. Predominantly, it is general practice and community health services that operate at this level and it these organisations that have been forming the core of primary care organisational developments through Primary Care Groups and Trusts in England (PCGs/PCTs), Local Health Groups (LHGs) in Wales, Scottish Primary Care Trusts (SPCTs) and more recently Primary Care Groups (PCGs) in Northern Ireland. Thus, it is pertinent to explore the relationship between public health and primary care.

The aim of this chapter, therefore, is to examine the relationship between public health and primary care. This will involve exploring the historical development of public health within a primary care context, setting out the current policy UK framework focusing on the intersection between public health and primary care policy and outlining the developing public health role of primary care organisations. The chapter will then go on to discuss the findings of a number of research projects which have explored the relationship between public health and primary care and examined how primary care organisations are tackling their public health role. In the preceding chapters the changes in primary care have been dealt with in some depth so it is perhaps useful to examine what is meant by public health and provide an overview of public health developments in the UK.

Defining Public Health

This section does not provide an exhaustive account of public health in the UK. Readers who would like to know more about the development of public health in the UK should read Lewis (1986), Ashton and Seymour (1988) and Baggott (2000). Essentially there have been four broad stages of public health development in the UK. The first was sanitation, the second was the shift in the Victorian period towards preventive medicine, the third was the medicalisation of public health in the twentieth century and the fourth the development of the New Public Health in the last decades of the twentieth century. Broadly speaking, the first public health efforts in the nineteenth century focused on clean water, better living spaces, improved working conditions and the control of diseases such as cholera and typhoid (Lewis 1986; Baggott 2000). The focus was very much on a social model of health which incorporated a range of social, environmental, biological and economic causes of ill-health (WHO/UNICEF 1978). At this time public health was an activity undertaken by a range of local authority-employed staff, including the Medical Officer for Health (MoH), community nurses and health visitors. However, from the mid to late nineteenth century onwards, particularly with the appointment of medically qualified MoHs, control of public health increasingly came under the control of medical professionals although they remained employed by local authorities up until the NHS reorganisation of 1974 (Ottewill and Wall, 1990; Baggott 2000).

The increasing medical domination of public health in the twentieth century has led to the definition of public health being drawn very narrowly, focusing on hygiene, epidemiology and disease control. As a discipline, public health medicine has focused mainly on epidemiological approaches, which identify health risks and use population approaches. For example, with coronary heart disease a medically dominated public health approach would be to determine those most at risk and focus prevention programmes on this population. Such an approach has been criticised by Ashton and Seymour (1989) who have argued for a broader approach to public health.

The literature on public health offers a range of definitions, from a pure epidemiological/communicable disease approach to an emphasis on changing health status (Harris 1995; Baggott 2000). In the latter part of the twentieth century, partly driven by definitions of health put forward by WHO contained within the Health for All programme and the Ottawa Charter for Health promotion (WHO 1986), there was a focus on the relationship between health promotion and other approaches to public health which has underpinned what is known as the New Public Health (Ashton and Seymour 1988). This approach is based on a wider definition of public health that encompasses social resources and all forms of health care, as has been defined as:

an approach which brings together environmental change and personal preventive measures with appropriate therapeutic interventions … [but] … goes beyond an understanding of human biology and recognizes the importance of those social aspects of health problems which are caused by life-styles. (*ibid*: 21)

The Health for All approach echoed this in its three main objectives:

1. promotion of life-styles conducive to health;
2. prevention of preventable conditions;
3. rehabilitation and health services.

From these objectives a range of goals or targets was developed for each WHO region and the UK was signatory to the European targets. A key aim of the European programme was to shift the emphasis away from a narrow medical view by:

- promoting self-care;
- integrating medical care with other related activities such as education, recreation, environmental improvements and social welfare (intersectoral action integrating the promotion of good health with preventive medicine, treatment and rehabilitation);
- meeting the needs of underserved groups;
- community participation.

It is perhaps worth pointing out that the integration of medical care with other related activities of this European approach is an objective that has been, by and large, unachieved, with health promotion remaining generally detached from clinical/treatment services.

This new approach to health promotion was to be based on the:

- active involvement of the population;
- direct action on the causes of ill-health;
- combination of a range of approaches aimed at improving health;
- dependence on public participation;
- recognition of the important role of all health workers.

The Ottawa Charter (WHO 1986) adopted these principles and also the broad approach developed within Health for All. In particular, it is possible to define three key elements to what a public health approach would be. These are:

1. equity (the focus on underserved groups, improving health *for all*);
2. collaboration (the need to work intersectorally);
3. participation (the need to involve the public in improving their health, strengthening community action).

These definitional elements are useful in providing a conceptual and policy framework for exploring primary care and public health (Macdonald 1992; Taylor *et al.* 1998). Drawing on key themes developed in earlier chapters it is possible to relate this framework to changes in primary care. For example, there is an increasing diversity of who delivers public health within primary care; there are changing boundaries between professional and organisational roles and the integration of primary care into central strategic public health policy. Integration can also be viewed as the organisational integration of public health and primary care which is currently been undertaken in England. These changes are being driven from the systemic level with an increasing focus on public health across government departments and also at the programmatic level with new priorities such as inequality targets. For primary care organisations there are changes at the organisational level with the integration of public health and primary care activities and also the emphasis on collaboration with local authorities and local communities. Finally, at the instrumental level public health is brought more into the everyday work of a wide range of health and other staff.

However, the integration of public health and primary care presents a challenge. As discussed in Chapter 2, primary care in the UK has been primarily focused on general practice, which has worked within a medical model of health. Public health, on the other hand, draws very much on a social model of health. Essentially the shift is one from primary medical care to primary health care. This can be seen visually by referring back to Figure 3.4 in Chapter 3 and imagining a shift from the top left-hand area of the figure to the bottom right-hand corner – from reactive, individual medicine to proactive, multi-sectoral, inter-professional health. This chapter will explore each of the three elements of public health in turn but first it is necessary to examine briefly the historical development and current policy context of public health in relation to primary care in the NHS.

Public Health and the NHS

Since 1974 responsibility for public health has been split between local authorities that have maintained an environmental health function and Health Authorities that have focused on identifying health need, commissioning health care services, and monitoring notifiable diseases. Since then these roles have developed but largely in an unco-ordinated way despite developments such as Health for All, the Healthy City Movement and Agenda 21 (Ranade 1998; Baggott 2000). With the election of a Labour Government in 1997, there has been a clearer recognition of the important roles played by health and local authorities in public health but central to government policy has been the call for greater co-ordination of strategy and action. Since 1998 primary care organisations have been given a public health responsibility that puts a much greater emphasis on local, community-based developments such as Health

Living Centres, Health Action Zones, Health Parks, and community-based regeneration projects (DoH 1999b). This change in the way the health of the public is addressed to secure healthier communities focuses attention on the local context of health services – an arena now clearly identified with primary care organisations. However, this refocusing of public health also requires a wider understanding of 'public health' – one that encompasses the circumstances and social reality of people's lives, and their perceptions and experiences of these as factors that contribute to their illness and their health. Both national policy and local action require that traditionally separate statutory organisations, including primary care, work jointly with each other, with other organisations, both private and voluntary, and with the individuals and groups comprising local communities. To date, little attention has been paid either to the public health role of primary care organisations (Le Grand *et al.* 1998; Mays *et al.* 1998) or, for that matter, to the role of communities in determining public health strategy and action (CMO 2001; DoH 1998b).

At its inception public health remained within local authorities integrated with welfare and community health services. The model was very much based on that of the Medical Officer of Health developed in the nineteenth century. It was only in 1974 that the public health function was brought into the NHS. This organisational shift was seen very much as going hand in hand with an increasing medical dominance of public health (Baggott 2000). The new NHS departments of community medicine became dominated by medical professionals creating strong divisions between public health medicine and activities such as health promotion. The advent of the New Public Health approach did find some support in the UK – particularly from local authorities and some health authorities – although at a national level the Conservative Government of the 1980s never fully backed the Health for All programme (Ranade 1998). However, at a definitional level some aspects of the New Public Health perspective were echoed in the Acheson Report (DHSS 1988) which set out the role of public health within the NHS. Acheson, for example, adopted a definition based on that developed by the World Health Authority in 1952, namely: 'the science and art of preventing disease, prolonging life and promoting health through organised efforts of society'.

Such a view was also endorsed five years later by the Abrams Committee (DoH 1993) which examined the public health role within the District Health Authorities in relation to the internal market arrangements introduced in 1991. The definition was also reflected in the *Health of the Nation* White Paper (DoH 1992) which was based on the promotion of health, prevention of disease, treatment of illness and social care. Yet despite these links to the New Public Health approach, public health within the NHS has remained predominantly within a medicalised model with a narrow focus.

By contrast, local authorities, which had maintained a somewhat more traditional, public health role in terms of sanitation, provision of housing, environmental issues and social welfare measures, embraced the new perspective. Community health services and the public health role were originally developed within local authorities and were only taken over by the NHS in 1974. This removal of community health services from local authorities severed the link between social care, housing and environment and focused public health towards the biomedical model (Tudor-Hart 1988). Despite this, many local authorities continued to maintain a health promotion role within the broad remit of their continuing responsibility for environmental health. For example, Brighton City Council has a health promotion unit, Coventry City Council has a Health Promotion Unit within its Environmental Health Division and works on a range of issues including sexual health, and Southampton City Council has a Health Policy Officer within its community services division and has a responsibility for Port Health as well as general environmental health issues.

With the advent of the WHO's Healthy Cities initiative and the linked Health for All programmes, many local authorities (notable firsts being Nottingham, Oxford and Sheffield) were able to reclaim a 'public health role' and worked with other agencies, including the NHS, to address health issues (Ashton and Seymour 1988). This was seemingly in contrast to the Conservative Government's agenda set out in *The Health of the Nation* which concentrated on the individual's own responsibility for their health, and their responsibility for avoiding unhealthy life-styles, with the professional role consisting largely in the offering of timely advice, although interagency collaboration was seen as an important element of public health practice.

Current Policy

The election of the Labour Government in 1997 stimulated a grater interest in both public health and primary care. Public health was identified as a key area for government action, with a clear recognition of the problems of health inequalities. Its plans for the improvement of public health in England were set out in the *The New NHS* (DoH 1997), a Green Paper on public health (DoH 1998a) and the subsequent White Paper, *Saving Lives: Our Healthier Nation* (DoH 1999b). Public health strategy focused on action at the national, local and individual levels with targets for improving health and establishing a framework for action in specific settings such as schools, workplaces and local communities. These aims have also been reflected in the policy developments for Northern Ireland, Scotland and Wales. However, there are important distinctions in relation to the role of the elected assemblies in these countries as well as the exact nature and responsibilities of their primary care organisations. One key weakness of national policy is the seeming lack of co-ordination between NHS organisational policy and public health, although government policy and guidance have been very clear about the central role of primary care in public health.

One key theme of the government's approach to public health has been the renewed emphasis on tackling health inequalities. Public health policy during the 1980s ignored the findings of key reports on structural influences on health, and in particular the Black Report and Whitehead's Health Divide (Townsend *et al.* 1992) on inequality and health. Until 1995 the then Conservative Government made no explicit recognition of socio-economic issues relating to variations in health of health inequalities. In the mid-1990s the government went some way to addressing these shortcomings with the acknowledgement that there are *variations* in health and a national research programme on variations in health was established (NHS CRD 1995; DoH 1995b). However, this only related to the contribution that can be made by the NHS and DoH and specifically avoids addressing the role of other areas of government policy such as the environment, transport, employment and welfare benefits.

Since 1997, the Labour Government has taken various steps associated with tackling health inequalities. One of its first actions was to commission an Independent Inquiry into Inequalities in Health, chaired by Sir Donald Acheson, the former Chief Medical Officer. The inquiry, which reported in November 1998 (Acheson 1998), reviewed the research evidence related to health inequalities and made 39 recommendations. Only three of the recommendations were directed to the NHS, thereby underlining the relative contribution of health care services to tacking health inequality compared to poverty, education, employment, housing, transport and nutrition. Primary care has an important contribution to all these areas (at least in theory) even though only two parts of the recommendations specifically mentioned primary care.

> 37.4. Performance management in relation to the national performance management framework is focused on achieving more equitable access, provision and targeting of effective services in relation to need in both primary and hospital sectors.

> 38.2. Extending the principle of needs-based weighting to non-cash limited GMS resources. The size and effectiveness of deprivation payments in meeting the needs and improving the outcomes amongst the most disadvantaged populations including ethnic minorities should be assessed. (Acheson 1998)

Subsequent policy documents have further emphasised the government's commitment to public health and tackling health inequality. *The New NHS* (1997) proposed to renew the NHS and to tackle the 'unfairness', 'unacceptable variations' and 'two-tierism' of the Conservative internal market (Powell and Exworthy 2000). To this end, *The New NHS* proposed the National Institute for Clinical Excellence (NICE) and the Commission for Health Improvement (CHI) to promote such equity. At the local level and in terms of primary care, *The New NHS* created PCGs and PCTs as vehicles by which local health improvement and health inequality strategies will be implemented. Whilst there is some sense in charging such organisations with this responsibility, there are currently doubts about their capacity to fulfil this task and also the relative priority accorded to it compared with commissioning and primary care development. This issue was identified by the Health Committee's inquiry into public health (House of Commons 2001).

The Green Paper on public health (DoH 1998a) was seen as a follow-up to *The Health of the Nation* (DoH 1992). The strategy aimed to improve the health of the population as a whole and to improve the health of the worst off in society to narrow the 'health gap'. It proposed four targets related to heart disease and stroke, accidents, cancer and mental health. The subsequent White Paper (DoH 1999b) reaffirmed the proposed targets but neither set national health inequality targets nor allocated specific monies to the task. Instead, local areas were to set their own targets. This position changed in February 2001 when two national health inequality targets were set, relating to life expectancy and infant mortality. Later in the same year the Department of Health published a consultation document on addressing health inequalities to stimulate debate about the relevancy of the targets and identify how these should be addressed (DoH 2001k). The document highlighted the role of primary care and the need to support disadvantaged communities.

The NHS National Plan was published in July 2000. Although it focused primarily on the structure and organisation of the NHS, it recognised that 'the wider inability to forge effective partnerships with local government, business and community organizations has inhibited the NHS's ability to prevent ill-health and tackle health inequalities' (DoH 2000: 29). This theme of partnership was discussed in Chapter 8 in relation to social care and is also addressed in relation to primary care and public health later in this chapter.

Initiatives begun in 2001 have increased further efforts to tackle health inequalities, including two national targets (on life expectancy and infant mortality), a DoH consultation exercise and a Treasury-led review on health inequalities. The effect of these has yet to be felt but the latter has the greatest potential since it could affect the spending programmes on all government departments over the next few years.

The effectiveness of these (and other) strategies to tackle health inequalities is not yet known since many of the mechanisms proposed in these documents have only been established within the last couple of years. Empirical evidence (at the local level) suggests that there is widespread support for such policies but their implementation is being hampered by competing priorities from central government and local partnerships difficulties (Exworthy and Powell 2000). Conceptually, the 'streams' of activity required to achieve effective policy implementation (see Chapter 2 for further discussion of 'streams' and policy implementation) have yet to be fully conjoined (Powell and Exworthy 2001; see also Challis *et al.* 1988; Kingdon 1995). The policy stream (dealing with ends and aims) is reasonably clear, although there is be a trade-off between improving the health of the population *and* improving the health of the worst off. The process stream (dealing with the means and mechanism to achieve policy goals) remains complex given the difficulties of establishing causation in health inequality and the subsequent (mainly up-stream) interventions required. Thus, issues of technical and political feasibility remain. Finally, the resource stream (dealing with the finances, time and support for policy goals and means) is problematic given the number of competing priorities that central government, through its silo approach, requires of each local agency. Moreover, many of the inequality initiatives (observed in the study by Exworthy and Powell) did not challenge existing mainstream budgets or services but were often non-recurrent projects. The challenge of delivery in Labour's second term may overshadow many such initiatives to address public health and to tackle health inequalities, thereby ensuring that the streams remain largely separate, although the Treasury has undertaken a cross-cutting review of health inequalities during 2002. There is an explicit emphasis within the policy and process streams on the role of primary care. The remainder of the chapter explores the role of primary care in public health within historical and policy contexts.

Developing a Public Health Approach in Primary Care

As has been discussed elsewhere in this book, over the last two decades of the twentieth century there was a growing recognition of the part played by primary care in the UK health service. In relation to public health it would be wrong, however, to see these links as a new phenomenon as public health and primary care share similar roots in developments in the nineteenth century in areas such as preventive medicine and community nursing. Health Visiting, for example, claims strong public health roots and has traditionally focused on the social model of health (Lindsay and Craig 2000). However, while community nursing in the UK retained links (organisationally and in its activities) with public health, general practice became more detached from its public health tradition during the past century. Thus the recent emphasis on public health in general practice has come as something of a rediscovery of the role. This rediscovery has not been a recent, sudden phenomenon but has gradually been introduced over the last 30 years.

The 1980s saw a number of government publications promoting the public health role in general practice and the wider primary health care team – *Promoting Better Health* (DHSS 1987), the House of Commons Social Services Committee report on primary health care (House of Commons 1987), Cumberlege Report (DHSS 1986b). These documents focused attention on primary care in a new way. The White Paper, with its emphasis on the promotion of health, led directly to changes to the GP contract in 1990. The Cumberlege Report on nursing within the community, with its a focus on geographical localities (Ottewill and Wall 1990), did not fit with the emphasis in the other documents on a GP-led primary health care team (PHCT) and a focus based on the practice list. It was this latter focus that was to survive the discussions about community nursing and the 1980s saw a rapid move towards practice-based teams with community nurse attachments, away from neighbourhood- and area-based approaches (*ibid.*). Twenty years on there is a slight irony in this given the move towards geographically based primary care organisations.

These policy developments in the 1970s and 1980s underpinned a growing emphasis on health promotion within the general practice and community setting. In general practice the new GP Contract in 1990 made payments to practices for health promotion activity encouraging a range of health promotion activities with individual patients and also, to a certain extent, with groups of patients. Such activity, particularly on an individual basis, had always been seen as an integral part of general practice. However, the contract formalised this area of work with banding payments related to the level of reported activity.

Alongside the change in the GP contract, the NHS reforms in 1991 introduced general practice fundholding identifying the GP in a key role as the patient's advocate or proxy and a new role for primary care in purchasing health care. As discussed in Chapter 6, this purchasing role was not simply related to fundholding, but included the development of non-fundholding approaches such as commissioning groups and the recent development of total purchasing (EL(94)79 (NHSE 1994)). These approaches had a stronger population focus than that traditionally conceived within general practice and occurred at a time when the size of health authorities was being increased following the mergers with Family Health Service Authorities (Health Authorities Act 1996) – leading to an increased emphasis on locality approaches to purchasing, and interest in new approaches to primary care (Meads 1996; Gordon and Hadley 1996). A number of issues emerged in the debate relating to definitions of the primary health care team: the role of primary care professionals; the role of primary care as purchers; relationships between primary care and secondary care; and the shift from a patient to a population focus (NHSE 1993; Peckham 1999; Pratt 1995). In the 1990s, it became increasingly clear that the relative isolation between public health and primary care was untenable and a growing debate emerged about the role of primary care in public health (Starfield 1998; Taylor *et al.* 1998). The growth of primary care commissioning in the 1990s provided some impetus to the debate through health needs assessment in primary care (A. Harris 1995) and it became clear that there needed to be more interconnection between primary care and public health. However, the focus of much public health specialist activity was on developing localised epidemiological data and providing Evidence based Medicine support – giving little recognition to the role of non-medics such as primary care nurses, or non-NHS approaches to primary care and public health developed by the Health for All and Healthy City initiatives (NHSE 1995; Peckham *et al.* 1996).

In England, PCOs have been given three main functions:

1. to improve the health of, and address health inequalities in, their community;
2. to develop primary care and community health services across their area (including improved integration of services);

3. to advise or take on the commissioning of hospital services for patients within their area to meet patient's needs appropriately (NHSE, 1998a).

These changes placed an emphasis on the primary care public health role in the NHS, raising important questions about roles and responsibilities. These were partly addressed by the Chief Medical Officer's report on the need for a multidisciplinary public health workforce (CMO 2001). This recognised the role of primary care staff and also other people working in local authorities and the wider community. With the development of primary care organisations into Trusts, the government announced in 2001 the intention to integrate public health functions within PCOs, with the new Strategic Health Authorities retaining a performance and review role. This represents a major reorganisation of public health in the NHS and presents challenges for primary care organisations in terms of creating a more diverse workforce, developing new relationships and partnerships between PCOs and with other organisations and examining the boundaries of professional expertise and activity (HDA 2001). PCOs will be required for the first time to address health inequalities, and develop broad partnerships and the participation of their local communities – perhaps moving primary care closer to primary health care (see Chapter 3).

Primary Care and Equity

If inequality in health is related to broader determinants such as income inequality and relative deprivation (Wilkinson 1998), what role can primary care play in achieving the health inequality targets outlined by the government? In relation to primary care, equity has traditionally been viewed as an access or service distribution issue (see Chapter 3). Concern here is, for example, with the 'inverse care law' (Tudor-Hart 1988), the distribution of general practitioners and other health care professionals or list size. However, these issues provide only a part of a broader structure of health inequalities. Yet, Starfield (1998) has argued that a robust primary care infrastructure has the potential for addressing broader health inequalities. She cites the example of Cuba where primary health care teams serve small populations adopting a public health approach including health surveillance, regular check-ups and reviewing medical records – an approach which has also been advocated, and adopted, in the UK (Tudor-Hart 1988).

Over the last 20 years there have been developments in UK primary care to address the determinants of inequalities in health. One approach has been the development of welfare advice in general practice with the support of Citizen Advice Bureau sessions in practices. These have been shown to improve the health status of patients (Abbott and Hobby 2000) and also encourage new clients, particularly those with a disability (Coppel *et al.* 1999). The use of advice workers in general practice has also shown benefits for families with young children, with positive benefits for maternal and child health (Reading *et al.* 2002). Research has also shown that GP advice on child safety coupled with the provision of low-cost safety equipment for families on means-tested benefits leads to increased use of safety equipment and other safe practices (Clamp and Kendrick 1998). There is also evidence to show that opportunistic GP advice to stop smoking is an effective way of reducing smoking rates (Butler *et al.* 1998) as is the sending of questionnaires and letters (Lennox *et al.* 2001). Approaches such as these suggest that there is much primary care can do to address inequalities in health linked to wider social interventions such as increasing income for people on benefits, or by providing appropriate advice and support on specific health issues.

Future involvement of PCOs on health inequalities is hard to determine at this point. In England many PCOs are finding it hard to tackle the broad public health agenda – especially alongside other changes and priorities. PCOs in Scotland and Wales have different functions and are being drawn more into the public health agenda but it is not clear beyond small, localised approaches what key role they will play in tackling health inequalities.

Primary Care and Partnerships for Public Health

As discussed above, developing partnerships is seen as an important cornerstone of tackling health inequalities. Post-1997, NHS Executive guidance in England identified the need for PCGs and PCTs to work with other local partners, including local authorities and housing agencies, to adopt community development approaches for reaching local people, to develop more one-to-one health promotion interventions and to work with all local stakeholders to address local health issues (NHS Executive 1998c). While the overall lead for public health remains with Health Authority Directors of Public Health, PCGs

> should . . . assess the public health capacity and capability available locally, to agree the
> best organisational arrangements, whilst ensuring clear lines of responsibility and
> accountability. (NHS Executive 1998c: para. 18)

It is interesting, therefore, that despite the prominence given to the development of primary care in the White Paper on the NHS and the aim set out by the NHSE, there was little reference to the role of Primary Care Groups in the Green Paper on public health for England (DoH 1998a). However, in *Saving Lives: Our Healthier Nation* White Paper, government policy is very clear about the centrality of the Health Improvement Programme (HImP) and the important role to be played in the development of local HImPs by PCGs

> Over time they will forge powerful local partnerships with local bodies . . . to deliver
> shared health goals. They will help shape the health improvement programme and

draw up their own plans for implementing it and for hitting the targets in it. (DoH 1999b: para 10.11)

Similarly in Scotland and Wales there is an increasing emphasis on drawing general practitioners and other primary care workers into local collaboration on public health action.

In Wales the emphasis on broader relationships with the voluntary and community sector and local authorities through greater LHG board membership and coterminosity between LHGs and local authorities may provide a more secure basis for developing public health partnerships. By contrast the organisational focus in England, as discussed in Chapter 9, is on health and social care partnerships. Yet, telephone interviews with chief executives and chairs of the majority of the 72 PCGs/PCTs in the Tracker Survey in England found that 44 PCGs had worked with departments of urban regeneration, 38 with leisure services, 31 with housing services and 29 with education (Gillam *et al.* 2001). While such links were described as rudimentary, consisting of membership of multi-agency groups, Gillam *et al.* argue that such links are a prerequisite of developing working relationships and back this with evidence showing that PCOs are beginning to allocate funding to health improvement activities. In Scotland there is a strong emphasis on public health. This may relate to the fact that the Scottish population has a poorer health status than that in England. Historically, both Scotland and Wales have been closely identified with health inequalities. During the inter-war period many of the most extreme examples of ill-health and social deprivation were found in the South-Wales valleys and in the industrial belt of central Scotland (Levitt 1988). Some areas of Glasgow have amongst the highest rates of infant mortality in Europe, and in the UK, 52 per cent of the 'worst off million people in terms of health live in Scotland' (Shaw *et al.* 1999). While at a policy level Scotland has followed the Model of *Our Healthier Nation* with a similarly focused White Paper, *Working Together for a Healthier Scotland* (Scottish Office 1998) there has been a more specific emphasis on developing strategies and action to address public health issues with a Health Improvement Fund, increasing public health intelligence but with the public function retained by the Scottish Health Boards which remain the key commissioning agencies. Thus, there are distinctive differences from the English and Welsh models.

In England and Wales PCOs are seen as being key local actors within public health, taking both a responsibility for addressing the local communities health needs but also collaborating with other local agencies on public health activities. While the links between public health and primary care are widely accepted, this indicates a significant change in the nature of primary care, and more specifically general practice. While the seeds of such a change were already sown before the Labour Government policy initiatives of the late 1990s, it is the post-1997 developments that placed the development of collaboration and partnership at the centre of public health development at a local level.

The importance of the role of PCGs and PCTs in England is likely to be further emphasised by the abolition of the NHSE Regions and Health Authorities and the establishment of Strategic Health Authorities (DoH 2001b; DoH 2002a). Larger health authorities will lead to more devolved public health functions, with Directors of Public Health taking a more strategic role through the development of regional public health networks that draw together NHS and local authorities. It is at the regional level of inter-organisational collaboration that the shape of public health will be formed in England, taking on the role that the assemblies in Northern Ireland, Scotland and Wales are beginning to perform. However, the assemblies in Wales and Scotland have committed themselves to a stronger public health focus and thus the framework for public health, where these democratically elected representatives provide a localised leadership, may provide a higher degree of political commitment than the more target-oriented, performance management approach in England. Such political leadership may provide a more conducive context for developing partnerships than the executive approach adopted in England.

Primary Care and Community Health

The third element of tackling public health at the local level is the need to develop and support local participation and engage with local communities. In the previous chapter the framework for public and patient involvement identified the need for participation in primary health care services and decision-making. While there has been little focus on public health in much of the recent development of policy on participation (DoH 2001j), community participation has always been an element of local public health action. Recent policy interest (DoH 1998b; CMO 2001) coincided with a broader interest within general practice and the wider context of primary care about public health and led to a range of formal and informal approaches to addressing public health issues – including an interest in the work of Julian Tudor-Hart, development of the arts and health movement, community health projects and the promotion of public health nursing (Peckham *et al.*1996). These generally developed on an ad hoc basis, although one approach, Community Oriented Primary Care (COPC), received more formal support through the King's Fund project.

COPC has been described as 'the continual process by which [primary health care teams] provide care to a defined community on the basis of its assessed health needs by the planned integration of public health with [primary care] practice' (Gillam and Miller 1997). The idea originated in South Africa and Israel (Kark and Kark 1983) but has been widely supported by the World Health Organisation and was adopted in the USA as the basis for many public health programmes (Nutting *et al.* 1985). Its introduction to the UK came in 1992 through the King's Fund which established eight pilot practices in four sites – Northumberland, Sheffield, Winchester and Haringey (Gillam and Miller 1997).

COPC is an approach which involves the whole primary health care team (PHCT). The team identifies local health problems (Community Diagnosis) and then prioritises these. The PHCT then selects one health problem which the team assesses in detail and then implements an action plan to deal with it. The pilot practices in the UK addressed a range of problems including hypertension, urinary incontinence and the health of young people. However, COPC has not been taken up in any comprehensive way in the UK, although the principles are embedded in current developments in local health needs assessment. The key strength of COPC lies in the way it brings together a range of primary care professionals to identify and address local health probems. However, there is little evidence from the UK experience to demonstrate that local communities were involved in the process and as such in this country COPC has tended to be a professionally led approach. This poor linkage between the community and general practice (the focus of COPC) has been identified in other studies and generally community participation has not been developed to any great extent within primary care (Peckham 1994; Peckham *et al.* 1996; Taylor *et al.* 1998).

Another approach adopted by primary care has been rapid appraisal, which was developed by the World Health Organisation for use in developing countries as a method of researching local communities (WHO 1991). Rapid appraisal involves identifying key local informants who have knowledge of their area. It has close links with the COPC approach and has been advocated by health professionals, including general practitioners, as one approach to identifying local health needs (Scott-Murray 1994). This is one step beyond the community diagnosis approach adopted in COPC but it still remains a professional-led exercise. Rapid appraisal has also predominantly been used as a method of local health needs assessment and with potential for planning local services, rather than being seen as a way of working with local commun- ities (Ong *et al.* 1991; Murray *et al.* 1994). However, many of these devel- opments emanating from general practice have not connected with other developments at a community level.

The concept of a community-based primary health care service has roots right back to the early days of general practice. Key developments occurred early in the twentieth century with the development of the health centre concept in many metropolitan areas such as London and, perhaps most importantly, the Peckham Health Centre (Kenner 1986). Such developments were, however, swept away with the establishment of the NHS in 1948. Nevertheless, the principles of primary health care, as we have discussed previously, are based on a community service (Macdonald 1992). Also of importance has been the development of community links through community health services. However, the latter half of the twentieth century has been characterised by a non-community-focused general practice service despite the growing strength of the community health movement.

For example, community health action developed in the late 1970s, with six community health projects set up in the UK in 1977 by the Foundation for

Alternatives. These were short-term funded neighbourhood health initiatives and all but one failed to survive beyond the first year of funding (Scott-Samuel 1989). Despite their being neighbourhood initiatives, Scott-Samuel has argued that this failure was due to their not being sufficiently rooted in the local community. From these beginnings a number of initiatives subsequently developed, focused either on geographical communities, or neighbourhoods such as the Stockwell Health Project (Kenner 1986), or on communities of interest such as the Avon Vietnamese Refugee Community Project and the Lambeth Women and Children's Health Project (Dun 1991).

Dun (1991) argued that the fundamental aspect of community health initiatives is that they are self-determining, developing their own view of health needs and how they should be met. For Rosenthal (1983), similarly, the key characteristic of the community health movement is that it is based firmly outside the health professions. By the mid-1980s there were thousands of local health groups across the country (Kenner 1986). These groups were often totally independent from health care services but in many cases worked alongside or with community and primary health care workers and health care professionals in hospitals. However, a key problem for many community-based health initiatives has been the lack, or problematic nature, of contacts with primary care organisations (Peckham *et al.* 1996; Taylor *et al.* 1998).

The community health approach was widely supported in the development of the new public health and the 'Healthy City' and 'Health for All' movements (Ashton and Seymour 1988). The principles of participation, which were made explicit in the World Health Organisation's document *Health for All 2000*, focused on the role of the community working with health care professionals (WHO 1978; 1991). Yet this policy was never given the formal support of the UK government and, while the 'Health for All' movement grew steadily in the 1980s (Scott-Samuel, 1989), there was no universal adoption of the approach across the country. The community health movement was also rooted in the democratic/citizen philosophy of participation and the real level of participation in formalised 'Healthy City'/'Health for All' projects was often very low and not achieved without considerable difficulties (Petersen and Lupton 1996). The focus on community or place – an approach advocated by proponents of the new public health (Ashton and Seymour 1988) – found some support in the NHS with experiments with PATCH (Planned Approach or Primary Action Towards Community Health) in places such as Pimlico and Lambeth (Dun 1989) although this very focus has been criticised by some writers as being manipulative of local communities (Peterson and Lupton 1996).

The community health movement also increasingly presented a challenge to government policy in the 1980s with its emphasis on self-defined needs and recognition of the broader environmental, material and social bases of inequalities in health (*The Black Report* (Townsend 1990); Townsend *et al.* 1987; Thunhurst 1991). Equity was a key plank of 'Health for All' and also of the community health movement. However, the government and the NHS did not take on this broader perspective of health. For example, Edwina Curry, the then Minister of Health, commented on the *Black Report:* 'I honestly don't think (health) has anything to do with poverty. The problem very often for many people is just ignorance ... and failing to realise they do have some control over their own lives (quoted in Townsend 1990: 383). This individual-istic approach to the public's health was formally reflected in *The Health of the Nation* (DoH 1992) which emphasised the importance of personal life-style choices (Ranade 1998). Many have highlighted the complacency of the govern-ment's response to the goals of 'Health for All', with no national strategy being developed and the issues of equity, community participation and intersectoral working being largely ignored in its response to the WHO (*ibid.* 1998).

Generally, then, the development of community health projects and the focus on new approaches to public health were not adopted into mainstream NHS activity in the 1980s and 1990s. The evidence on the relationship between community health projects and the NHS is poor, but overall it would appear that such activity was marginalised and remained dependent on the goodwill and activity of individual health care workers, particularly those in community health units (Ottewill and Wall 1990). Many initiatives were piecemeal and/or short-lived. The role of community and place has, therefore, developed alongside the NHS rather than as a constituent part of health care services. Nevertheless, the growth in the 1980s of such initiatives (numbered in their thousands) demonstrates the ability of communities to engage in public health action outside the formal public health sphere. Where such initiatives worked alongside primary care, innovative responses to individual and com-munity health have been developed. An early example of this is the Wells Park Health Project (see Box 11.1) which had a dramatic impact on the health of patients from the Wells Park Practice (Fisher 1994). More recent examples include the Bromley by Bow Centre in East London (see Box 11.2).

More recently, the development of welfare advisory sessions has been supported by many practices as a way of dealing with individual patient prob-lems but using a broader community perspective (Coppel *et al.* 1999; Abbott and Hobby 2000). There has in fact been a real resurgence in community-based and -led initiatives (Smithies and Webster 1998) and a growing interest in community-based strategies (Demos 1997; New Economics Foundation undated; Gillam and Brooks 2001). New developments, both policy and in practice, highlight community ownership and a holistic approach to health (Gaskin *et al.* 1998) which go beyond health services developments to incorpor-ate strategies such as Building Better Communities, community co-ops, com-munity cafes, LETS and 'time bank' schemes (Cowe 2000). Other recent policy initiatives which draw very much on the community-based model include Healthy Living Centres and Sure Start. In fact, the Secretary of State for Health, Alan Milburn, highlighted Sure Start as making one of the most important contributions to health improvement in the UK (Milburn 2000). Sure Start is one of many community partnership approaches being developed around the country that seek to address individual problems through community-based responses, but by working with the local communities involved.

Box 11.1 Wells Park Health Project

The project started in 1991 in the basement of the Wells Park Practice in Sydenham, Kent. The goals of the project were to promote health awareness and develop new approaches to primary care. While organisationally separate from the NHS the community health project and practice have formal and informal links through joint management committee and staff meetings.

The health project addressed health needs in different ways from the practice, using community-based solutions such as a reminiscence group for older people with depression and campaigning for a bus to the local supermarket as a response to problems of angina. The practice has seen the project as an effective vehicle for health needs assessment. The project, by working with the practice, has also provided a basis for community participation and patient-centred care rooted in a wider social model of health than the medical model.

(Fisher 1994)

Box 11.2 Bromley by Bow Centre

The Bromley by Bow Centre is a community organisation which runs a variety of projects in an integrated way – linking health with education and enterprise, for example, or environment with training and family support – to serve as a focus for that energy and ability and so to help regenerate the area. It incorporates a health centre and is integrating the work of GPs and other health professionals with community projects. There is a café, nursery and park and the Centre runs a wide range of activities including art training, employment skills, community care services and sports. The Centre is funded from regeneration monies and also the new Opportunities Fund, with statutory agency revenue provided from normal sources.

The Role of PCOs in Promoting Community Participation

As argued above, the implementation of government policy on public health will increasingly fall to primary care organisations and thus their role, and the role of communities, in determining public health strategy and action will come under increasing scrutiny. Irrespective of their exact functions in the different countries of the UK, primary care organisations are responsible for developing their own strategies for addressing local public health and including local communities. Some may have a history of joint working with other organisations to meet community needs; however, many more do not. Involving the community in local public health issues within the context of developing local partnerships may be difficult and time-consuming. The government does not appear to want to be prescriptive about how the public is involved in public health activity, although there are more detailed guidelines and structures relating to health care services (DoH 2001b; DoH 2001h; DoH 2001j). The key issue here seems to be that primary care organisations need to develop a clearer understanding of public health and how to engage local people (Gillam *et al.* 2002). This will take time, as will the subsequent development work. The time-scales set by the government for this work do not appear to allow the work required.

Primary care organisations are expected by the government to take a lead in public health action. Further, primary care organisations are expected to demonstrate that they have involved the public in their plans, and that these plans are sensitive to local need as well as meeting government targets. However, policy documents offer little guidance about how this can be achieved or about how primary care might fulfil its role as one of the partners in Health Action Zone activity. In addition, the rhetoric in primary care organisations plans about involving the community may not be reflected in actions. To date, primary care organisations have not found it easy to address this aspect of public involvement (Wilkin *et al.* 2000; Anderson and Florin 2000; Anderson *et al.* 2002). When primary care organisations do attempt to involve the public it is from a consumerist rather than a participative perspective, for example as patients giving feedback on existing services rather than being involved in a wider dialogue on health issues (Lupton *et al.* 1998).

The emphasis on medical knowledge, medical, reactive approaches to health, and the dominance of medical culture and organisation within the NHS, suggest that primary care organisations may find it difficult to work collaboratively with either professional partners or with the public on wider public health issues. Such a focus may also lead to a poor understanding of public health beyond the confines of the medical model.

The public health activity of primary care organisations may be located in the community but primary care professionals do not necessarily engage with the community about public health issues and the relevance of their activity to the community's priorities. Generally, the organisational structures and cultures of primary care organisations reflect the predominant medical model and the fact that this inhibits the development of community perspectives on health (Taylor *et al.* 1998). Therefore, professionals may confine their public health activity to a strictly medical agenda. Others, however, may go beyond their formal role to engage with the community on wider public health issues (Heather Elliot 2000, personal communication). This suggests that some primary care organisations may not formally sanction some forms of public health activity in the community.

Findings from Taylor *et al.* (1998) suggest that engaging with the community about local public health issues means, amongst other things, addressing equity in the roles and relationships of professionals and community members. A number of factors may make this difficult. In the past, communities have not had a statutory right of access to the processes that would allow them to influence decisions about health. The current changes in primary care have yet to identify clear processes and mechanisms for such involvement and guidance for public involvement has yet to be published. Professionals may not engage with the public about the concerns of the community, may not agree with their concerns, or may not consider communication with the public on these matters as part of their role.

PCOs and Public Health: Moving Forward?

Thus the history of primary care in the UK would appear to demonstrate a move from primary medical care (general practice) to primary health care with a public health focus. It also charts the shift of primary care from the policy sideline, in the early years of the NHS, to its current central place in health policy. This shift is summarised in Table 11.1.

Table 11.1 An Historical Framework for Developments in Primary Care and Public Health in the UK

	The local context	*The national context*	*Dominant themes*
Pre NHS	The Peckham Health Centre – debates about establishing local health centres	GPs establish private practice or panel practices	Dominance of municipal health services but with growing national regulation of the organisation of health care services
1940s	GPs established as independent contractors with patient lists	NHS established in 1948	Ascendancy of hospital medicine over aims of NHS
1950s	GPs start to form partnerships in increasing numbers		General practice starts to develop as a profession dominated by a medical model of health
1960s	First quality framework for general practice; primary health care teams start to develop	Recognition of the need to co-ordinate health and social care services	Increasing professionalisation within the welfare state The rediscovery of poverty
1970s	Public health and community health services brought into NHS	Unification of community health and secondary services in the NHS	Crisis in health denotes shift from acute to chronic disease management

Table 11.1   (*continued*)

	The local context	The national context	Dominant themes
1980s	GPs dominate community nursing through practice attachments	Government concerned about the quality and role of primary care services	Ascendance of managerialism and concerns about controlling professionals and resources within the NHS
	'Health for All' and the Healthy City movements		
	Community health movement		Recognition, but official suppression of growing evidence and debate about health inequalities
1990s	Primary care purchasing and commissioning	1990 – GP contract	Integration of health promotion activity
		1992 – *The Health of the Nation*	
	Grouping general practices – multi-funds and Total Purchasing	1996 – *Primary Care: The Future*	Mid-1990s official recognition of 'health variations'
	Primary care organisations – PCGs, LHGs	1997 – *The New NHS*	Re-emphasis on health inequalities
		1999 – *Saving Lives: Our Healthier Nation*	
	Health Action Zones, healthy living centres, health parks		
2000	Primary Care Trusts and Care Trusts – combined health and social care organisations	2000 – NHS Plan – health inequalities targets	Focus on 'modernisation' of the NHS
		England – shifting the balance of power	Multi-agency action and integration of public health and primary care
	England – public health function to move to PCTs	Scotland and Wales – increasing role of National Assembly/ Parliament	

However, these developments highlight the tensions between the models of health that underpin developments in health and health care. The dominance of the medical model in UK primary care practice must, therefore, raise important questions about the potential of primary care to take on key public health roles – to transform itself from primary *medical* to primary *health* care (Macdonald 1992). It is also pertinent to ask whether such a public health role is new in terms of wider definitions of primary care (e.g. WHO 1978; WHO 1991) which recognise different models and practice of primary care and public health. For example, what has been the contribution of 'Health for All', the community health movement and, with specific relevance to the UK, community health services (Ottewill and Wall 1990; Turton *et al.* 2000).

Research in the late 1990s highlighted some of the key problems associated with developing public health within a primary care setting. Taylor *et al.* (1998) identified a number of barriers to effective public health activity including:

- lack of a 'shared language', i.e. shared definitions of public health, between primary care practitioners, and other stakeholders, including members of the community;
- poor understanding of collaborative working both within primary health care teams, and between GPs and other agencies;
- the dominance of a medical model of primary care with its emphasis on general practice, and medically dominated organisation and values;
- poor understanding of the key principles of public health among primary care professionals.

Research with developing PCG organisations in England by Meads *et al.* (1999) also identified a number of organisational blocks to developing public health in primary care. Key findings related to the need for primary care organisation to develop a public health perspective involving the acquiring of public health skills, developing organisational links with local authorities, communities, and developing organisational capacity. In addition Meads *et al.* also concluded that primary care organisations need to change their outlook:

> Primary care groups are a fundamental 'mindset' change for individuals as well as organisations. The biggest obstacles are attitudinal not structural. (Health authority director of public health quoted in Meads *et al.* 1999: 47)

Yet the new policy context is for primary care to play an active role in public health. Professor Jennie Popay in her evidence to the House of Commons Health Committee referred to the 'awesome' expectations now laid upon primary care to deliver the public health agenda and to address inequalities in health, that 'there is little if any evidence from research or practice that past primary care organisations or primary care medical professions have the capacity or the inclination to do this' (Popay 2001).

Problems are further exacerbated by the increasing focus on health inequalities (DoH 1999b) and we need to understand what role primary care organisations can play in addressing health inequalities within the public health agenda. Research evidence, from as far back as the *Black Report* (Townsend 1987) has demonstrated that poorer people are more likely to experience poor physical and mental health and have a lower than average life expectancy. Over the past two decades in the UK there has been an increasing gap between high and low incomes. People on lower incomes often live in poor and undesirable neighbourhoods. Primary care organisations are expected to take a lead in activities to address these problems.

However, local people, especially those experiencing social deprivation, may not be able to prioritise public health issues, and may lack resources to participate actively in their communities. If they do get involved they may find it difficult to participate in conventional ways without support. There is a need to empower people in these communities if they are to contribute as the government wishes. Primary care organisations will need to develop specific skills, and work together with other organisations including Local Authorities if they are to facilitate community contributions to public health. As Gillam *et al.* (2001) argue, the development of PCOs provides an opportunity to develop partnerships and take a population approach which was not possible from an individual practice approach. However, PCOs are being asked to operate within an increasingly crowded policy arena responding either singularly or in partnership with others to a range of policy streams emanating within the health policy and local authority policy arenas. This requires dealing with substantial complexity and involves developing new skills. Considering the tendency of general practice in the past not to become involved in such activities and notwithstanding the experience of community health services which are now being integrated into PCOs (in England at least), developing public health within primary care will require a cultural as well as organisational shift. As PCTs in England absorb public health specialists from the dismantled health authorities we may see an increased emphasis on medical approaches which may be at odds with the need to develop a multidisciplinary public health workforce (HDA 2001) which works with local communities rather than delivers public health to them. There may also be opportunities gained by drawing on the wider primary care workforce. In Scotland, the Executive has proposed extending the role of public health nurses (Scottish Executive 2001) – also envisaged in England and Wales by the Standing Nursing and Midwifery Advisory Committee (DoH 1995a) but yet to be fulfilled.

PART III

Primary Care: The Future

In this final part we look to the future. This last chapter draws on the policy perspectives that have been discussed previously and offers some signposts for understanding future developments. It also sets out some alternative scenarios of the ways primary care may develop in the early part of the twenty-first century.

CHAPTER 12

Conclusions: Directions for Primary Care

After eleven chapters of this book, we have hopefully shown the ways in which primary care has become a complex and dynamic sector of health policy, organisation and management in the UK. The need to document, understand and interpret the significance of primary care in UK health policy has underpinned the purpose of this book. However, given the ever-changing face of primary care, it would be a mistake if this book did not, at least, attempt to provide an indication of the direction in which primary care might travel over the next few years. This chapter provides such a direction but, inevitably, this is a dangerous undertaking because the only certainty is that the exact pace and destination of travel can never be precisely defined. However, drawing on the policy perspectives that we have presented in this book, we can offer some of the signposts or landmarks upon this journey. Using the various frameworks and concepts presented here, the evolution of primary care can thus be better understood, interpreted and acted upon.

This final chapter draws together many of the disparate themes discussed in the book since the first two opening chapters. These opening chapters set the context for primary care and provided some definitions and concepts. This set the basis for subsequent chapters which examined different facets of primary care. The final chapter will review the past and present state of primary care, highlighting two salient themes. The drivers for change are identified and some scenarios for/of future policy development will then be discussed.

Where has Primary Care Come From and Where is it Now?

The elements of primary care, in the form of generalist medical services and community health services, have long existed in various forms and under different organisational structures. However, for much of the first half of the twentieth century these two strands remained separate in organisational and administrative/managerial terms such that it was not possible to identify a *de facto* or *de jure* policy towards primary care. This reflected the largely hap-hazard way in which these services had become established and the degree of self-regulation which professions, notably medicine, enjoyed.

Even after the creation of the NHS, policy towards primary care was, at best, nascent, its development being a function of the 'opt-out' which GPs had secured in 1948 and the local authority control of most community health services. This situation set the pattern for much of the first 20–30 years of the NHS, a period in which primary care was 'detached' from the mainstream of the NHS. A concomitant aspect was that policy towards primary care was similarly 'detached'. Policy, such as it was, was marked by stasis and conservatism. Even if policy-makers and administrators had wanted to take a more interventionist stance in/on primary care (and for the most part, they did not want to), the levers available to them were few and weak.

The point of emergence of a separate sphere of health policy which addressed primary care is difficult to define precisely but the Family Doctor Charter of 1965 and the transfer of control of community health services in 1974 mark, in their different ways, watersheds for primary care policy in the UK. Governments in the UK (and elsewhere) began to see the need to address primary care in a more systematic and structured way than hitherto. Although changes were wrought by the crisis of the Welfare State in the 1970s, primary care remained detached and, to some extent, insulated against the wider reform. Primary care had yet to become seen as a problem in itself or a solution to structural crises elsewhere.

Primary care did become seen as both an issue ('problem') to be tackled and also as that solution to 'difficulties' elsewhere in the NHS during the 1980s and especially the 1990s. As the recognition of the contribution of primary care to the wider NHS became increasingly recognised, there was thus a greater need to integrate it into the NHS's organisation and management. Perhaps the most significant trigger for this was a process of managerialisation which took place right across the public sector – the rise of New Public Management (NPM). It established new patterns of policy, organisation and management. Although it initially had a marginal effect on primary care, NPM began to permeate primary care through the introduction of managerialism in community health services and other providers, the shift in focus from FPCs to FHSAs and the more managerial approaches (often associated with IT) within individual general practices.

The process of integration – making primary care less detached – continued into the 1990s with a series of reforms which were designed both as an attempt to reorganise primary care and to act as an additional lever upon secondary care. This was most clearly evident in the GP fundholding scheme and Trust status but also through a series of policy statements. Although the internal market had profound inter- and intra-professional consequences, the policy direction continued to move towards further integration with the introduction of PCGs and PCTs (and LHGs and SPCTs), not least because these were not voluntary schemes. Once community health services had been reorganised into PCGs and PCTs, primary care was effectively integrated into the NHS. A process which began some 30 years earlier had been realised.

However, such integration has not been absolute and nor is it complete. Primary care has always been noted for its diversity, in terms of service provision and quality. Despite many initiatives oriented around quality improvement (often associated with NPM) in the 1980s and 1990s, the linkage between management and quality has formally become established only with the introduction of clinical governance since 1997. Whilst primary care has long been noted for diversity in provision and quality, it is also becoming increasingly characterised by diversity in its organisational form. Integration has not been, and is unlikely to be, a uniform process applying to all areas and to all services equally. This characteristic derives from two aspects.

First, as we discussed in Chapter 2, the nature of policy-making has changed. Policy is far more emergent and, by implication, much less certain and more complicated than it once was, say, 20 years ago. No single policy blueprint exists in a drawer in Whitehall. Moreover, the emergent strategy involves the deliberately uneven spread of policy innovations (particularly in a devolved political system such as the UK); initiatives are launched or piloted in particular areas before being implemented further afield. Whilst this partly relates to the voluntary nature of these initiatives (such as GP fundholding or PMS pilots) and the selective uptake of innovations, much of it derives from the competitive, bidding nature of policy-making. Areas are required to bid for additional funding or 'flexibilities'. This not only increases the control from the centre but also changes the character of managers and clinicians in relating to the policy (through the use of performance indicators, for example). Organisations and individuals, in turn, become 'calculating selves': that is, they are subject *to* and subjects *of* this new system (Miller 1992). Many question whether the experience and practice of 'leading edge' sites can be replicated in other areas; the leaders are qualitatively different from the laggards. Although the policy may apparently be the same in each area, the context is likely to be sufficiently different to ensure a significant range of (policy) outcomes (Pettigrew *et al.* 1992; Pawson and Tilley 1997; Davies 2001).

Second, primary care organisations are responding to the needs and exigencies of their local health needs and organisational context, and to the policy-making environment, by seeking new organisational responses. These multiple options are entailing new organisational configurations, new mixes of professional staff and new interagency partnerships. For example, some organisations are seeking to employ the flexibilities offered by PMS schemes whilst some still have merged with other agencies.

A by-product of both factors has been the increasing scale of primary care organisations. The independent contractor status of GPs has long shaped policy towards general practice, not least in emphasising the diminutive scale of this 'small' business component of health care. Not only was their status a hindrance to a more integrative policy towards primary care but so was its scale. Schemes which specifically involved community health services (such as Cumberlege's neighbourhood nursing [DHSS 1986b]) were equally small scale.

The increasing scale of primary care organisations was evident in the variants of the GP fundholding schemes such as multi-funds and GP consortia. Here, increasing organisational scale brought economies of scale (especially in management costs) and significantly in power *vis-à-vis* the secondary care and other agencies (such as health and local authorities). These reasons have underlain the process of organisational enlargements which has continued through PCGs and PCTs. The original intention had been to form PCGs from communities of 100 000 but in reality this ranged from 46 000 to 255 000. Furthermore, PCTs have seen a successive population increase of about 15 000 with the second and third wave. Many such PCTs resemble the former DHAs in size. Arguably, given PCTs' triple functions, they also resemble them in other ways too. Retaining a local dimension and local responsiveness will undoubtedly become a significant issue for PCTs as they grow in scale. The introduction of locality schemes (similar to commissioning in the 1990s) is therefore likely, not least because size does not necessarily deliver its supposed benefits (Bojke *et al.* 2001). Failure to retain a 'local feel' will leave primary care organisations (and the policy which begat them) open to claims that they have become like any other health care organisation; primary care would thus have lost its organisational distinctiveness. In turn, the nature of primary care is itself changed as such organisations develop 'internal' specialisms, provide more than a straightfoward gatekeeping service, place managers in a stronger position *vis-à-vis* individual professional groups and have a more remote relationship with its population. Such organisations may, however, satisfy the policy goals of the wider NHS more readily or easily. Budget constraint and partnerships with other agencies may be among the advantages of the increasing scale. The resolution of these policy trade-offs or compromises will reveal much about direction and destination of travel for primary care.

What are the Salient Themes within Primary Care Now?

Klein's (1990) acute observation that the NHS resembles an opera with recurring melodies and changing characters has some relevance in the primary care policy context. Since the late 1980s, the notable change in the 'NHS opera' has been the scene shifting in which primary care has moved 'centre stage'. This has necessitated a fundamental review of the plot and the role of the characters. To continue (perhaps unwisely!) this metaphor, there are now many more singers on the policy stage (or, at least, with access to the policy-making machinery). One such group of actors come from primary care. Whilst some groups of actors (like doctors) have remained central throughout, others have begun to play an increasing role. The role of primary care nurses on PCGs and their public health role exemplify this.

This section tries to interpret some of the melodies and decipher the refrains coming from the primary care singers in the NHS opera stage. As outlined above, the key themes within primary care are integration and diversity. At first glance, these might appear to be in contradiction. Integration implies that the scope for independent action in and by primary care has been substantially minimised as primary care organisations fall more centrally within the NHS systems. However, the nature of policy formulation and implementation has changed such that there is greater scope for organisational and geographical difference in policy process and policy outcome. For example, this is manifest in political devolution (with competencies for health a central component of devolved territories), in the levels of PCGs/PCTs (and possibly Care Trusts) and in the experimental nature of implementation (such as pilot and beacon sites).

Furthermore, these dual themes have been running at different speeds and for different lengths of time. The process of integration of primary care has had a longer trajectory than attempts to address its diversity. However, the significance of the current phase of primary care policy is the close interrelation between these. It should not be assumed that the process of integration or efforts to address diversity have stopped; if anything, the pace of change is accelerating. The process of integration has not stopped with the introduction of PCTs or even Care Trusts. PCTs at levels 5, 6 and beyond may yet materialise, new forms of partnerships with secondary care are already emerging and the perennial issue of integration with local authorities (especially social services) may yet reappear. Diversity in quantity and quality has been a hallmark in primary care. In 1998, Alan Milburn, then Minister of Health, said:

> It is important to understand that the variations in quality in secondary care are *as nothing* compared to variations in quality in primary care. (Milburn 1999. Evidence to Health Select committee, 12 November 1998, qu. 32 emphasis added)

This diversity was a function of the certainties of policy-making prevalent in the NHS until the 1990s. Professional inputs into policy-making were guaranteed, standards of performance were largely set by the profession, private sector involvement was limited and managerial roles often reinforced the status quo (rather than challenged it). The scope for diversity has remained in the sense of the potential for local organisational and managerial responses but has also diminished (at least, in theory) in terms of service quality and quantity. The reforms over the last 20 years have provided the platform for such an equivocal position. This situation puts the government in a strong position; it is able to hold the reins over the entire spectrum of health care much more easily than before. Freedoms are apparently granted local areas but within tighter limits held by government. The new institutions of NICE and CHI and the mechanisms of NSFs are helping to reinforce this situation. This development needs to be understood in terms of the wider context in which governments generally have 'greater control over less' as a result of privatisation and NPM (Rhodes 1997). This may increasingly apply to primary care as and when PFI/ PPP schemes become established. Hence, some commentators claim that PCOs will become like American HMOs (Pollock 2001).

Diversity may also become increasingly apparent with the stratification within and between professions, especially medicine and nursing. Managerial and organisational change coupled with patient and political pressure for greater accountability are having the effect of exposing and widening inter- and intra-professional divisions. These divisions may be according to the degree of specialisation, along hierarchical lines (in terms of senior and junior clinicians) but may also be manifest in terms of knowledge (according to producers and consumers of the evidence-base) or of managerialism (according to super-ordinate and subordinate staff). A division between NHS and private sector clinicians or between 'core' and 'periphery' staff (Pinch 1997) may be evident in future. The effect is to erode further the notion of equality of competence (Causer and Exworthy 1999), although the longer-term impact of such change is debatable (Freidson 1994; Exworthy and Halford 1999).

Yet, at the same time we are increasingly seeing a blurring of boundaries between organisations and professionals. Central to the current development of primary care is the expansion of the area of activity of primary care integrating health and social care commissioning, public health and the provision of social care. The developments have been encouraged through policy and an emphasis on the development of partnerships such as Care Trusts in England, LHGs in Wales and partnership organisations in Scotland. Thus the boundary of primary care has grown to integrate other agencies and professional roles. This also challenges the professional roles of those working in such agencies and we are seeing the blurring of professional roles (e.g. nurse practitioners, the joint learning disability nurse/social worker). There is also a blurring of managerial and professional roles as GP and nurses take on new managerial roles in the PCOs. Finally, there is a blurring of roles between patients, carers and professionals with an increased emphasis on involving patients and using their experience (The Expert Patient Programme) and an increasing recognition of the role of carers as being experts in their own right. In Table 12.1 we have mapped these themes of integration, diversity and shifting boundaries across the other broad themes of this book – policy, organisation and management.

From a conceptual point of view, the twin themes of integration and diversity are instructive about the state of primary care policy itself. Several aspects are pertinent to understanding primary care in the early years of the twenty-first century. Traditionally, primary care has had a limited power-base with respect to secondary care and despite the relative dominance of GPs within it. The small business tradition of general practice has made it easier to inculcate the tenets of NPM but perhaps less easy to introduce standards and improve quality. Primary care has acted as the intermediary (in its gatekeeper role) between patients/public and secondary care providers. Primary care thus plays multiple roles of patient advocate, service provider and professional collaborator, among others. Across each of these dimensions, primary care is evolving rapidly to the extent that former power-bases and relationships are no longer applicable as once they were. Indeed, it is likely that the notion of a separate entity called 'primary care' may no longer be evident or recognisable in, say, 10 years. The evolution of primary care is changing the very nature of primary care.

Table 12.1 Cross-cutting Themes in UK Primary Care

	Integration	*Diversity*	*Changing Boundaries*
Policy	National standards – NICE, NSFs, with inspection (CHI) Shifting the Balance of Power – New shape for English NHS, PCTs are mandatory	Devolution – different approaches in England, NI, Scotland and Wales Public–private partnerships (PPP)	Changing professional roles – nurse practitioners, primary care nurses, GP specialists Redefining professional roles – dual nursing and social work qualifications
Organisation	Primary Care Trusts Care Trusts Local Health Groups Scottish Partnership Agencies	Range of organisational approaches to primary care organisations – PCTs, Care Trusts, LHGs, SPCTs Commissioning and providing mixed in different combinations Note: range of size, style and composition of PCOs across UK New forms of primary care – NHS Direct, Walk-In Centres	Integrated services – rapid response, one stop shops Care Trusts
Management	Performance management and earned autonomy Governance: board structure with lay chair and non-executive directors Practice-band contracts	PPP/PFI PMS LIFT DPH and Executive Committee Chair both on PCT board (England); reflects multiple role of PCOs	New management options for primary care professionals New career paths route for primary care managers Management/professional boundary more exposed Clinical governance

A note of caution should, however, be entered here. Power-bases within the health sector remain largely intact, the independent contractor status of GPs is still in place and primary care continues to play the pivotal role in access to other services. We should not be too hasty to rewrite the entire NHS script because structural interests are, by their nature, entrenched (Alford, 1975). For example, casting back 10 years, the introduction of the GP fundholding scheme associated with the NHS internal market was thought to herald such significant change that the NHS and primary care would be unrecognisable by 2002. That it remains such a potent political and organisational symbol is testament to the enduring features of professional capture, public affection and electoral saliency. However, the centrality of the NHS in the June 2001 election and the vote in May 2001 by GPs to consider resignation reinforces these features.

Policy analysis teaches us to view such developments in a wider framework of understanding. The strength of power-bases and the disjointed and incremental nature of policy-making denote that change will not happen overnight. However, this should not blind us to the changes that are happening because the drivers of change are clearly evident. It is these that enable us to sketch the possible scenarios for primary care in the coming years. This exercise in crystal-ball gazing is the subject of the concluding section of this final chapter.

Where is Primary Care Going?

The direction of travel for primary care may be evident but the destination is not entirely clear. Indeed, destination may not be the most suitable metaphor as it implies a finished state. Primary care policy is in a continual state of flux; it should not be assumed that there will be a time when policy development stands still. It will continually need to adapt to changing professional capabilities, public expectations, technological capabilities and political imperatives, among others. Furthermore, primary care is faced with multiple futures, not a single one. The drivers for change thus need to be understood in order to make the policy trade-offs. This section outlines such drivers and trade-offs before proposing some possible scenarios which might characterise primary care over the next few years.

Drivers of Change

The current drivers for change in primary care policy in the UK emerge from the range of issues discussed in this book. (Attention is specifically focused on internal drivers here rather than wider societal forces). First, PCTs and Care Trusts will develop over the next few years to the extent that all PCGs should be PCTs by 2004 and that Care Trusts will be introduced from 2002. (The introduction of the latter is expected to be much more piecemeal as only certain places that have good working relationships with social services are likely to become Care Trusts. They are not seen as a universal option). The reunification of providing and commissioning functions in PCTs will herald new ways of meeting health needs and new organisational forms beyond primary care. The governance issues that arise with the move to Care Trusts will be substantial as this organisational form mixes NHS and local authority systems of accountability. While on the one hand early attempts at service integration have produced positive outcomes (Peck *et al.* 2001) there will be major organisational and professional obstacles to overcome – not least union opposition.

Second, political devolution will test the robustness of the *National* Health Service, notably in the ways in which it deals with institutionalised diversity. To date, diversity has been the result of administrative (cf. political) devolution. The balance between commissioning, provision and health improvement functions will reflect the territorial policy networks (involving managers, clinicians and policy-makers/ politicians). Although political devolution may generate a desire to be different from England, the mechanisms of NICE and CHI may, however, counter the devolved competences. For example, Scotland may wish to 'subscribe' to NICE's decisions.

Third, the second Labour term of government (from June 2001) has signalled the intention to introduce private sector involvement more widely. This will surely apply to primary care but probably through smaller-scale schemes than have developed thus far. Improvements to the state of premises in primary care may be one of the first targets for such schemes. This process may facilitate the search for greater managerial control over quality and quantity of primary care provision delivered and may also precipitate the more intensive use of such premises for other forms of service provision. The latter may be in the form of more flexible use of space or longer opening hours, for example.

Fourth, new relationships are emerging from local collaborations between primary care and other partner agencies (such as social services). The representation of social services on PCG boards helped to develop existing collaborations and foster one where they were previously absent. Care Trusts will extend this process further but how much further before integration takes place? New central–local (or inter-governmental) relations are being forged. Not only has the centre taken a more interventionist role *vis-à-vis* local agencies but it has, to some degree, used primary care to act as a lever upon the area of highest health care spending – secondary care. As with the experience of general managers, this strategy of using local agents (managers or primary care) as agents of central government policy has only been partly successful. The importance of the PMS experience has been a major influence on policy development at a general practice level. Proposals agreed between GP negotiators and the Government in April 2002 propose a new practice based contract which would appear to draw directly on the experience of PMS. Of particular interest will be the shift in England where the contracts will be held between practices and PCTs. This will change local relationships and bring them more squarely in to the role of policy implementers on behalf of the Government. How this will develop in the future will depend on whether GPs vote to accept the new contract framework and then how the detail of such a contract is developed during 2002 and 2003. Local discretion (Lipsky 1980), implementation failure (Pressman and Wildavsky 1973) and collusion (Hunter 1992) have long been recognised as ways in which national policy is undermined at the local level.

Fifth, the changing balance within and between professions is creating new patterns of service delivery. General practice is re-forming itself in the light of changing perceptions of the generalist role within medicine, recruitment difficulties and revalidation as a means of professional development. Primary care nursing has been pursuing a professionalisation strategy which is challenging other professions and expanding its role especially in the public health field. Nursing roles are also being readjusted as new groups of nurses are introduced. Moreover, the state–profession relations are in flux as both come to terms with the declining authority of professionals, the degree of self-regulation and autonomy, and the problem of how to secure accountability. In Klein's terms, the 'politics of the double bed' is seeing a shifting in the relative positions of its occupants – both are fighting for control of the duvet! In addition, new professions are emerging (such as complementary therapists), alongside a renewed interest in the role of those professions allied to medicine (such as physiotherapists and occupational therapists). An increasingly broader range of services are being offered through primary care. More formal links with community pharmacists are developing and it is possible that in future more links may develop with community dentistry and ophthalmology services. The first moves in this direction will come with PCTs in England where responsibility for these services is taken on alongside other community health services. It is possible that such developments may provide a bridge for building stronger links with independent/private pharmacists, dentists and opticians.

Sixth, the increasing emphasis on partnerships with patients and carers will challenge both traditional working patterns and the role of health care and other professionals. Current NSFs place an emphasis both on involving patients in their own health care and ensuring that carers are recognised as a carer and also someone with their own health and social care needs (e.g. Older Persons NSF, Mental Health NSF). To what extent patients and carers themselves, or indeed the wider public, can influence policy is still, perhaps, open to discussion. Current proposals for public and patient involvement will require time to develop but clearly there is government support for developing structures and mechanisms for a greater lay involvement in policy development. The boundary between professional and lay expertise and practice will be one they may have to be fought over despite government policy to support lay involvement and a seemingly receptive professional view of the importance of patient participation (Wilson 2001).

Finally, the increasing emphasis being placed on public health and tackling health inequalities is providing primary care with new challenges to existing boundaries of practice and increasing diversity of roles. Central to this debate is the extent to which UK primary care can develop into a primary health care approach. This requires a reassessment of the role of primary care and a change in culture. Recent research (Taylor *et al.* 1998; Meads *et al.* 1999; Gillam *et al.* 2001) has raised a range of questions about whether UK primary care can take on such a public health role and has demonstrated that, where it has, such efforts are limited. This does not mean that there are not proponents of such a development – indeed many people see primary health care as providing an important way forward in the UK and also other countries (Starfield 1998). The key question is the extent to which the other pressures identified above support or mitigate against such a development.

Policy Trade-offs

The trade-offs or compromises that will need to be resolved in constructing and responding to the emerging policy towards primary care will determine the *de facto* shape and size of primary care's futures. Here, these trade-offs are presented as simple bipolar divisions (either/or options) whereas, in practice, shades of grey will undoubtedly be more prevalent.

- Certainty versus uncertainty;
- Centre versus local;
- Integration versus detachment;
- Diversity versus uniformity;
- Control versus autonomy;
- Generalist versus specialist;
- Financial efficiencies versus patient responsiveness;
- Medical versus a public health model.

These tensions have been apparent in the discussion throughout this book. In looking to the future we would argue that such divisions represent contested areas of policy direction. Currently it is possible to identify movements across the broad spectrum of these dichotomies – a desire for local determination mixed with a strong sense of central control or the need to address public health issues but a clear focus on medical practice, clinical systems, commissioning secondary care and, of course, tackling waiting lists.

It would be wrong to assume that such tensions or dichotomies are either new or unique to the UK. Tensions such as that between central and local are resonant throughout the UK NHS and also in other countries with public health care systems such as Canada and New Zealand. In the USA there are clear moves by insurance companies to control the activities of practitioners, thus reducing autonomy, and in Canada there are moves in some provinces (such as Ontario) to standardise the organisation and structure of primary care by developing a group practice model (similar to UK group practices). Such moves will eradicate the diversity of current primary care organisation.

Having addressed the drivers of change and presented the trade-offs, it is possible to construct some scenarios that are likely to characterise primary care's futures given current and expected trends. (We state only what we think might happen, not our own preferences.) The scenarios are:

- Dynamic conservatism;
- Corporate organisation;
- Specialisation;
- Integration;
- Public health PCO.

It is interesting to contrast these scenarios with those developed by Meads *et al.* (1999). Their scenarios related to Primary Care Groups and the development of Primary Care Trusts in England. While time has moved forward by a couple of years the policy and organisational environment has significantly altered. However, two of their models – for PCTs (executive and franchised company) – provide the basis for two of our own scenarios.

These scenarios are not predictors of the future. Combinations of them may occur and hence they need to be seen as heuristic devices which enable the outcomes that do result to be interpreted and understood. We start from the standpoint which assumes that, if the primary care-led NHS is to become meaningful, then it is no longer possible for it to remain detached or on the edge of policy-making, organisational configuration or service delivery. We do, however, assume that policy, organisation and management is still able to address an identifiable entity called 'primary care'. (This is, by no means, assured.)

Scenario 1: dynamic conservatism

This scenario is based on the expected extension of current policy developments; the process of integration would continue, diversity would be maintained and the organisational scale would increase. All PCGs would become PCTs, though larger in population coverage and, hence, smaller in number than currently envisaged. New alliances would be formed between these large-scale PCOs and local authorities and secondary care trusts on an equal basis. PCOs would retain commissioning and provision roles. The public health/health improvement function would be transferred to local authorities.

A degree of specialisation would further highlight the diversity between and within PCOs in terms of their quality of service provision and clinical outcomes. Diversity would be more tightly managed through local and national mechanisms (such as performance management and more extensive use of clinical outcome measures). Diversity between the devolved territories would undermine the notion of a *national* health service but would be moderated by the continued development of an evidence-based approach to NICE and the transfer of 'good' practice throughout the UK by CHI.

Scenario 2: corporate organisation

PFI is widespread with a building programme to renovate/expand premises but with tighter control of staff/resources. The organisation is similar to the HMO model. Patients have a choice of HMO (e.g. specialist needs such as maternity). Management teams are franchised to private/public teams. PCOs provide accredited services to their patients.

In the second scenario, PCOs would become part of the corporatisation of the NHS, involving greater application of private sector finance and management. This would mean a competitive process of patient registration and of management. Competition (such as it) would be different from the form of competition introduced during the internal market; it would be less about competition for provision but more about substitution. Particular emphasis in this scenario is, by implication, upon health care delivery (rather than, say, health improvement).

PFI/PPP schemes would be introduced throughout primary care. Although the ostensible basis would be to improve the number, quality and condition of primary care premises, it would have the effect of precipitating a more intensive use of these and remaining premises. It would also provide the basis for alliances with other PFI/PPP schemes such as hospitals. This would provide cross-agency/sector initiatives (such as those outlined in scenario 3).

Patient 'choice' would be extended through an ability to register with any PCO which would become like an American HMO. Patient registration would be non-geographical though it would probably retain a city-wide or county-wide focus. This might be especially appealing to those with particular needs, such as diabetics.

The management of PCOs would be periodically franchised to public or private sector teams. Although this franchise process may not initially affect clinical staff, management franchises and PFI/PPP schemes would provide greater leverage over 'poorly' performing clinical staff.

The regulation of this competitive model would demand a strengthened role of accreditation for national bodies such as CHI. Governmental control would thus be retained and even increased.

Scenario 3: specialisation

This scenario would entail primary care taking a subordinate role in local health care communities. As such, the power of secondary care (in terms of budgets and professional clout) would dominate. Specialist staff and specialist services would move into primary care settings (e.g. health centres and surgeries). The notion of primary care would be augmented through more fluid alliances with secondary care or local authorities.

Under this scenario, policy towards primary care would become a component of a broader agenda such as an emphasis upon service delivery. Service provision would be organised around clinical episodes of care (rather than based around organisational boundaries), possibly in terms of NSFs (namely older people or mental health, etc.). However, the ability of primary care to achieve specific goals related to health care (such as patient responsiveness or increasing activity) or even the public health agenda (such as tackling health inequalities) may be less feasible as a result. Patients would be able to gain direct access to specialists; the gatekeeper model of general practice would be scrapped. However, such an approach may lead to more integrated care. Such models exist embryonically in some areas for services for older people where staff work across hospital and community boundaries. Also, for many people with specific illnesses such as HIV/AIDS specialist hospital services provide primary as well as secondary care.

Scenario 4: integration

This scenario sees a growing development of primary care and social services (and possibly other LA services) alliances, evolving from integrated structures such as Care Trusts or the Scottish integrated management structures. While such a model represents real challenges to local government accountability and to social work practice as it has developed in the UK, current reorganisation of local government political structures and a reassessment of social work may facilitate such developments.

Such a development would open up primary care to greater local political involvement and provide new policy contexts and processes. Local authorities would become key policy players in primary care, forcing a redefinition of what is meant by primary care itself. Primary care may become a policy football – caught between central and local government. Conversely, weakened accountability structures may provide professionals with greater opportunity to develop and shape local policy agendas (and possibly national ones). Such an approach will also lead to changes in education and training and the redefinition of professional boundaries – such as that already happening between learning disability nursing and social work.

Scenario 5: public health PCO

In this scenario PCOs would develop their local community roots, establishing strong partnerships with other local statutory and voluntary agencies and placing public health as central to the organisations aims. Similar models have existed in North America (Community Health Centres), although these are increasingly under threat in the USA from for-profit HMOs and in Canada through a desire for a more standardised primary care structure.

A public health PCO would place importance on community ownership, public involvement and closer integration of lay and professional workers. Organisationally the PCO may develop as a charity or voluntary organisation interwoven with the statutory PCO. Healthy Living Centres and Health Parks may provide embryonic models for such developments. Such a model is closest to the idea of primary health care but also raises the greatest challenges for both the community and primary care professionals. However, such an approach would transcend traditional agency boundaries in more ways than the Care Trust scenario above as it would integrate a much wider range of local health and welfare agencies looking beyond current NHS and LA services.

In this scenario policy would flow upwards from the community as well as down from central government. The PCO would be placed in a position of brokering local/national tensions to a greater degree than currently envisaged. The policy community would also be expanded, creating more uncertainty on policy-making and implementation but potentially achieving better local policy outcomes.

Conclusions

Where primary care has come from is easier to decipher than where it is heading. Its futures will be contested and not just by those groups within what is currently called primary care. Politicians, hospital clinicians, managers, local authorities and, of course, patients as well as those working in primary care will all shape its future direction. It is rapidly apparent that multiple primary cares will be evident in the UK. This reflects the interaction between the political devolution, organisational reform, technological change, shifting inter-professional relations, local health needs, patient preferences and involvement.

As this book has demonstrated, primary care in the UK is experiencing three seismic shifts – integration, diversity and changing boundaries. Each is changing primary care fundamentally, either breaking down the notion of a distinct sphere of health care or reforming into the centre-piece of health policy. The changes may be documented but the interpretations will be contested. These changes are illustrated by current policy initiatives and organisational developments. The continued emphasis on national inspection, regulation, NSFs, and the vote of approval in July 2002 by GPs to negotiate practice-based contracts demonstrates continued integration. At the same time, primary care in the UK is becoming more diverse as devolution is leading to different organisational and management arrangements in England, Scotland, Wales and Northern Ireland. Even in England, different approaches to Care Trusts and local agreements on areas for service development emphasise increasing diversity. Finally, boundaries continue to change and blur through, for example, the continued extension of nursing roles, joint local authority and primary care organisation appointments and, in England, the appointment of Directors of Public Health in PCTs.

At the moment, governments appear to tolerate and even encourage different forms of primary care. This is partly because policy has used primary care as a convenient vehicle to achieve other health policy objectives such as cost containment or leverage of reform in secondary care. However, primary care is not simply a means to another end but, to some extent, it can also be seen as a goal which is based upon continuity of care, patient-centred care, gatekeeping, and community-based care. Seen in this light, primary care (divorced from organisational conceptions) can represent a distinctive approach to health (as opposed to just health care). However, this goal is likely to be lost in the plethora of new organisational configurations in the UK health care system.

It is debatable whether primary care policy will be a distinctive component of UK health policy as primary care becomes integrated, as it becomes ever more diverse and as its boundaries are re-formed. If so, primary care policy will be no different from any other aspect of health policy. Yet, as we have hopefully shown in this book, primary care is different; its particular contribution to health and health care deserves to be recognised. Equally, analysis of primary care policy, organisation and management needs to recognise multiple frameworks and concepts. Our description and explanation of a policy perspective upon primary care in the UK has been but a small contribution to understanding the changing face of primary care.

References

Abel-Smith, B. (1964) *The Hospitals 1800–1948*, Heinemann: London.

Abel-Smith, B. (1994) *An Introduction to Health Policy, Planning and Finance*, London: Longman.

Abbott, S. and Hobby, L. (2000) 'Welfare benefits advice in primary care: evidence of improvements in health', *Public Health*, 114(5), pp. 324–7.

Acheson, D. (chair) (1981) *Primary Health Care in Inner London*, Report of a study commissioned by the London Health Planning Consortium.

Acheson, D. (chair) (1998) *Independent Inquiry into Inequalities in Health*, the Acheson Report, London: TSO.

Ackroyd, S., Hughes, J. and Soothill, K. (1989) 'Public sector services and their management', *Journal of Management Studies*, 26(6), pp. 603–19.

Adams, J. and Tovey, P. (2000) 'Complementary medicine and primary care: towards a grassroots focus', Chapter 10 (pp. 167–82) in Tovey, P. (ed.) *Contemporary Primary Care: the Challenges of Chang*, Buckingham: Open University Press.

Agass, M., Coulter, A., Mant, D. and Fuller, A. (1991) 'Patient participation in general practice: who participates?', *British Journal of General Practice* 41, pp. 198–201.

Alford, R.R. (1975) *Health Care Politics*, Chicago: University of Chicago Press.

Allsop, J. (1995) *Health Policies and the NHS towards 2000*, London: Longman.

Allsop, J. (1986) 'Primary health care – the politics of change', *Journal of Social Policy*, 15, pp. 489–96

Allsop, J. and May, A. (1986) *The Emperor's New Clothes: Family Practitioner committees in the 1980s*. London: King Edward's Hospital Fund for London.

Allsop, J., Baggott, R. and Jones, K. (2002) 'Health consumer groups and the national policy process', in Henderson, S. and Petersen, A. (eds), *Consuming Health: The Commodification of Health Care*. London: Routledge.

Anderson, W. and Florin, D. (2000) *Involving the Public – One of Many Priorities*, London: King's Fund.

Anderson, W., Florin, D., Mountford, L. and Gillan, S. (2002) *Every Voice Counts: Primary Care Organisation and Public Involvement*, London: King's Fund.

Anderson, T.F. and Mooney, G. (1990) *The Challenge of Medical Practice Variations*, Basingstoke: Macmillan.

Armstrong, P. and Armstrong, H. (1999) 'Decentralised health care in Canada', *British Medical Journal*, 318, pp. 1201–4.

Arnstein, S. (1969) 'A ladder of participation', *Journal of the Royal Town Planning Institute*, 57 (April), pp. 176–182.

Ashton, J. and Seymour, H. (1988) *The New Public Health*, Milton Keynes: Open University Press.

Atkin, K. and Lunt, N. (1996) 'Negotiating the role of the practice nurse in general practice', *Journal of Advanced Nursing*, 24(3), pp. 498–505.

Audit Commission (1995) *What the Doctored Ordered? GP Fundholding*, London: HMSO.

Audit Commission (2000) *Local Health Groups in Wales: The First Year*, London: Audit Commission.

Bacharach, P. and Baratz, M.S. (1970) *Power and Poverty: Theory and Practice*, London: Oxford University Press.

Baggott, R. (1998) The politics of health care reform in Britain: a moving consensus?', ch. 9 (pp. 155–72) in Field, D. and Taylor, S. (eds), *Sociological Perspectives on Health, Illness and Health Care*. Oxford, Blackwell.

Baggott, R. (2000) *The Politics of Public Health*, Basingstoke: Palgrave – now Palgrave Macmillan.

Bailey, J., Glendinning, C. and Gould, H. (1997) *Better Buildings for Better Services: Innovative Developments in Primary Care*, Oxford: Radcliffe Medical Press.

Balint, M. (1964) *The Doctor, his Patient and the Illness*, London: Pitman Medical.

Balogh, R. (1996) 'Exploring the role of localities in health commissioning: a review of the literature', *Social Policy and Administration*, 30(2), pp. 99–113.

Bartlett, W. and Le Grand, J. (eds) (1993) *Quasi-markets and Social Policy*, London: Macmillan – now Palgrave Macmillan.

Bartlett, W., Roberts, J. and Le Grand, J. (eds) (1998) *A Revolution in Social Policy: Quasi-market Reforms in the 1990s'*, Bristol: Policy Press.

Benzeval, M., Judge, K. and Whitehead, M. (1995) *Tackling Inequalities in Health*, London: King's Fund.

Beveridge, W. (1942) *Social Insurance and Allied Services*, Report by Sir William Beveridge CMd 6404. London: HMSO.

Biggs, S. (1997) 'User Voice, Interprofessionalism and Postmodernity', *Journal of Interprofessional Care*, 11(2), pp. 195–203.

Biles, A., Mornement, A. and Palmer, H. (2001) 'From the ballot box to the real world', *Regeneration and Renewal* (8 June), pp. 14–15.

Bindman, A.B. (2001) 'Challenges on the road to clinical governance: the UK's strategy for health care quality improvement', ch. 3 (pp. 29–36) in Davies, H.T.O., Tavakoli, M. and Malek, M. (eds), *Quality in Health Care: Strategic Issues in Health Care Management*, Aldershot: Ashgate.

Bloor, K. and Maynard, A. (1999) *Primary Care in the UK: Evolution or Revolution?*, London: Institute of Health Services Management.

Bloor, M. (2001) 'On the Consulting Room Couch with Citizen Science', Paper to the Medical Sociology Conference, York.

Boaden, N. (1997) *Primary Care*, Buckingham: Open University Press.

Bojke, C., Gravell, H. and Wilkin, D. (2001) 'Is bigger better for primary groups and trusts?', *British Medical Journal*, 322 (10 March) pp. 599–602.

Bond, C. (2001) 'Pharmacists and the multi-disciplinary health care team', ch. 15 (pp. 249–69) in Taylor, K. and Harding, G. (eds), *Pharmacy Practice*, London: Taylor and Francis.

Bond, J., Cartlidge, A.M., Gregson, B.A., Baeton, A.G., Philips, P.R., Armitage, P., Brown, A.M. and Ready, B. (1987) 'Inter-professional collaboration in primary health care', *Journal of the Royal College of General Practitioners*, 37, pp. 158–61.

Boyne, G. and Powell, M. (2001) 'The spatial strategy of equality and the spatial division of welfare', *Social Policy and Administration*, 35(2 May 2001), pp. 181–94.

Bradshaw, J. (1972) 'A taxonomy of social need', in G. McLachlan (ed.), *Problems and Progress in Medical Care: Essays on Current Research*, Seventh series, Oxford: Oxford University Press for Nuffield Provincial Hospitals Trust.

Buchanan, J. (1965) *The Inconsistencies of the National Health Service*, London: Institute of Economic Affairs.

Bulpitt, J. (1983) *Territory and Power in the United Kingdom*, Manchester: Manchester University Press.

Burns, D., Hambleton, R. and Hoggett, P. (1994) *The Politics of Decentralisation*, Basingstoke: Macmillan – now Palgrave Macmillan.

Burrows, R. and Loader, B. (eds) (1994) *Towards a Post-Fordist Welfare State?*, London: Routledge.

Butler, C.C., Pill, R. and Stott, N.C.H. (1998) 'Qualitative study of patients' perceptions of doctors' advice to quit smoking: implications for opportunistic health promotion', *British Medical Journal*, 316, pp. 1878–81.

Butler, J. (1973) *Family Doctors and Public Policy: a Study of Manpower Distribution*, London: RKP.

Butler, J. (1994) 'Origins and early development', ch. 2 (pp. 13–23) in R. Robinson and J. Le Grand (eds), *Evaluating the NHS Reforms*, London: King's Fund Institute.

Calgary Regional Health Authority (1996) 'Primary Health Care Report: "A Work in Progress"', Calgary: Calgary Regional Health Authority.

Callaghan, G., Exworthy, M., Hudson, B. and Peckham, S. (2000) 'Prospects for collaboration in primary care: relationships between social services and the new PCGs', *Journal of Inter-Professional Care*, 14(1), pp. 19–26.

Calman, K. and Smith, D. (2001) 'Works in theory but not in practice? The role of the precautionary principle in public health policy', *Public Administration*, 79(1), pp. 185–204.

Calnan, M. and Gabe, J. (1991) 'Recent developments in general practice: a sociological analysis', ch. in J. Gabe, J., Calnan and M. Bury (eds), *The Sociology of the Health Service*, London: Routledge.

Carter, N., Klein, R. and Day, P. (1992) *How Organisations Measure Success: the Use of Performance Indicators in Government*, London: Routledge.

Castells, M. (1996) *The Rise of the Networked Society*, Oxford: Blackwells.

Causer, G. and Exworthy, M. (1999) 'Professionals as managers across the public sector', ch. 6 (pp. 83–101) in M. Exworthy and S. Halford (eds), *Professionals and the New Managerialism in the Public Sector*, Buckingham: Open University Press.

Cernik, K. and Wearne, M. (1994) 'Promoting the integration of primary care and public health', *Nursing Times*, 90(43), pp. 44–5.

Challis, L., Fuller, S. Henwood, M., Klein, R., Plowden, W. and Webb, A. (1988) *Joint Approaches to Social Policy*, Cambridge: Cambridge University Press.

Clamp, M. and Kendrick, D. (1998) 'A randomised controlled trial of general practitioner safety advice for families with children under 5 years', *British Medical Journal*, 316, pp. 1576–9.

Clarence, E. and Painter, C. (1998) 'Public services under new Labour: collaborative discourses and local networking', *Public Policy and Administration*, 13(3), pp. 8–22.

Clarke, J., Cochrane, A. and McLoughlin, E. (eds) (1994) *Managing Social Policy*, London: Sage.

Clegg, S. (1989) *Frameworks of Power*, London: Sage.

CMA (1996) *Medical Data and Statistics*, CMA: Cambridge.

CMO (2001) *The Report of the Chief Medical Officer's Project to Strengthen the Public Health Function*, London: DoH.

Cohen, J.M. and Uphoff, N.T. (1977) *Rural Development Participation: Concepts and measures for Project Design, Implementation and Evaluation*, Ithaca: Cornell University.

Cohen, J.M. and Uphoff, N.T. (1980) 'Participation's place in rural development: seeking clarity through specificity', *World Development*, 8, pp. 213–35.

Colin-Thome, D. (1996) 'The total fundholder', ch. 4 (pp. 53–78) in G. Meads (ed.), *Future Options for General Practice*, Oxford: Radcliffe Medical Press.

Coppel, D.H., Packham, C.J. and Varnam, M.A. (1999) 'Providing welfare rights in primary care', *Public Health*, 113(3), pp. 131–5.

Coulter, A. (1997) 'Partnership with patients: the pros and cons of shared clinical decision making', *Journal of Health Services Research and Policy*, 2(2), pp. 112–20.

Coulter, A., Entwistle, V. and Gilbert, D. 'Sharing decisions with patients: is the information good enough?', *British Medical Journal*, 318(7179), pp. 318–22.

Cowe, R. (2000) 'Swap shop', *The Guardian*, August 2000.

Cowley, S. (2002) *Public Health in Policy and Practice: A Course Book for Health and Community Services*, London: Baillière Tindall.

Cumberledge (1986) (see DHSS 1986b).

Cutler, T. and Waine, B. (1994) *Managing the Welfare State*, Oxford: Berg.

Dargie, C. (1998) 'The role of public sector chief executives', *Public Administration*, 76 (spring), pp. 161–77.

Davies, C. (1998) 'Care and the transformation of professionalism', in Knight and Sevenhuijsen (eds) *Care, Citizenship and Social Cohesion*, Utrecht, Netherlands School of Social and Economic Policy Research.

Davies, H.T.O.. (2001) 'Transformational change in health care quality: systemic reorientation – not magic bullets', ch. 8 (pp. 91–103) in Davies, Tavakoli and Malek (eds), *Quality in Health Care: Strategic Issues in Health Care Management*, Aldershot: Ashgate.

Davies, H.T.O., Crombie, I.K. and Mannion, R. (1999) 'Performance indicators in health care: guiding lights or wreckers lanterns', ch. in H.T.O. Davies, M. Malek, A. Neilson and M. Tavakoli (eds), *Managing Quality and Controlling Costs: Strategic Issues in Health Care Management*, Ashgate: Aldershot.

Davies, H.T.O., Nutley, S.M. and Smith, P.C. (2000) *What works? Evidence-based Policy and Practice in the Public Services*, Bristol: Policy Press.

Dawson, Lord (1920) *Interim Report in the Future Provision of Medical Services and Allied Services*, Report of Consultative Council on Medical and Allied Services CMD693, London: HMSO.

Day, P. and Klein, R. (1983) 'Mobilisation of consent versus the management of conflict: decoding the Griffiths report.', *British Medical Journal*, 287, pp. 1813–15.

Demos (1997) *Escaping Poverty. From Safety Nets to Networks of Opportunity*, London: Demos.

DETR (2000) *Our Towns and Cities*, London: DETR.

DETR (2001) *Local Strategic Partnerships: Government Guidance*, London: DETR.

Devlin, N., Maynard, A.. and Mays, N. (2001) 'New Zealand's new health sector reforms: back to the future?', *British Medical Journal*, 322, pp. 1171–74.

DHSS (1971) *The National Health Service Reorganisation*, Consultative Document, London: HMSO.

DHSS (1983) *Health Care and the Costs, The Development of the National Health Service in England*, London: HMSO.

DHSS (1986a) *Primary Health Care: An Agenda for Discussion*, Cmnd. 9771, London: HMSO.

DHSS (1986b) *Neighbourhood Nursing: A Focus for Care*, The Cumberlege Report, London: HMSO.

DHSS (1987) *Promoting Better Health: The Government's Programme for Improving Primary Health Care*. Cmnd. 249, London: HMSO.

DHSS (1988) *Public Health in England. The Report of the Committee of Inquiry into the Future Development of the Public Health Function*, The Acheson Report, London: HMSO.

Dietz, T. and Burns, T.R. (1992) 'Human agency and the evolutionary dynamics of culture', *Acta Sociologica*, 35(3), pp. 187–200.

Dixon, J. (1998) 'The context', ch. 1 (pp. 1–14) in Le Grand *et al.* (eds), *Learning from the NHS Internal Market*, London: King's Fund.

Dixon, J. and Mays, N. (1997) 'New Labour: New NHS?', *British Medical Journal*, 315(7123), pp. 1639–40.

Dixon, J., Inglis, S. and Klein, R. (1999) 'Is the English NHS Underfunded?', *British Medical Journal*, 318(7182), pp. 522–26.

DoH (1989a) *Working for Patients*, White Paper. Cm 555, London: HMSO.

DoH (1989b) *Caring for People*, Cm 849. London: HMSO.

DoH (1991) *Welfare of Children and Young People in Hospital*, London: HMSO.

DoH (1992) *The Health of the Nation: A Strategy for Health in England*, Cm 1986, London: HMSO.

DoH (1993) *Public Health Responsibilities of the NHS and Others*, London: DoH.

DoH (1994) *The Government's Expenditure Plans 1994–95 to 1996–97*, London: DoH.

DoH (1995a) *Making it Happen: Public Health – the Contribution, Role and Development of Nurses, Midwives and Health Visitors*, Report of the Standing Nursing and Midwifery Advisory Committee, London: DoH.

DoH (1995b) *The Health of the Nation: Variations in Health. What Can the Department of Health and the NHS Do?*, London: HMSO.

DoH (1995c) *Workbook on Joint Commissioning*, London: DoH.

DoH (1996a) *Primary Care: Delivering the Future*, London: HMSO.

DoH (1996b) *Primary Care: Choice and Opportunity*, London: DoH.

DoH (1996c) *Patient Partnership*, London: DoH.

DoH (1997) *The New NHS: Modern, Dependable*, Cm 3807, London: HMSO.

DoH (1998a) *Our Healthier Nation*, Green Paper 3852, London: HMSO.

DoH (1998b) *Partnership in Action*, London: DoH.

DoH (1998c) *Modernising Social Services*, Cm 4169, London: HMSO.

DoH (1999a) *Practice Nurses' Level of Job Satisfaction*, London: DoH.

DoH (1999b) *Saving Lives: Our Healthier Nation*, White Paper, Cm 4386, London: TSO.

DoH (1999c) *National Service Framework for Mental Health: Modern Standards and Service Models*, London: TSO.

DoH (2000) *The NHS Plan*, London: TSO.

DoH (2001a) *National Service Framework for Older People*, London: TSO.

DoH (2001b) *Shifting the Balance of Power: Securing Delivery*, London: DoH.

DoH (2001c) *Shifting the Balance: Creating Strategic Health Authorities*, London: DoH.

DoH (2001d) *The Report of the Public Inquiry into Children's Heart Surgery at the Bristol Royal Infirmary 1984–1995*, Cm 5207(II), London: TSO.

DoH (2001e) *Care Trusts: an Emerging Framework*, London: TSO.

DoH (2001f) *Guidance on Integrated Services*, London, HMSO.

DoH (2001g) *Modernising Regulation in the Health Care Professions*, London: TSO.

DoH (2001h) *Involving Patients and the Public in Healthcare: A Discussion Document*, London: DoH.

DoH (2001i) *The Expert Patient: A New Approach to Chronic Disease Management for the 21st Century*, London: DoH.

DoH (2001j) *Involving Patients and the Public in Healthcare: Response to the Listening Exercise*, London: DoH.

DoH (2001k) *Tackling Health Inequalities: Consultation on a Plan for Delivery*, London: DoH.

DoH (2002a) *Shifting the Balance: Next Steps*, London: TSO.

DoH (2002b) *Keys to Partnership*, London: DoH.

Doyal, L. (1979) *Political Economy of Health*, London: Pluto Press.

Duggan, M. (1995) *Primary Health Care: the Prognosis*, London: IPFR.

Dun, R. (1989) *Pictures of Health*, London: West Lambeth HA.

Dun, R. (1991) 'Working with the voluntary sector', in McNaught A. (ed.), *Managing Community Health Services*, London: Chapman & Hall.

Dunning, M., Abi-Aal, G. and Gilbert, D. (1998) Turning evidence into everyday practice, *Nursing Times*, 94(47): 60.

Dunsire, A. (1978) *Implementation in a Bureaucracy*, Oxford: Martin Robertson.

Edelman, M. (1971) *Politics as Symbolic Action*, Chicago: Markham Publishing.

Elston, M.-A. (1991) 'The politics of professional power: medicine in a changing health service', ch. 3 (pp. 58–88) in Gabe, Calnan and Bury (eds), *The Sociology of the Health Service*', London: Routledge.

Elston, S. and Holloway, I. (2001) 'The impact of recent primary care reforms in the UK on inter-professional working in primary care centres', *Journal of Inter-Professional Care*, 15(1), pp. 19–27.

Elwyn, G., Edwards, A., Kinnersley, P. (1999) 'Shared decision-making in primary care: the neglected second half of the consultation', *British Journal of General Practice*, 49(443), pp. 477–82.

Enthoven, A. (1985) *Reflections on Management of the NHS*, London: Nuffield Provincial Hospitals Trust.

European Observatory on Health Care Systems (EOHCS)(1999) *The United Kingdom*, London: LSE Health and Social Care.

Evans, D. and Exworthy, M. (1996) 'The changing dynamic of power in British primary care: towards a critical analysis', Paper presented to BSA medical sociology conference, Edinburgh, September 1996.

Exworthy, M. (1993a) 'A review of recent structural changes to district health authorities as purchasing organisations', *Environment and Planning C: Government and Policy*, 11, pp. 279–89.

Exworthy, M. (1993b) 'The development of purchasing: liaison with GPs', *Primary Care Management*, 3(5), pp. 9–10

Exworthy, M. (1994a) 'The contest for control in community health services: professionals and managers dispute decentralisation', *Policy and Politics*, 22(1), 17–29.

Exworthy, M. (1994b) 'Medical practice areas: discussion and development of MPAs for primary care', Briefing paper no. 11, Southampton: IHPS, University of Southampton.

Exworthy, M. (1998a) 'Localism in the NHS quasi-market', *Environment and Planning C: government and Policy*, 16, 449–62.

Exworthy, M. (1998b) 'Clinical audit in the NHS internal market: from peer review to external monitoring', *Public Policy and Administration*, 13(2, summer), pp. 40–53.

Exworthy, M., Robison, J., Gantley, M. and Evans, D. (1996) 'Power points', *Health Service Journal*, 106(5504, 23 May 1996), pp. 24–5.

Exworthy, M. and Moon, G. (1998c) 'The shape of things to come', *Health Service Journal*, 108(5618), pp. 20–22.

Exworthy, M. and Peckham, S. (1998) 'The contribution of coterminosity to joint purchasing health and social care', *Health and Place*, 4(3), pp. 233–43.

Exworthy, M. and Halford, S. (eds) (1999) *Professionals and the New Managerialism in the Public Sector*, Buckingham: Open University.

Exworthy, M. and Peckham, S. (1999) 'Collaboration between health and social care: coterminosity in the "New NHS"', *Health and Social Care in the Community*, 7(3, May 1999), pp. 229–32.

Exworthy, M., Powell, M. and Mohan, J. (1999) 'The NHS: quasi-market, quasi-hierarchy and quasi-network?,' *Public Money and Management*, 19(4), pp. 15–22.

Exworthy, M. and Powell, M. (2000) 'Variations on a theme: new Labour, health inequalities and policy failure', ch. 4 (pp. 45–62) in A. Hann (ed.), *Analysing Health Policy*, Aldershot: Ashgate.

Exworthy, M. (2001) 'Primary care in the UK: understanding the dynamics of devolution', *Health and Social Care in the Community*, 9(5), pp. 266–78.

Exworthy, M., Berney, L. and Powell, M. (2002a) '"How great expectations in Westminster may be dashed locally": the local implementation of national policy on health inequalities', *Policy and Politics*, 30(1), pp. 79–97.

Exworthy, M., Wilkinson, E.K., McColl, A., Moore, M., Roderick, P., Smith, H. and Gabbay, J. (2002b) 'The role of performance indicators in changing the autonomy of the general practice profession in the UK', *Social Science and Medicine*, (2002).

Farrell, C. and Law, J. (1998) 'Regional policy differences in the UK: education in Wales', *Public Policy and Administration*, 13(2), pp. 54–69.

Ferlie, E., Ashburner, L., Fitzgerald, L. and Pettigrew, A. (1996) *The New Public Management in Action*, Oxford: Oxford University Press.

Ferlie, E. and Pettigrew, A. (1996) 'Managing through networks: some issues and implications for the NHS', *British Journal of Management*, 7 (special issue), pp. s81–s99.

Fernie, K. and McCarthy, J. (2001) 'Partnership and Community Involvement: Institutional Morphing in Dundee', *Local Economy*, 16(4), pp. 299–311.

Fisher, B. (1994) 'The Wells Park Heath Project', in Heritage, Z. (ed.) *Community Participation in Primary Care*, Occasional Paper 64, London: RCGP.

Flynn, R. *et al.* (1996) *Markets and Networks in Community Health Services*, Buckingham: Open University Press.

Flynn, R. (1999) 'Managerialism, professionalism and quasi-markets', ch. 2 (pp. 18–36) in Exworthy and Halford (eds), *Professionals and the New Managerialism in the Public Sector*, Buckingham: Open University Press.

Foucault, M. (1973) *The Birth of the Clinic. An Archaeology of Medical Perception*, London: Tavistock.

Freidson, E. (1994) *Professionalism Reborn: Theory, Prophecy and Policy*, Cambridge: Polity Press.

Friedson, E. (1970) *Profesional Dominance: the Social Structure of Medical Care*, New York: Aldine.

Frenk, J. (1994) 'Dimensions of health system reform', *Health Policy*, 27, pp. 19–34.

Fry, J. (1993) *General Practice – The Facts*, Oxford: Radcliffe Medical Press.

Fry, J. and Hodder, J.P. (1994) *Primary Health Care in an International Context*, London: Nuffield Provincial Hospitals Trust.

Gabe J., Calnan, M. and Bury, M. (eds) (1991) *The Sociology of the Health Service*, London: Routledge.

Garside, P. (1999) 'Evidence based mergers', *British Medical Journal*, 318, pp. 345–6.

Gaskin, K., Vincent, J. and Miles, A. (1998) *Healthy Living Centres. Practical Illustrations of Key Principles*, Loughborough: CRSP, Loughborough University.

Giddens, A. (2001) *Sociology*, Cambridge: Polity.

Gillam, S. and Brooks, F. (eds) (2001) *New Beginnings: Towards Patient and Public Involvement in Primary Health Care*, London: King's Fund.

Gillam, S. and Irvine, S. (2000) 'Collaboration in the new NHS', *Journal of Inter-Professional Care*, 14(1), pp. 5–6.

Gillam, S. and Miller, R. (1997) *COPC – A Public Health Experiment in Primary Care*, London: King's Fund.

Gillam, S. and Pencheon, D. (1998) 'Managing demand in general practice', *British Medical Journal*, 316, pp. 1895–8.

Gillam, S., Abbott, S., Banks-Smith, J. (2001) 'Can primary care groups and trusts improve health?', *British Medical Journal*, 323, pp. 89–92.

Glendinning, C. (1998) 'From general practice to primary care: development in primary care services 1990–1998', ch. 8 (pp. 137–64) in E. Brunsden, H. Dean and R. Woods, *Social Policy Review 10*, London: Social Policy Association.

Glendinning, C. (1999) 'GPs and contracts: bringing general practice into primary care', *Social Policy and Administration*, 33(2), June, pp. 115–31.

Glendinning, C., Chew, C. and Wilkin, D. (1994) 'Professional power and managerial control: the case of GP assessments of the over-75s', *Social Policy and Administration*, 28, pp. 317–323.

Glendinning, C., Coleman, A., Shipman, C. and Malbon, G. (2001) 'Primary Care Groups: Progress in partnerships', *British Medical Journal*, 323, pp. 28–31.

Glendinning, C., Rummery, K. and Clarke, R. (1998) 'From collaboration to commissioning: developing relationships between primary health and social services', *British Medical Journal*, 317, pp. 122–5.

Glennerster, H., Matasaganis, M., Owens, S. and Hancock, P. (1994) *Implementing GP Fundholding*, Buckingham: Open University Press.

Godber, E., Robinson, R. and Steiner, A. (1997) 'Economic evaluation and the shifting balance towards primary care: definitions, evidence and methodological issues', *Health Economics*, 6(3), pp. 275–94.

Goddard, M., Mannion, R. and Smith, P.C. (1999) 'Assessing the performance of NHS hospital trusts: the role of hard and soft information', *Health Policy*, 48 (2, August), pp. 119–34.

Goodwin, N. (1998) 'GP fundholding', ch. 4 (pp. 43–68) in J. Le Grand, N. Mays and J.-A. Muligan (eds), *Learning from the NHS Internal Market: a Review of Evidence*, London: King's Fund.

Goodwin, N., Leese, B., Baxter, K., Abbott, S. Malbon, G. and Killoran, A. (2001) 'Developing primary care organizations', ch. 3 (pp. 46–63) in N. Mays, S., Wyke, G., Malbon and N. Goodwin (eds) *The Purchasing of Health Care by Primary Care Organizations*, Buckingham: Open University Press.

Gordon, P. and Hadley, J. (eds) (1996) *Extending Primary Care*, Oxford: Radcliffe Medical Press.

Gordon, P. and Plampling, D. (1996) 'Primary healthcare: its characterization and potential', in Gordon and Huckley (eds).

Graffy, J. and Williams, J. (1994) 'Purchasing for all: an alternative to fundholding', *British Medical Journal*, 308, pp. 391–4.

Graham, H. (ed) (2000) *Understanding Health Inequalities'*, Buckingham: Open University Press.

Granovetter, M. (1992) 'Economic action and social structure: the problem of embeddedness', ch. (pp. 53–81) in M. Granovetter and R. Swedberg (eds), *The Sociology of Economic Life*, Boulder, CO: Westview Press.

Green, J. (1993) 'The views of single-handed general practitioners: a qualitative study', *British Medical Journal*, 290, pp. 823–6.

Green, J. and Britten, N. (1999) 'Putting the theory back in primary care organisation as an example of the potential contribution of sociology to health services research.' Paper presented to the BSA Medical Sociology Conference, York University, September 1999.

Green, J. and Thorogood, N. (1998) *Analysing Health Policy: a Sociological Approach*, London: Longman.

Greenwood, E. (1957) 'Attributes of a profession', *Social Work*, 14, p. 2.

Griffiths, L. and Hughes, D. (2000) 'Talking contracts and taking care: managers and professionals in the British National Health Service internal market', *Social Science and Medicine*, 51(2), pp. 209–22.

Griffiths, R. (1983) *NHS Management Inquiry: report*, London: DHSS.

Gunn, L. (1978) 'Why is implementation so difficult?', *Management Services in Government*, issue 33, pp. 169–76.

Guzzo, R. and Shea, G. (1992) 'Group performance and inter-group relations' (pp. 269–313) in M. Dunnette and L. Hough (eds), *Handbook of Indusrial and Organizational Psychology*, Palo Alto, CA: Consulting Psychologists Press, Second edn, vol. 3.

Gwyn, R. and Elwyn, G. (1999) 'When is a shared decision not (quite) a shared decision? Negotiating preferences in a general practice encounter'. *Social Science and Medicine*, 49(4), pp. 437–47.

Ham, C. (1992) *Health Policy in Britain*, 2nd edn, Basingstoke: Macmillan – now Palgrave Macmillan.

Ham, C. (1996) 'Contestability: a middle path for health care', *British Medical Journal*, January, 312(7023), pp. 70–1.

Ham, C. and Hill, M. (1993) *The Policy Process in the Modern Capitalist State*, London: Harvester Wheatsheaf.

Ham, C. and Hunter, D.J. (1988) *Managing Clinical Activity in the NHS*. London: King's Fund Institute.

Ham, C., Hunter, D.J. and Robinson, R. (1995) 'Evidence-based policy-making', *British Medical Journal*, January 1995, 310, 71–2.

Handy, C. (1994) *The Empty Raincoat*, London: Arrow.

Hardey, M. (1999) 'Doctor in the house: the internet as a source of lay knowledge and the challenge to expertise', *Sociology of Health and Illness*, 21(6), pp. 82–835.

Hardy, B., Leedham, I. and Wistow, G. (1996) 'Care manager co-location in GP practices', ch. in R. Bland (ed.), *Developing Services for Older People and their Families*, London: Jessica Kingsley Publishing.

Harris, A. (1995) 'Fresh fields: the relationship between public health medicine and general medical practice', *Primary Care Management*, 5(7), pp. 3–9.

Harrison, A. (1993) *From Hierarchy to Contract'*, Newbury: Policy Journals.

Harrison, S. (1988) *Managing the National Health Service: Shifting the Frontier?*, London: Chapman & Hall.

Harrison, S. (1998) 'The policy of evidence based medicine in the United Kingdom, *Policy and Politics*, 26(1), pp. 15–31.

Harrison, S. (1999) 'Clinical autonomy and health policy: past and futures', ch. 4 (pp. 49–61) in M. Exworthy and S. Halford (eds), *Professionals and the New Managerialism in the Public Sector*, Buckingham: Open University Press.

Harrison, S. (2001) *New Labour, Modernisation and the Medical Labour Process*, City University, March.

Harrison, S., Hunter, D.J. and Pollitt, C. (1990) *The Dynamics of British Health Policy*, London: Unwin.

Harrison, S., Hunter, D., Marnoch, G. and Pollitt, C. (1992) *Just Managing: Power and Culture in the National Health Service*, Basingstoke: Macmillan – now Palgrave Macmillan.

Harrison, S. and Pollitt, C. (1994) *Controlling Health Professionals*, Buckingham: Open University Press.

Harrison, S. and Lachmann, P. (1996) *Towards a High Trust NHS*, London: IPPR.

Harrison, S. and Wood, B. (1999) 'Designing health service organization in the UK 1968–1998: from blueprint to bright idea and 'manipulated emergence'', *Public Administration*, winter, 77(4), pp. 751–68.

Harrison, S., Ahmad, W., Milewa, T., Heywood, T. and Tovey, P. (2000) *Public and Patient Involvement in Primary Care Groups: an Interim Report to the Department of Health*, London: NHS Executive.

Hayter, P., Peckham, S. and Robinson, R. (1996) *Morale in General Practice*, Southampton: Institute for Health Policy Studies, University of Southampton.

Hazell, R. and Jervis, P. (1998) *Devolution and Health*, Nuffield Trust Series No. 3, University College: London and the Nuffield Trust: London.

HDA (2001) *Public Health Skills Audit*, London: HDA.

Heclo, H. and Wildavksy, A. (1974) *The Private Government of Public Money*, London, Macmillan – now Palgrave Macmillan.

Heritage, Z. (1994) *Community Participation in Primary Care*, London: RCGP.

Hill, M. (1997) 'Implementation: yesterday's issue?', *Policy and Politics*, 25(4), pp. 375–85.

Hill, M. (1998) *The Policy Process in the Modern State*, London: Prentice-Hall.

Hirschman, A. (1970) *Exit, Voice and Loyalty*, Cambridge, MA: Harvard University Press.

Hogg, C. and Graham, G. (2001) *Patient and Public Involvement in the NHS*, Report of a scoping study commissioned by the College of Health, the Long-term Medical Conditions Alliance and the Patient's Forum.

Hoggett, P. (1996) 'New modes of control in the public service', *Public Administration*, 74, pp. 9–32.

Hogwood, B.W. and Gunn, L.A. (1989) *Policy Analysis for the Real World*, Oxford: Oxford University Press.

Holliday, I. (1995) *The NHS Transformed*, Manchester: Baseline.

Honigsbaum, F. (1979) *The Division in British Medicine: a History of the Separation of General Practice from Hospital Care, 1911–1968*, London: Kogan Page.

Hood, C. (1991) 'A public management for all seasons?', *Public Administration*, 69, spring, pp. 3–19.

House of Commons, Social Services Committee (1987) *Primary Health Care HC37, Session 1986–87*, London: HMSO.

House of Commons Select Committee on Health (1998) *The Relationship Between Health and Social Services, First Report 1998/99 Session*, London: HMSO.

House of Commons Health Select Committee on Health (2001) *Public Health. Second Report, Volume I. Report and Proceedings of the Committee*, London: TSO.

Hudson, B. (1999a) 'Primary health care and social care: working across professional boundaries', *Managing Community Care*, 7(2), April, pp. 15–20.

Hudson, B. (1999b) 'Joint commissioning across the primary health care–social care boundaries: can it work?', *Health and Social Care in the Community*, 7(5), pp. 358–66.

Hudson, B. (1999c) *Primary Care Group and Partnership, Report for ADSS*, Leeds: Nuffield Institute for Health.

Hudson, B. (2002) 'Interprofessionality in health and social care: the Achilles heel of partnership?,' *Journal of Inter-professional Care*, 16(1), pp. 7–17.

Hudson, B., Hardy, B., Henwood, M. and Wistow, G. (1997) *Inter-agency collaboration: Primary Health Care Sub-study, Final report*, University of Leeds: Nuffield Institute for Health.

Hudson, B., Exworthy, M. and Peckham, S. (1998) *The Integration of Localised and Collaborative Purchasing: A Review of the Literature and a Framework for Analysis*, Nuffield Institute for Health, University of Leeds/Institute for Health Policy Studies, University of Southampton.

Hudson, B., Exworthy, M., Peckham, S. and Callaghan, G. (1999) *Locality partnerships: the Early PCG Experience*, Leeds: Nuffield Institute for Health.

Hudson, B. and Hardy, B. (2001) 'Localization and partnership in the "New National Health Service": England and Scotland compared', *Public Administration*, 79(2), pp. 225–315.

Hughes, D. and Griffiths, L. (1999) 'Access to public documents in a study of the NHS internal market: openness vs. secrecy in contracting for clinical services', *International Journal of Social Research Methodology: Theory and Practice*, Jan–Mar, 2(1), pp. 1–16.

Hunter, D.J. (1980) *Coping with Uncertainty: Policy and Politics in the NHS*, Chichester: John Wiley & Sons.

Hunter, D.J. (1992) 'Doctors as managers: poachers turned gamekeepers?', *Social Science and Medicine*, 35(4), pp. 557–66.

Hunter, D.J. (1994) 'From tribalism to corporatism: the managerial challenge to medical dominance', in J. Gabe, D. Kelleher and G. Williams (eds), *Challenging Medicine*, London: Routledge.

Hunter, D.J. (1998) *Desperately Seeking Solutions: Rationing Health Care*, London: Longman.

Hunter, D.J. and Wistow, G. (1987) *Community Care in Britain: Variations on a Theme*, London: King Edward's Hospital Fund for London.

Huxham, C. and Macdonald, D. (1992) 'Introducing collaborative advantage', *Management Decision*, 30(3), pp. 50–6.

Iliffe, S. (2001) 'The national plan for Britain's National Health Service: Toward a managed market', *International Journal of Health Services Research and Policy*, 31(1), 105–10.

Immergut, E. (1992) *Health Politics*, Cambridge: Cambridge University Press.

James, J.H. (1994) *Transforming the NHS: the View from Inside*, Bath Social Policy Papers no.19, Bath: University of Bath.

Janovsky, K. (ed.) (1996) *Health Policy and Systems Development: an Agenda for Research*, Geneva: WHO.

Janovsky, K. and Cassells, A. (1996) 'Health policy and systems research: Issues, methods and priorities', ch. 3 (pp. 11–24) in K. Janovsky (ed.), *Health Policy and Systems Development*, Geneva: WHO.

Jarman, B. (1983) 'Identification of underprivileged areas', *British Medical Journal*, 286, pp. 1705–9.

Jenkins-Clarke, S., Carr-Hill, R.A. and Dixon, P. (1998) 'Teams and seams: skill mix in primary care', *Journal of Advanced Nursing*, 28, pp. 1120–6.

Jervis, P. and Plowden, W. (2000) *Devolution and Health: First Annual Report of a Project to Monitor the Impact of Devolution on the UK's Health Service*, London: UCL Constitution Unit.

John, P. (2000) *Analysing Public Policy*, London: Continuum.

Jones, K., Baggott, R. and Allsop, J. (2000) 'Under the Influence', *Health Service Journal*, (5731), pp. 28–9.

Kark, S.L. and Kark, E. (1983) 'An alternative strategy in community-health care – community-oriented primary health-care', *Israel Journal of Medical Sciences*, 19(8), pp. 707–13.

Kavanagh, D. and Richards, D. (2001) 'Departmentalism and joined-up government: back to the future', *Parliamentary Affairs*, 54, pp. 1–18.

Kellas, J. (1975) *The Scottish Political System*, Cambridge: Cambridge University Press.

Kendall, J. (2000) 'The mainstreaming of the third sector into public policy in England: whys and wherefores', *Policy and Politics*, 28(4), pp. 541–62.

Kent, A. and Kumar, A. (1999) *The Development Needs of Primary Care Groups*, Chichester: AENEAS ERC.

Kennedy, T.E. (1999) *European Union of General Practitioners (UEMO) Reference book 1999/2000*, 6th edn, London: Kensington Publications Ltd.

Kenner, C. (1986) *Whose Needs Count?*, London: Bedford Square Press.

Kickert, W., Klijn, E-H. and Koppenjan, F.M. (1997) *Managing Complex Network*, London: Sage.

Kind, P., Leese, B. and Hardman, G. (1993) *Evaluating the Fundholding Initiative: the Views of Patients*, York: Centre for Health Economics, York University.

Kingdon, J. (1995) *Agendas, Alternative and Public Policies*, Boston: Little, Brown.

King's Fund Centre (1988) *Patching In*, No. 5, July 1988, pp. 1–7.

Kirk, S. (1999) Caring for children with specialized health care needs in the community: the challenges for primary care', *Health and Social Care in the Community*, 7(5), pp. 350–7.

Kirk, S. and Glendinning. C. (1998) 'Trends in community care and patient participation: implications for the roles of informal carers and community nurses in the UK', *Journal of Advanced Nursing*, 28(2), pp. 370–81.

Klein, R. (1990) 'The state and the profession: the politics of the double bed', *British Medical Journal*, 301, pp. 700–2.

Klein, R. (1989) *The Politics of the NHS*, London: Longman, 2nd edn.

Klein, R. (1995) *The New Politics of the NHS*, London: Longman, 3rd edn.

Klein, R. (2000) 'Governing the Health Care System: a comparative study of the United Kingdom, the United States and Germany', *Journal of Social Policy*, 29(3), pp. 527–8.

Klein, R. and Day, R. (1997) *Steering but now Rowing: the Transformation of the DoH. A Case Study*, Bristol: Policy Press.

Lattimer, V., Sassi, F., George, S., Moore, M., Turnbull, J., Mullee, M. and Smith, H. (2000) 'Cost analysis of nurse telephone consultation in out-of-hours primary care: evidence from a randomised controlled trial', *British Medical Journal*, 320, pp. 1053–7.

Laughlin, S. and Black, D. (1995) *Poverty and Health: Tools for Change*, Birmingham: Public Health Alliance.

Le Grand, J., Mays, N. and Mulligan, J.-A. (eds) (1998) *Learning from the NHS Internal Market: a Review of Evidence*', London: King's Fund.

Lennox, A.S., Osman, L.M., Reiter, E,.Robertson, R., Friend, J., McCann, I., Skatun, D. and Donnan, P.T. (2001) 'Cost effectiveness of computer tailored and non-tailored smoking cessation letters in general practice: randomised controlled trial', *British Medical Journal*, 322, p. 1396.

Leopold, N., Cooper, J. and Clancy, C. (1996) 'Sustained partnership in primary care', *Journal of Family Practice*, 42, pp. 129–37.

Levitt, I. (1988) *Poverty and Welfare in Scotland*, Edinburgh University Press.

Lewis, J. (1986) *What Price Community Medicine? The Philosophy, Practice and Politics of Public Health Since 1919*, Brighton: Wheatsheaf.

Lewis, J. (1997) *Independent Contractors: GPs and the GP Contract in the Post-war Period*, Debates in Primary Care 1, Manchester: National Primary Care Research and Development Centre.

Lewis, J. (1998) 'What is primary care? Developments in Britain since 1960s', *Health Care Analysis*, 6(4), pp. 324–9

Lewis, J. (1999) 'The concepts of community care and primary care in the UK: the 1960s to the 1990s', *Health and Social Care in the Community*, 7(5), 333–41.

Lindblom, C. (1959) 'The science of "muddling through"', *Public Administration Review*, 19, 79–88.

Lindblom, C. (1965) *The Intelligence of Democracy*, New York: Free Press.

Lindblom, C. (1977) *Politics and Markets*, New York: Basic Books.

Lindsay, J. and Craig, P. (2000) *Nursing for Public Health: Population-based Care*, Edinburgh: Churchill Livingstone.

Lipsky, M. (1980) *Street Level Bureaucracy*, New York: Russell Sage Foundation.

Little, P., Everitt, H., Williamson, I., Warner, M., Gould, C. *et al.* (2001) 'Preferences of patients for patient centred approach to consultation in primary care: observational study', *British Medical Journal*, 322, pp. 468–72.

Loader, B. and Burrows, R. (1994) *Towards a Post-Fordist Welfare State*, London: Routledge.

Longley, D. (1993) *Public Law and Health Service Accountability*, Buckingham: Open University Press.

Lorig, K., Stewart, A., Ritter, P., Gonzàlez, V., Laurent, D. and Lynch, J. (1996) *Outcome Measures for Health Education and Other Health Care Interventions*, Thousand Oaks, CA: Sage.

Lukes, S. (1974) *Power: a Radical View*, London: Macmillan – now Palgrave Macmillan.

Lupton, C., Buckland, S. and Moon, G. (1995) 'Consumer involvement in health care purchasing: the role and influence of CHCs', *Health and Social Care in the Community*, 3(4), pp. 215–26.

Lupton, C., Peckham, S. and Taylor, P. (1998) *Managing Public Involvement in Healthcare Purchasing*, Buckingham: Open University Press.

Lupton, D. (1994) *Medicine As Culture*, London: Sage.

Macdonald, J. (1992) *Primary Health Care: Medicine in its Place*, London: Earthscan.

McColl, A., Roderick, P., Gabbay, J., Smith, H. and Moore, M. (1998) 'Performance indicators for primary care groups: an evidence-based approach', *British Medical Journal*, 317, pp. 1354–60.

McColl, A., Roderick, P., Wilkinson, E.K., Smith, H., Moore, M., Exworthy, M. and Gabbay, J. (2000) 'Clinical governance in primary care groups: the feasibility of deriving evidence-based performance indicators', *Quality in Health Care*, 9(2), pp. 90–7.

McKeown, T. (1976) *The Role of Medicine*, London: Nuffield Provincial Hospitals Trust.

Mahon, A., Wilkin, D. and Whitehouse, C. (1994) 'Choice of hospital for elective surgery referrals: GPs' and patients' views', ch. 5 (pp. 108–29) in R. Robinson and J. Le Grand, (eds), *Evaluating the NHS Reforms*, London: King's Fund.

Malcolm, L. and Powell, M. (1996) 'The development of independent practice association in New Zealand, *New Zealand Medical Journal*, 109, pp. 184–7.

Marks, L. and Hunter, D. (1998) *The Development of Primary Care Groups: Policy into Practice*, Birmingham: NHS Confederation.

Marmor, T. (2001) *Fads and Fashion in Health Policy*, Rock Carling lecture, London: Nuffield Trust.

Marshall, M.N., Shekelle, P., Brook, B. and Leatherman, S. (2000) *Dying to Know*. Public release of information about quality of health care services, Series no. 12, London: Nuffield Trust.

Mayston, E.L. (1969) *Report of the Working Party on Management Structures in the Local Authority Nursing Services* (Chair, Mayston). DHSS, Scottish Home and Health Departments and Welsh Office.

Maxwell, R. (1984) 'Quality assessment in health', *British Medical Journal*, 300, pp. 919–22.

Mays, N. and Dixon, J. (1996) *Purchaser Plurality in UK Health Care*, London: King's Fund.

Mays, N. and Dixon, J. (1998) 'Purchaser plurality in UK health care: is a consensus emerging and is it the right one?', ch. 9 (pp. 175–200) in W. Bartlett, J. Roberts and J. Le Grand (eds) *A Revolution in Social Policy: Quasi-market Reforms in the 1990s*, Bristol: Policy Press.

Mays, N., Goodwin, N., Killoran, A. and Malbon, G. (1998) *Total Purchasing. A Step Towards Primary Care Groups*, London: King's Fund.

Mays, N., Mulligan, J.-A. and Goodwin, N. (2000) 'The British quasi-market in health care: a balance sheet of the evidence', *Journal of Health Services Research and Policy*, 5(1), pp. 49–58.

Mays, N., Wyke, S., Malbon, G., Killoran, A. and Goodwin, N. (eds) (2001a) *The Purchasing of Health Care by Primary Care Organizations*, Buckingham: Open University Press.

Mays, N., Wyke, S., Malbon, G., Killoran, A. and Goodwin, N. (2001b) 'The total purchasing experiment: a guide to future policy development?', ch. 14 (pp. 278–97) in Mays, Wyke, Malbon and Goodwin (eds), *The Purchasing of Health Care by Primary Care Organizations*, Buckingham: Open University Press.

Meads, G. (ed.) (1996) *A Primary Care-Led NHS: Putting it into Practice*, London: Churchill Livingstone.

Meads, G., Killoran, A., Ashcroft, J. and Cornish, Y. (1999) *Mixing Oil and Water: How can Primary Care Organisations Improve Health as Well as Deliver Effective Health Care?*, London: HEA.

Medical Practices Committee (MPC) (1993) *The London Initiative Zone: A Discussion Draft of a General Medical Manpower Planning Model*, London: MPC.

MPC (1999) *Annual Report 1998/9*, London: MPC.

Medical Practice Committee (MPC) (2002) *Final Annual Report: 1948–2002*, London: MPC.

Melesis, A. (1992) 'Community participation and involvement: theoretical and empirical issues', *Health Services Management Research*, 5, pp. 5–16.

Milburn, A. (1999) *Evidence to the House of Commons Select Committee on Health Report on Primary Group Care*, Hc 153, London: TSO.

Milburn, A. (2000) *A Healthier Nation and a Healthier Economy: the contribution of a modern NHS*, LSE Health Annual Lecture, 8 March, London.

Miller, F. (1992) 'Competition law and anti-competitive professional behaviour affecting health care', *The Modern Law Review*, 55(4), pp. 453–81.

MoH (1962) *A Hospital Plan for England and Wales*, CMD 1604, London: HMSO.

Mohan, J. (1995) *A National Health Service?*, Basingstoke: Macmillan – now Palgrave Macmillan.

Moon, G. and Lupton, C. (1995) 'Within acceptable limits: health care provider perspectives on community health councils in the reformed NHS', *Policy and Politics*, 23(4), pp. 335–46.

Moon, G. and North, N. (2000) *Policy and Place: General Medical Practice in the UK*, Basingstoke: Macmillan – now Palgrave Macmillan.

Moran, M. and Wood, B. (1993) *States, Regulation and the Medical Profession*, Buckingham: Open University Press.

Mulligan, J.-A. (1998) 'Health authority purchasing', ch. 3 (pp. 20–42) in Le Grand, Mays and Mulligan (eds), *Learning from the NHS Internal Market: a Review of Evidence*, London: King's Fund.

Murray, S.A., Tapson, J., Turnbull, L., McCallum, J. and Little, A. (1994) 'Listening to local voices: adapting rapid appraisal to assess health and social needs in general practice', *British Medical Journal*, 308, pp. 698–700.

Myles, S., Wyke, S., Popay, J., Scott, J., Campbell, A. and Girling, J. (1998) *Total Purchasing and Community and Continuing Care: Lessons for Future Policy Developments in the NHS*, London: King's Fund.

National Assembly for Wales (2001) 'New democratic structure proposed for NHS', Press release, 18 July 2001.

New Economics Foundation (Undated) Participation Works! 21 Techniques of Community Participation for the 21st Century. London: NEF with UK Community Participation Network.

Newman, P. (1995) 'Interview with Alain Enthoven: is there convergence between Britain and the United states in the organisation of health services?', *British Medical Journal*, 310, 24 June, pp. 1652–55.

NHS Centre for Reviews and Dissemination (CRD) (1995) *Review of the Research on the Effectiveness of Health Service Interventions to reduce Variations in Health*, York: University of York.

NHS Executive (1994) *Developing NHS Purchasing and GP Fundholding. Towards a Primary Care-led NHS*, Leeds: NHS Executive Published in conjunction with EL(94)79.

NHS Executive (1993) *Better Living – Better Lives*, Leeds: NUSR.

NHS Executive (1995) *Accountability Framework for GP Fundholding*, Leeds: NHS Executive.

NHS Executive (1996) *Primary Care: The Future*, Leeds: NHS Executive.

NHS Executive (1998a) *Establishing Primary Care Group*, HSC 1998/065, Leeds NHS Executive.

NHS Executive (1998b) *In the Public Interest*, Leeds: NHS Executive.

NHS Executive (1999) *PCGs: Taking the Next Steps*, HSC 1999/246, Leeds: NHS Executive.

NHS Management Executive (1992) *Local Voices*, Leeds: NHSME.

Nichols, A. (1996) 'Making it happen: community nurses' public health role', *Health Visitor*, 69(1), pp. 28–9.

North, N. (1995) 'Alford revisited: the professional monopolisers, corporate rationalisers, community and markets,' *Policy and Politics*, 23(2) pp. 115–25.

North, N., Lupton, C. and Khan, P. (1999) 'Going with the grain? GPs and the New NHS', *Health and Social Care in the Community*, 7(6), pp. 409–17.

North, N. and Peckham. S. (2001) 'Analysing structural interests in Primary Care Groups', *Social Policy and Administration*, 35(4), pp. 426–40.

Nutting, P.A., Wood, M. and Cowner, E.M. (1985) Community-orientated primary care in the United States. A status report. *JAMA*, 253(12), pp. 1763–66.

Office of Commissioner for Public Appointments (OCPA) (2000) *Public appointments to NHS Trusts and Health Authorities. A report by the Commissioner for Public Appointments*, March, London: OCPA.

Office of Health Economics (OHE) (1997) *10th Compendium of Health Statistics*, London: Office of Health Economics, Table 4.21.

Office for National Statistics (1996) *Living in Britain: Results from the 1995 General Household Survey*, London: TSO.

OHE (1995) *Compendium of Health Statistics*, London: TSO.

Ong, B.N., Humphris, G., Annett, H. and Rifkin, S. (1991) 'Rapid appraisal in an urban setting an example from the developed world', *Social Science and Medicine*, 32(8), pp. 909–15.

Osbourne, D. and Gaebler, T. (1992) *Re-inventing Government: How the Entrepreneurial Spirit is Transforming the Public Sector*, Reading MA: Addison-Wesley.

Ottewill, R. and Wall, A. (1990) *The Growth and Development of Community Health Services*, Sunderland: Business Education Publishers Ltd.

Ovretveit, J. (1995) *Purchasing for Health*, Buckingham: Open University Press.

Packwood, T., Keen, J. and Buxton, B. (1991) *Hospitals in Transition: the Resouorce Management Experiment*, Milton Keynes: Open University Press.

Parkin, P.A.C. (1995) 'Nursing the future: a re-examination of the professionalization thesis in the light of some recent developments', *Journal of Advanced Nursing*, 21, pp. 561–7.

Parson, D. (1989) 'Why the government will not abolish the Medical Practices Committee' (letter), *British Medical Journal*, 298, 14 January, p. 120.

Parsons, T. (1951) 'Social structure and dynamic process: the case of modern medical practice', in Parsons, T. (ed.), *The Social System*, New York: Free Press.

Pater, J.E. (1981) *The Making of the National Health Service*, London: King Edward's Hospital Fund for London.

Pawson, N. and Tilley, R. (1997) *Realistic Evaluation*, London: Sage.

Pearson, P. and Jones, K. (1994) 'The primary health care non-team', *British Medical Journal*, 309, pp. 1387–8.

Peck, E., Towell, D. and Gullier, P. (2001) 'The meaning of "culture" in health and social care: a case study of the combined grant in Somerset', *Journal of Interprofessional Care*, 15(4), pp. 319–27.

Peckham, S. (1994) 'Local voices and primary health care', *Critical Public Health*, 5(2), pp. 36–40.

Peckham, S. (1999) 'Primary care purchasing: Are integrated primary care providers/purchasers the way forward?', *PharmacoEconomics*, 15(3), pp. 209–16.

Peckham, S., Macdonald, J. and Taylor, P. (1996) *Towards a Public Health Model of Primary Care, First Report of the Public Health and Primary Care Project*, Birmingham: Public Health Alliance.

Peckham, S., Turton, P. and Tayor, P. (1998) 'The missing link Health Service', *Journal*, 108(5606), pp. 22–3.

Peckham, S. and Exworthy, M. (1999) 'Health and social care collaboration: early lessons for primary care groups', *British Journal of Health Care Management*, 5(3), pp. 101–103.

Peckham, S., Taylor, P. and Turton, P. (2000) 'Integrating primary care and public health', in Lindsay, J. and Craig, P. *Nursing for Public Health: Population-based Care*, Edinburgh: Churchill Livingstone.

Pendleton, D. and Vouler, J. (1983) *Doctor–Patient Communication*, London: Academic Press.

Pereira Gray, D. (1992) *Forty Years On: the Story of the First Forty Years of the Royal College of General Practitioners*, London: Atalink.

Petchey, R. (1995) 'General practice fundholding: weighing the evidence', *Lancet*, 346, pp. 1139–42.

Petchey, R. (1996) 'From stableboys to jockeys? The prospects for a primary care-led NHS', ch. 9 (pp. 157–83) in S. May, E. Brunsden and G. Craig (eds), *Social Policy Review 8*, London: Social Policy Association.

Peters, T. and Waterman, R. (1982) *In Search of Excellence*, New York: Harper Row.

Petersen, A. and Lupton, D. (1996) *The New Public Health*, London: Sage.

Pettigrew, A., Ferlie, E. and McKee, L. (1992) *Shaping Strategic Change – Make Change in Large Organisation: the Case of the NHS*, London: Sage.

Pickard, S. (1998) 'Citizenship and consumerism in health care: a critique of citizens' juries', *Social Policy and Administration*, 32(3), pp. 226–44.

Pickard, S., Williams, G., Flynn, R. (1995) 'Local voices in an internal market: the case of community health services', *Social Policy and Administration*, 29(2), pp. 135–49.

Pietroni, P. (1996). 'The integrated community care practice: General practice, citizenship and community care', ch. 9 (pp. 133–48) in G. Meads (ed.), *Future Options for General Practice*, Oxford: Radcliffe Medical Press.

Pinch, S. (1997) *Worlds of Welfare*, London: Routledge.

Pollock, A. (2001) 'Will Primary Care Trusts lead to US-style health care?' *British Medical Journal*, 322, pp. 964–7.

Popay, J. (2001) *Evidence to the House of Commons Health Committee Report on Public Health*, Volume II, Minutes of Evidence and Appendices, HC30-II, London, TSO.

Powell, M. (1997) *Evaluating the NHS*, Buckingham: Open University Press.

Powell, M. (1998) *New Labour, New Welfare State?: The 'Third Way' in British Social Policy*, Bristol: Policy Press.

Powell, M. (ed.) (2002) *New Labour's Welfare Reform*, Bristol: Policy Press.

Powell, M. (1999) 'In what sense a national health service?', *Public Policy and Administration*, 13(3), pp. 56–69.

Powell, M. and Exworthy, M. (2001) 'Joined-up solutions to address health inequalities analysing policy, process and resource streams', *Public Money and Management*, January–March, pp. 21–6.

Powell, M. and Exworthy, M. (2002) 'Quasi-networks and social policy', ch. in Glendenning, C., Powell, M. and Rummery, K. (eds) *Partnerships: New Labour and the Governance of Welfare*, Bristol: Policy Press.

Power, M. (1999) *The Audit Society: Rituals of Verification*, Oxford: Oxford University Press.

Pratt, J. (1995) *Practitioner and Practices: a Conflect of Values*, Oxford: Radcliffe Medical Press.

Pressman, J. and Wildavsky, I. (1973) *Implementation: How Great Expectations in Washington are Dashed in Oakland*, Berkeley: University of California Press.

Pringle, M. (ed.) (1998) *Primary Care: Core Values*, London: BMJ Books.

Pritchard, P. (1994) 'Community Involvement in a changing world', in *Heritage, Z. (ed.), Commuunity Participation in Primary Care*.

Public Accounts Committee (2000) *Appointments to NHS bodies. July 2000*, London: TSO.

Rachlis, M. and Kushner, N. (1994) *Strong Medicine*, Toronto: HarperCollins.

Ranade, W. (1998) *A Future for the NHS? Health Care for the Millennium*, Harlow: Longman.

RCGP (1996) *The Nature of General Practice, Report No. 27*, London: RCGP.

RCGP (1998) *Information Sheet 21: The Primary Health Care Team*, London: RCGP.

Reading, R., Steel, S. and Reynolds, S. (2002) 'Citizens advice in primary care for families with young children', *Child Care Health Development*, 28(1), pp. 39–45.

Redmayne, S. (1995) *Reshaping the NHS: Strategies, Priorities and Resource Allocation*, Research Paper No 16, Birmingham: National Association of Health Authorities and Trusts.

Reed, M. (1989) *The Sociology of Management*, Hemel Hempstead: Harvester Wheatsheaf.

Revans, L. (2001) *Party Politics: Community Care*, 27/09.

Rhodes, R.A.W. (1997) *Understanding Governance*, Buckingham: Open University Press.

Richards, A., Carley, J., Jenkins-Clarke, S. and Richards, D.A. (2000) 'Skill mix between nurses and doctors working in primary care: delegation or allocation. A review of the literature', *International Journal of Nursing Studies*, 37, pp. 185–97.

Richardson, G., Maynard, A., Cullum, N. and Kindig, D. (1998) 'Skill mix changes: substitution or service development?', *Health Policy*, 45, pp. 119–32.

Robison, J. and Exworthy, M. (1995) 'Primary care nursing: approaches and opportunities', *Primary Care Management*, 5(1), pp. 11–14.

Robinson, B. (1996) 'Primary managed care: the Lyme alternative', in *Future Options for General Practice*, pp. 201–10, Oxford: Radcliffe Medical Press.

Robinson, R., Evans, D. and Exworthy, M. (1994) *Health and the Economy*, Research paper no.14. Birmingham: National Association of Health Authorities and Trusts.

Robinson, R. and Hayter, P. (1995) *Why do GPs Choose Not to Apply for Fundholding*, Southampton: Institute for Health Policy Studies.

Robinson, R. and Le Grand, J. (eds) (1994) *Evaluating the NHS Reforms*, London: King's Fund.

Robinson, R. and Steiner, A. (1998) *Managed Health Care*, Buckingham: Open University Press.

Robinson, R. and Exworthy, M. (2000) *Three at the Top: Preliminary Report on Chief Executives and Board Chairs at First Wave Primary Care Trusts*, London: LSE.

Rogers, A., Hassell, K. and Nicolaas, G. (1999) Demanding *Patients? Analysing the Use of Primary Care*, Buckingham: Open University Press.

Roland, M. and Shapiro, J. (eds) (1998) *Specialist Outreach Clinics in General Practice*, Oxford: Radcliffe Medical Press.

Rose, R. (1982) *Understanding the United Kingdom: the Territorial Dimension*, Harlow: Longman.

Rosenthal, M.M. (1983) 'Neighbourhood health projects some new approaches to health and community work in parts of the UK', *Community Development Journal*, 18(2), pp. 120–31.

Rosenthal, M. (1995) *The Incompetent Doctor: Behind Closed Doors*, Buckingham: Open University Press.

Rothstein, B. (1998) *Just Institutions Matter*, Cambridge: Cambridge University Press.

Rummery, K. and Glendinning, C. (1997) *Working Together: Primary Care Involvement in Commissioning Social Care Services. Debates in Primary Care No. 2*, Manchester: NPCRDC, University of Manchester.

Sabatier, P. (1991) 'Towards better theories of the policy process', *Political science and politics*, 24, pp. 147–56.

Saks (1995) *Professions and the Public Interest, Medical Power, Aftercare and Alternative Medicine*, London: Routledge.

Salter, B. (1998) *The Politics of Change in the Health Service*, Basingstoke: Macmillan – now Palgrave Macmillan.

Saltman, R. (1997) 'Equity and distributive justice in European health care reform', *International Journal of Health Services*, 27(3), pp. 443–53.

Saltman, R. and Von Otter, C. (1992) *Planned Markets in Health Care*, Buckingham: Open University Press.

Saltman, R. and Figueras, J. (1997) *European Health Care Reform: Analysis of Current Strategies*, Copenhagen: Regional Office for Europe, WHO.

Savage, M., Barlow, J., Dickens, P. and Fielding, A. (1992) *Property, Bureaucracy and Culture: Middle Class Formation in Contemporary Britain*, London: Routledge.

Scott-Murray, S.A., Tapan, J., Turnbrill, G., McCallum, J. and Little, A. (1994) 'Listening to local voices: adapting rapid appraisal to access health and social needs in general practice', *British Medical Journal*, 308, pp. 698–700.

Scott-Samuel, A. (1989) 'The new public health? Speke neighbourhood health group', in D. Seedhouse and A. Cribb (eds), *Changing Ideas in Healthcare*, London: John Wiley.

Scottish Office (1998) *Working Together for a Healthier Scotland*, Cm 3854. Edinburgh: HMSO.

Scottish Executive (2001) *Joint Resourcing and Joint Management of Community Care Services*, ECD7/2001, Edinburgh: Scottish Executive.

Secretary of State for Northern Ireland (1998) *Fit for the Future: A Consultation Document on the Government's Proposals for the Future of Health and Personal Social Services in Northern Ireland*, Belfast: TSO.

Secretary of State for Scotland (1997) *Designed to Care: Renewing the National Health Service in Scotland*, CMB 3811, Edinburgh: TSO.

Secretary of State for Wales (1998) *NHS Wales: Putting Patients First*, CMB 3841, Cardiff: TSO.

Seebohm (1968) *Local Authorities and Allied Social Services*, London: HMSO.

Senior, M. (1991) 'Deprivation payments to GPs: not what the doctor ordered', *Environment and Planning C: Government and Policy*, 9, pp. 70–94.

Shaw, M., Dorling, D., Gordon, D. and Davey Smith, G. (1999) *The Widening Gap: Health Inequalities and Policy in Britain*, Bristol: The Policy Press.

Sibbald, B. (2000) 'Primary care: background and policy issues', ch. 1 (pp. 14–26) in Williams, A., *Nursing, Medicine and Primary Care*, Buckingham: Open University Press.

Silverman (1987) *Communication and Medical Practice*, London: Sage.

Skelcher, C. (2000) 'Changing images of the state: overloaded, hollowed-out and congested', *Public Policy and Administration*, 15(3), pp. 3–19.

Smith, F.J. (1990) 'The extended role of the community pharmacist: implications for the primary health care team', *Journal of Social and Administrative Pharmacy*, 7, pp. 101–10.

Smith, J. and Barnes, M. (2000) 'Developing primary care groups in the New NHS: towards diversity or uniformity?', *Public Money and Management*, January–March, pp. 45–52.

Smith, J., Regen, E., Goodwin, N., McLoed, H. and Shapiro, J. (2000) *Getting into Their Stride: Interim Report of a National Evaluation of Primary Care Groups*, University of Birmingham: Health Services Management Centre.

Smith, K., Leese, B., Pickard, S. and Chapple, A. (2000) 'Involving Stakeholders', in Wilkin, D., Gillam, S. and Leese, B. (eds), *The National Tracker Survey of Primary Care Groups Progress and Challenges, 1999/2000*, University of Manchester: National Primary Care Research and Development Centre.

Smith, R. (1998) 'All changed, utterly changed', *British Medical Journal*, 316, pp. 1917–18.

Smithies, J. and Webster, G. (1998) *Community Involvement and Health: from Passive Recipients to Active Participants*, Aldershot: Chem.

SSI (1999) *Of Primary Importance*, London: SSI.

Starfield, B. (1998) *Primary Care: Balancing Health Needs, Services and Technology*, New York: Oxford University Press.

Stevens, A. and Gabbay, J. (1991) 'Needs assessment needs assessment', *Health Trends*, 23(1), pp. 20–23.

Stewart, M. (2001) 'Towards a global definition of patient centred care', *British Medical Journal*, 322, pp. 444–5.

Stewart, M., Brown, J.B., Donner, A., McWhinney, J.R., McWilliam, C.L. and Freeman, T.R. (1995) *Patient-centred Medicine Transforming the Clinical Outcome*, Thousand Oaks, CA: Sage.

Summerton, N. (1999) 'Accrediting research practices', *British Journal of General Practice*, 49(438), pp. 63–4.

Sutters, C. and Nathan, A. (1993) 'The community pharmacist's extended role: GPs' and pharmacists' attitudes towards collaboration', *Journal of Social and Administrative Pharmacy*, 10, pp. 70–84.

Tarimo, E. and Creese, A. (1988) *Achieving Health for All by the Year 2000*, Geneva: WHO.

Taylor, D. (1991) *Developing Primary Care: Opportunities for the 1990s*, London: King's Fund

Taylor, P. and Lupton, C. (1997) *Public Involvement in Health Care Purchasing, Phase 2, Reprint No. 44*, Portsmouth: Social Services Renewal and Information Unit.

Taylor, P. and Lupton, C. (1995) *Consumer Involvement in Healthcare Commissioning. Report No. 30*, Portsmouth: Social Services Research and Information Unit, University of Portsmouth.

Taylor, P., Peckham, S. and Turton, P. (1998) *A Public Health Model of Primary Care: from Concept to Reality*, Birmingham: Public Health Alliance.

Thomas (1995) 'There is hope yet for the development of health care in deprived areas', *British Journal of General Practices*, 45, pp. 572–4.

Thompson, G., Frances, J., Levacic, R. and Mitchell, J. (1991) *Markets, Hierarchies and Networks*, London: Sage.

Thunhurst, C. (1991) 'Information and Public Health', in P. Draper (ed.), *Health through Public Policy*, London: Merlin Press.

Timmins, N. (1995) *The Five Giants*, London: Fontana.

Titmuss, R. (1974) *Social Policy*, London: Allen & Unwin.

Tomlinson, B. (1992) *Report of the Inquiry into London's Health Services, Medical Education and Research. Presented to Secretaries of State for Health and Education*, London: HMSO.

Toop, L. (1998) 'Primary care: core values. Patient centred primary care', *British Medical Journal*, 316(7148), pp. 1882–3.

Townsend, P., Phillimore, P. and Beattie, A. (1987) *Health and Deprivation: Inequality and the North*, London: Croom Helm.

Townsend, P., Davidson, N. and Whitehead, M. (eds) (1992) *Inequalities in Health*, London: Penguin.

Townsend, P. (1990) 'Individual or social responsibility for premature death? The current controversies in the British debate about health', *International Journal of Health Services*, 20(3), pp. 373–92.

Tranter, G. and Sullivan, S. (1996) 'Service planning. Whose shout?', *Health Service Journal*, 106(5501), p. 31.

Tudor-Hart, J. (1988) *A New Kind of Doctor*, London: Merlin Press.

Tuohy, C.H. (1999) *Accidental Logics: the Dynamics of Change in the Health Care Arena in the United States*, Britain and Canada. Cambridge: Cambridge University Press.

Turton, P., Peckham, S. and Taylor, P. (2000) 'Integrating primary care and public health', in Lindsay, J. and Craig, P. *Nursing for Public Health: Population Borad Care*, Edinburgh: Churchill Livingstone.

UNRISD (1979) *Enquiry into Participation – a Research Approach*, Geneva: UNRISD.

Vuori, H. (1985) 'The role of public health in the development of primary health care', *Health Policy*, 4, pp. 221–30.

Wagner, J., Power, E.J. and Fox, H. (1988) 'Technology-dependent children: hospital versus home care', *Office of Technology Assessment Task Force*, Philadelphia, PA: J.P. Lippincott.

Wainwright, D. (1998) 'Disenchantment, ambivalence and the precautionary principle: the becalming of British health policy', *International Journal of Health Services*, 28(3), pp. 407–26.

Walby, S. and Greenwell, J. (with Mackay, L. and Soothill, K.) (1994) *Medicine and Nursing: Professions in a Changing Health Service*, London: Sage.

Walsh, N., Allen, L., Baines, D. and Barnes, M. (1999) *Taking Off: a First Year Report of Primary Medical Services Pilots in England*, Birmingham: Health Services Management Centre.

Walsh, N., Andre, C., Barnes, M., Huntington, J., Rogers, H., McLeod, H. and Hendron, C. (2001) *First Wave PMS Pilots: Opening Pandora's Box*, Project Report No. 18, Birmingham: University of Birmingham, Health Services Management Centre.

Walt, G. (1994) *Health Policy: An Introduction to Process and Power*, London: Zed Books.

Wanless, D. (2002) *Securing our Future Health: Taking a Long Term View. Final Report. November 2001*, London: HM Treasury.

Webb, A. and Wistow, G. (1986) *Planning, Need and Scarcity*, London: Allen & Unwin.

Weber, M. (1949) *The Methodology of the Social Sciences*, New York: Free Press.

Webster, C. (1991) *Aneurin Bevan on the National Health Service*, Oxford: Wellcome Unit for the History of Medicine.

Webster, C. (1998) *The National Health Service: a Political History*, Oxford: Oxford University Press.

WHO (1986) *Ottawa Charter* for Health Promotion, Geneva: WHO.

WHO (1991) *Community Involvement in Health Development. Report of a WHO Study Group*, WHO Technical Report Series No. 809, Geneva: WHO.

WHO/UNICEF (1978) *Primary Health Care: The Alma Ata Conference*, Geneva: WHO.

Widgery, D. (1991) *Some Lives! A GP's East End*, London: Sinclair-Stevenson.

Wildavsky, A. (1979) *Speaking Truth to Power: The Art and Craft of Policy Analysis*, Boston: Little, Brown.

Wiles, R. and Robison, J. (1994) 'Teamwork in primary care: the views and experiences of nurses, midwives and health visitors', *Journal of Advanced Nursing*, 20(2), pp. 324–30.

Wilkin, D., Gillam, S. and Leese, B. (eds) (2000) *The National Tracker Survey of Primary Care Groups Progress and Challenges, 1999/2000*, University of Manchester: National Primary Care Research and Development Centre.

Wilkin, D., Gillam, S. and Coleman, A. (eds) (2001) *The National Tracker Survey of Primary Care Groups and Trusts 2000/2001: Modernising the NHS?*, University of Manchester: National Primary Care Research and Development Centre.

Wilkinson, R. (1998) *Unhealthy Societies*, London: Routledge.

Wilkinson, E.K., McColl, A., Exworthy, M., Roderick, P., Smith, H., Moore, M. and Gabbay, J. (2000) 'Reactions to the use of evidence-based performance indicators in primary care: a qualitative study', *Quality in Health Care*, 9(3), pp. 166–74

Williams, A. (2000) *Nursing, Medicine and Primary Care*, Buckingham: Open University Press.

Williamson, O.E. (1975) *Markets and Hierarchies*, New York: Free Press.

Williamson, C. (1992) *Whose Standards? Consumer and Professional Standards in Health Care*, Buckingham: Open University Press.

Wilsford, D. (1994) 'Path dependency or why history makes it difficult but not impossible to reform health care in a big way', *Journal of Public Policy*, 14(3), pp. 251–84.

Wilson, A.E. (2000) 'The changing nature of primary health care teams and interprofessional relationships', ch. 3 (pp. 43–60) in P. Tovey (ed.), *Contemporary Primary Care: the Challenge of Care*, Buckingham: Open University Press.

Wilson, P.M. (2001) 'A policy analysis of the Expert Patient in the United Kingdom: self-care as an expression of pastoral power?', *Health and Social Care in the Community*, 9(3), pp. 134–42.

Wistow, G. (1982) 'Collaboration between health and local authorities: why is it necessary', *Social Policy and Administration*, 16(1), pp. 44–52.

Wistow, G. and Fuller, S. (1983) 'Joint planning and perspective', *The NAUA Survey of Collaboration 1976–1982*, London: National Association of Health Authorities.

Wistow, G. and Harrison, S. (1998) 'Rationality and rhetoric: the contribution to social care policy-making of Sir Roy Griffiths 1986–1991', *Public Administration*, winter, 76(4), pp. 649–68.

Witz, A. (1994) 'The challenge of nursing', ch. 2 (pp. 23–45) in J. Gabe, D. Kelleher and G. Williams (eds), *Challenging Medicine*, London: Routledge.

Wolman, H. (1981) 'The determinants of program success and failure', *Journal of Public Policy*, 1(4), pp. 433–64.

Wood, B. (2000) *Patient Power? The Politics of Patient's Associations in Britain and America*, Buckingham: Open University Press.

Woodruffe, C., Glichman, M., Barker, M. and Power, C. (1993) *Children, Teenagers and Health: the Key Data*, Buckingham: Open University Press.

Wright, K. (1998) *The New NHS White Papers*, House of Commons Research paper, 98/15, London: House of Commons Library.

Index